2014
YEAR BOOK OF
**HAND AND UPPER
LIMB SURGERY**®

The 2014 Year Book Series

Year Book of Endocrinology®: Drs Schott, Clarke, Eugster, Khaodhiar, Meikle, Oetjen, Petersenn, Toth, and Willenberg

Year Book of Hand and Upper Limb Surgery®: Drs Yao, Adams, and Rizzo

Year Book of Medicine®: Drs Barker, DeVault, Garrick, Gold, Khardori, Lawton, LeRoith, and Pearson

Year Book of Neonatal and Perinatal Medicine®: Drs Fanaroff, Benitz, Donn, Neu, Papile, and Van Marter

Year Book of Ophthalmology®: Drs Rapuano, Fudemberg, Gupta, Hammersmith, Milman, Nagra, Nelson, Penne, Pyfer, Sergott, Shields, and Talekar

Year Book of Orthopedics®: Drs Morrey, Huddleston, Rose, Swiontkowski, and Trigg

Year Book of Pathology and Laboratory Medicine®: Drs Raab and Bissell

Year Book of Pediatrics®: Dr Cabana

Year Book of Plastic and Aesthetic Surgery™: Drs Miller, Gutowski, and Smith

Year Book of Pulmonary Disease®: Drs Barker, Jones, Maurer, Spradley, Tanoue, and Willsie

Year Book of Surgery®: Drs Behrns, Daly, Fahey, Hines, Howe, Huber, Klodell, Mozingo, and Pruett

Year Book of Urology®: Drs Andriole and Coplen

Year Book of Vascular Surgery®: Drs Gillespie, Bush, Passman, Starnes, and Watkins

2014

The Year Book of HAND AND UPPER LIMB SURGERY®

Editor-in-Chief

Jeffrey Yao, MD

Associate Professor of Orthopaedic Surgery, Robert A. Chase Hand and Upper Limb Center, Stanford University Medical Center, Redwood City, California

Associate Editors

Julie Adams, MD

Associate Professor of Orthopedic Surgery, University of Minnesota, Minneapolis, Minnesota

Marco Rizzo, MD

Professor, Department of Orthopedic Surgery, Mayo Clinic College of Medicine, Rochester, Minnesota

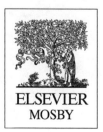

ELSEVIER
MOSBY

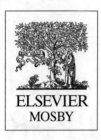

ELSEVIER
MOSBY

VP Global Medical Reference: Mary E. Gatsch
Senior Clinics Editor: Jennifer Flynn-Briggs
Developmental Editor: Stephanie Carter
Production Supervisor, Electronic Year Books: Donna M. Skelton
Electronic Article Manager: Mike Sheets
Illustrations and Permissions Coordinator: Dawn Vohsen

2014 EDITION

Printed in the United States of America
Composition by TNQ Books and Journals Pvt Ltd, India
Printing/binding by Sheridan Books, Inc.

Editorial Office:
Elsevier
Suite 1800
1600 John F. Kennedy Blvd.
Philadelphia, PA 19103-2899

International Standard Serial Number: 1551-7977
International Standard Book Number: 978-0-323-26467-9

Contributing Editors

Julie E. Adams, MD
Associate Professor, Orthopaedic Surgery, University of Minnesota, Minneapolis, Minnesota

Philip Blazar, MD
Assistant Professor, Department of Orthopaedic Surgery, Brigham and Women's Hospital, Boston, Massachusetts

Deborah Bohn, MD
Hand Surgeon, TRIA Orthopaedic Center, Bloomington, Minnesota

Jonathan Braman, MD
Associate Professor, Orthopaedic Surgery, University of Minnesota, Minneapolis, Minnesota

Jeff Brault, MD
Assistant Professor, Department of Physical Medicine and Rehabilitation, Mayo Clinic, Rochester, Minnesota

Llewella Brooke, OTR/L, CHT
Certified Hand Therapist, Stanford University Medical Center, Redwood City, California

Charles Carroll IV, MD
Associate Professor of Clinical Orthopedic Surgery, Feinberg School of Medicine, Northwestern University, Chicago, Illinois

James Chang, MD
Chief, Division of Plastic & Reconstructive Surgery, Professor of Surgery (Plastic Surgery) & Orthopedic Surgery, Stanford University Medical Center, Palo Alto, California

Emilie Cheung, MD
Assistant Professor, Robert A. Chase Hand & Upper Limb Center, Department of Orthopaedic Surgery, Redwood City, California

Harvey Chim, MD
Assistant Professor, Department of Plastic Surgery, University of Miami Medical Center, Miami, Florida

Matthew Seung Suk Choi, MD
Associate Professor, Chief, Department of Plastic and Reconstructive Surgery, Hanyang University Guri Hospital, Guri, Gyunggi-do, Korea

Alphonsus KS Chong, MD
Head and Senior Consultant, Department of Hand and Reconstructive Microsurgery; Assistant Professor, Department of Orthopaedic Surgery, Yong Loo Lin School of Medicine, National University Hospital, Singapore

Susan J. Clark, OTR/L, CHT
Certified Hand Therapist, Stanford University Medical Center, Redwood City, California

Catherine Curtin, MD
Assistant Professor, Robert A. Chase Hand & Upper Limb Center, Division of Plastic Surgery Stanford University Medical Center, Stanford, California

Piotr Czarnecki, MD, PhD
Hand Surgery Department, Poznan University of Medical Sciences, Poznan, Poland

Aaron Daluiski, MD
Assistant Professor of Orthopaedic Surgery, Weill Cornell Medical College, Hospital for Special Surgery, New York, New York

Johnny Elfar, MD
Assistant Professor, Department of Orthopaedic Surgery, University of Rochester Medical Center, Rochester, New York

Ryan Endress, MD
Assistant Professor, Department of Plastic Surgery, University of Kansas Medical Center, Kansas City, Kansas

Felicity G. Fishman, MD
Assistant Professor, Department of Orthopaedics and Rehabilitation, Yale University School of Medicine, New Haven, Connecticut

John M. Froelich, MD
Assistant Professor, Department of Orthopaedics, University of Colorado, School of Medicine, Aurora, Colorado

Glenn Gaston, MD
OrthoCarolina, Chief of Hand Surgery, Carolinas Medical Center, Department Orthopedic Surgery, Charlotte, North Carolina

Carolyn Gordon, OTR/L, CHT
Certified Hand Therapist, Stanford University Medical Center, Redwood City, California

Ruby Grewal, MD, MSc, FRCS
Assistant Professor, The Hand and Upper Limb Centre, St Joseph's Health Centre, London, Ontario, Canada

Warren C. Hammert, MD
University of Rochester Medical Center, Department of Orthopaedic Surgery, Rochester, New York

Cherrie Heinrich, MD
Plastic Surgeon, Regions Hospital, St Paul, MN

Vincent R. Hentz, MD
Professor of Surgery, Robert A. Chase Hand & Upper Limb Center, Division of Plastic Surgery Stanford University Medical Center, Stanford, California

Yi-Chao Huang, MD
Department of Orthopedics, Taipei Veterans General Hospital, Taipei City, Taiwan

Thomas Hughes, MD
Assistant Professor, AGH Department of Orthopedics, Allegheny Orthopedics Associates, Pittsburgh, Pennsylvania

Sidney M. Jacoby, MD
Associate Professor in Orthopaedic Surgery, Thomas Jefferson University Hospital, The Philadelphia Hand Center, P.C., Philadelphia, Pennsylvania

Ryosuke Kakinoki, MD, PhD
Associate Professor, Chief, Hand Surgery and Microsurgery, Department of Orthopedic Surgery and Rehabilitation Medicine, Graduate School of Medicine, Kyoto University, Kyoto, Japan

Sonja Kranz, OT, CHT
Department of Physical Medicine and Rehabilitation, Mayo Clinic, Rochester, Minnesota

Amy L. Ladd, MD
Editor-in-Chief, Emeritus, Yearbook of Hand & Upper Limb Surgery, Professor of Orthopaedic Surgery & Plastic Surgery, Robert A. Chase Hand & Upper Limb Center at Stanford University, Palo Alto, California

Jeffrey Macalena, MD
Assistant Professor, Orthopaedic Surgery, University of Minnesota, Minneapolis, Minnesota

Dan Mastella, MD
Assistant Clinical Professor, Department of Orthopaedic Surgery, University of Connecticut, Hartford, Connecticut

Kai Megerle, MD
Assistant Professor, Department of Plastic Surgery and Hand Surgery, Technical University of Munich, Munich, Germany

Amy T. Moeller, MD
Assistant Professor, Orthopaedic Surgery, University of Minnesota, Minneapolis, Minnesota

Peter Murray, MD
Professor, Department of Orthopedic Surgery, Mayo Clinic, Jacksonville, Florida

Michael Nicoson, MD
Assistant Professor, Department of Plastic Surgery, University of Louisville Medical Center, Louisville, Kentucky

Virginia H. O'Brien, OTD, OTR/L, CHT
Supervisor, Hand and Physical Therapy, Fairview Hand Center, University Orthopaedics Therapy Center, University of Minnesota Medical Center, Fairview, Minneapolis, Minnesota

William Payne, MD
Assistant Professor, Department of Orthopaedics, University of Colorado, Aurora, Colorado

Marco Rizzo, MD
Professor, Department of Orthopedic Surgery, Mayo Clinic, Rochester, Minnesota

Tamara Rozental, MD
Assistant Professor of Orthopaedic Surgery, Harvard Medical School, Beth Israel Deaconess Medical Center, Carl J. Shapiro Department of Orthopaedics, Boston, Massachusetts

Steven S. Shin, MD
Chief of Hand Surgery, Kerlan-Jobe Orthopaedic Clinic, Los Angeles, California

Jin Bo Tang, MD
Professor and Chair, Department of Hand Surgery, Affiliated Hospital of Nantong University, Chair, Hand Surgery Research Center, Nantong University, Jiangsu, China

Julia Toto, MD
Hand and Plastic Surgeon, Advanced Hand Surgery, Danbury, Connecticut

Johnathan Tueting, MD
Chief, Hand and Upper Extremity Surgery, Department of Orthopedics and Rehabilitation Medicine, University of Wisconsin School of Medicine and Public Health

Eric Wagner, MD
Department of Orthopedic Surgery, Mayo Clinic, Rochester, Minnesota

Abhijeet L. Wahegaonkar, MD
Consultant, Department of Upper Extremity, Hand and Microvascular Reconstructive Surgery, Brachial Plexus and Peripheral Nerve Surgery, Sancheti Institute for Orthopaedics and Rehabilitation, Jehangir Hospital, Oyster & Pearl General Hospital, Pune, India

Christina M. Ward, MD
Assistant Professor, Orthopaedic Surgery, University of Minnesota, Regions Hospital, St Paul, Minnesota

David Zelouf, MD
Assistant Clinical Professor, Department of Orthopaedic Surgery, Thomas Jefferson University Hospital and The Philadelphia Hand Center, King of Prussia, Pennsylvania

Dan Zlotolow, MD
Associate Professor, Department of Orthopaedic Surgery, Shriner's Children's Hospital, Philadelphia, Pennsylvania

Table of Contents

Journals Represented

Journals represented in this YEAR BOOK are listed below.

Acta Orthopaedica
American Journal of Sports Medicine
Anesthesia & Analgesia
Annals of Plastic Surgery
Annals of Vascular Surgery
Archives of Physical Medicine and Rehabilitation
Arthroscopy
Bone and Joint Journal
British Journal of Surgery
Burns
Clinical Orthopaedics and Related Research
European Journal of Plastic Surgery
Injury
Journal of Athletic Training
Journal of Bone Mineral Research
Journal of Clinical Investigation
Journal of Hand Surgery
Journal of Hand Surgery (American)
Journal of Hand Therapy
Journal of Neurology, Neurosurgery, and Psychiatry
Journal of Neurosurgery
Journal of Orthopaedic Research
Journal of Orthopaedic Trauma
Journal of Pain
Journal of Pediatric Orthopedics
Journal of Plastic, Reconstructive & Aesthetic Surgery
Journal of Reconstructive Microsurgery
Journal of Rheumatology
Journal of Ultrasound in Medicine
Medicine and Science in Sports and Exercise
Neurosurgery
Orthopedics
Pediatric Neurology
Plastic and Reconstructive Surgery
Skeletal Radiology
World Neurosurgery

STANDARD ABBREVIATIONS

The following terms are abbreviated in this edition: acquired immunodeficiency syndrome (AIDS), cardiopulmonary resuscitation (CPR), central nervous system (CNS), cerebrospinal fluid (CSF), computed tomography (CT), deoxyribonucleic acid (DNA), electrocardiography (ECG), health maintenance organization (HMO), human immunodeficiency virus (HIV), intensive care unit (ICU), intramuscular

(IM), intravenous (IV), magnetic resonance (MR) imaging (MRI), ribonucleic acid (RNA), and ultrasound (US).

NOTE

The YEAR BOOK OF HAND AND UPPER LIMB SURGERY® is a literature survey service providing abstracts of articles published in the professional literature. Every effort is made to assure the accuracy of the information presented in these pages. Neither the editors nor the publisher of the YEAR BOOK OF HAND AND UPPER LIMB SURGERY® can be responsible for errors in the original materials. The editors' comments are their own opinions. Mention of specific products within this publication does not constitute endorsement.

To facilitate the use of the YEAR BOOK OF HAND AND UPPER LIMB SURGERY® as a reference tool, all illustrations and tables included in this publication are now identified as they appear in the original article. This change is meant to help the reader recognize that any illustration or table appearing in the YEAR BOOK OF HAND AND UPPER LIMB SURGERY® may be only one of many in the original article. For this reason, figure and table numbers will often appear to be out of sequence within the YEAR BOOK OF HAND AND UPPER LIMB SURGERY®.

Introduction

We are proud to present the 30th edition of the YEAR BOOK OF HAND AND UPPER LIMB SURGERY. It is our honor to continue a Mayo Clinic and Stanford University collaborative editorial tradition begun by Drs James Dobyns and Robert Chase and continued by Drs Peter Amadio and Vincent Hentz, and most recently, by Drs Richard Berger, Amy Ladd, James Chang, and Scott Steinmann.

This is the third year the YEAR BOOK has enlisted an editorial board, with associate editors chosen for their expertise in the field of upper limb surgery. Dr Jeffrey Yao remains the editor-in-chief and is indebted to the editorial board (Drs Julie Adams and Marco Rizzo) for their contributions.

We are deep within the Internet generation, with information readily at a surgeon's fingertips. As the number of available sources of information regarding upper limb surgery or the busy surgeon increases, the goal of the YEAR BOOK is to distill the previous year's most salient journal articles into a shorter, more digestible form, all in one place. Upper limb surgeons continue to express interest in pathology of the entire limb, including the shoulder, elbow, wrist, and hand. The content of this year's YEAR BOOK of HAND AND UPPER LIMB SURGERY continues to reflect this trend. The literature surveyed by this year's YEAR BOOK covers a diverse subject matter, stretching from the brachial plexus to the fingertip. Many articles have addressed current concepts and the cutting edge regarding topics ranging from arthroplasty, reconstruction, trauma, arthroscopy, diagnostic imaging, and congenital conditions of the entire upper limb.

As with every year, we would like to acknowledge the immense effort of the contributing editors to the YEAR BOOK, without whom this edition would not be possible. All of the contributing editors have been personally selected for their national and international expertise in particular areas of the upper limb. The contributing editors have been enlisted from all around the world, and we are indebted to them for their commentaries printed on these pages.

Finally, we would like to thank Jennifer Flynn-Briggs and Stephanie Carter from Elsevier for their stewardship in helping guide us through this edition, and into the future.

Enjoy!

Jeffrey Yao, MD

1 Hand and Wrist Arthritis

Salvage Options for Flexor Carpi Radialis Tendon Disruption During Ligament Reconstruction and Tendon Interposition or Suspension Arthroplasty of the Trapeziometacarpal Joint

Jones DB Jr, Rhee PC, Shin AY, et al (Mayo Clinic, Rochester, MN)
J Hand Surg 38:1806-1811, 2013

Several techniques of thumb basilar joint arthroplasty depend on an intact flexor carpi radialis (FCR) tendon. There are situations, however, when the FCR tendon may be attenuated or iatrogenically injured, which make these techniques difficult or unfeasible. Familiarity with intraoperative salvage techniques in this setting is imperative. We present techniques for stabilizing the base of the thumb metacarpal when the FCR is deficient or injured.

▶ This surgical technique report presents a modification of a previously described technique for thumb metacarpal stabilization after complete trapeziectomy, in which the flexor carpi radialis (FCR) is either deficient or injured, or in revision cases with proximal migration of the first metacarpal. The authors recommend using a distally based strip of extensor carpi radialis longus (ECRL) tendon approximately 4 mm wide by 13 cm long. This strip is passed dorsal to volar through a drill hole 1 cm distal to the base of the second metacarpal. It is then routed either through the base of the first metacarpal or through the abductor pollicis longus tendon. They also recommend consideration for utilization of a suture button between the thumb and index metacarpals in the revision setting.

The authors report a useful technical pearl when one is faced with either an iatrogenic injury to the FCR or when the FCR is deficient as a result of attrition over an arthritic scaphotrapezial joint. I believe the modification of the prior reported technique whereby the ECRL strip is routed dorsal to palmar through a drill hole in the second metacarpal more closely approximates the FCR vector and may be useful in the described settings.

D. Zelouf, MD

Clinical and Radiological Results of Radiolunate Arthrodesis for Rheumatoid Arthritis: 22 Wrists Followed for an Average of 7 Years

Motomiya M, Iwasaki N, Minami A, et al (Hokkaido Univ Graduate School of Medicine, Sapporo; Hokkaido Chuo Rosai Hosp Spinal Cord Injury Ctr, Bibai, Japan)
J Hand Surg 38A:1484-1491, 2013

Purpose.—To evaluate the clinical and radiological results of radiolunate (RL) arthrodesis for rheumatoid arthritis (RA) patients treated with disease-modifying antirheumatic drugs and/or biologicals with an average of 7 years of follow-up. In addition, we compared the results in advanced stages with those in less advanced stages in patients with comparatively low disease activity of RA.

Methods.—This study included RL arthrodesis for 22 wrists in 19 patients with comparatively low disease activity of RA. The mean follow-up period was 7 years (range, 2-16 y). Fourteen wrists with Larsen classification grade III and 8 wrists with grade IV were included in this study. The range of motion was calculated, and clinical scores were graded using the Mayo wrist score and the Stanley classification. The carpal height ratio (CHR) and ulnar translation (UT) were determined from the radiographs.

Results.—All wrists achieved radiographic fusion. Clinical scores were markedly improved, although there was a decrease in flexion. The Larsen grade did not deteriorate during follow-up. CHR and UT improved immediately after operation and remained good through the final follow-up. Although the flexion/extension range of motion of the grade IV wrists was smaller than that of the grade III wrists at follow-up, both groups obtained good clinical results.

Conclusions.—Our results for RL arthrodesis were clinically and radiologically better than those of previous reports. Control of the disease activity of RA could theoretically be a factor in obtaining good long-term clinical and radiographic outcomes. RL arthrodesis is our recommended procedure for the RA wrist even in the advanced stage.

Level of Evidence.—Therapeutic IV.

▶ Radiolunate arthrodesis is an effective surgical procedure for the treatment of rheumatoid patients having painful radiocarpal arthritis and carpal malalignment. Radiolunate arthrodesis has the benefit of preserving the wrist flexion-extension arc in opposition to a standard total wrist arthrodesis. This study aims to assess the midterm results of rheumatoid patients being treated with biologicals or disease-modifying antirheumatic drugs undergoing radiolunate arthrodesis.

The authors have a considerable published experience treating rheumatoid hand patients and again have executed a well-designed study with adequate patient numbers. Their surgical procedure for radiolunate arthrodesis is based on that of Stanley, with the utilized bone graft coming from the resected distal ulna specimen. Bony fixation is done with a cannulated compression screw from the radius to the lunate and supplemented with K-wires from the trique-trum to the radius.

Based on the results of this study, it is evident that radiolunate arthrodesis is an excellent option for patients with rheumatoid arthritis having painful radiocarpal arthritis, wanting to maintain the flexion-extension arc of their wrist. Addition-ally, this study provides evidence that medical management of rheumatoid dis-ease activity may be correlated with obtaining good long-term radiologic and clinical results. One limitation of this study is the short patient follow-up. It would be interesting to have the authors report again on the longer-term results of these same patients to see their clinical outcomes at 15 years.

M. Nicoson, MD

Suture-Button Suspensionplasty for Thumb Carpometacarpal Arthritis: A Minimum 2-Year Follow-Up

Yao J, Song Y (Stanford Univ Med Ctr, Redwood City, CA)
J Hand Surg 38A:1161-1165, 2013

Purpose.—To retrospectively review the results at a minimum of 2 years of suture-button plasty with partial or full trapeziectomy and suture-button suspensionplasty.

Methods.—We evaluated 21 patients who received suture-button sus-pensionplasty at least 2 years after surgery. We measured postoperative pinch strength, grip strength, range of motion, and metacarpal height. All patients also completed the *Quick* Disabilities of the Arm, Shoulder, and Hand questionnaire.

Results.—At an average follow-up of 2.8 ± 0.7 years, the mean *Quick* Disabilities of the Arm, Shoulder, and Hand score was 10 ± 9. Pinch and grip strengths were 86% and 89% of the contralateral limb, respec-tively. Average first trapezial height was 74% of the contralateral trapezial height. There were no major complications.

Conclusions.—The favorable results of the suture-button suspension-plasty procedure confirm its usefulness in treating thumb carpometacarpal arthritis with minimal risk of complications, ineffective fixation, or loss of function. Subjective and objective outcomes measures are similar to previ-ously described techniques. The benefit of this technique results from the implanted nature of the suspensionplasty elements that require no time to heal, so rehabilitation is begun as early as 10 days postoperatively.

Type of Study/Level of Evidence.—Therapeutic IV.

▶ Thumb carpometacarpal (CMC) arthritis represents one of the most common degenerative conditions seen in the outpatient hand clinic. The authors provide 2-year follow-up of suture-button suspensionplasty for thumb CMC arthritis. This novel technique uses the principle of suture button suspension of the thumb to index metacarpal to prevent thumb metacarpal subsidence following partial or full trapeziectomy. Numerous studies have verified that the critical component of thumb CMC surgery is removal of at least a portion of the degenerative trapezium. What remains elusive is the superiority of one technique over the other.

The authors provide objective data including pinch and grip strength, range of motion, metacarpal height and Quick Dash to demonstrate outstanding results with their efficiently described technique.

Key benefits to thumb CMC suture button suspensionplasty is the earlier movement afforded by stable fixation, which does not require healing time associated with K-wire fixation or other soft-tissue reconstructive procedures. Earlier rehabilitation often leads to quicker recovery time and increased patient satisfaction. The authors correctly point out the cost associated with the implant (currently $495) but opine that diminished period of immobilization and accelerated rehabilitation are variables that justify the added cost associated with the implant.

In sum, the authors present encouraging objective and patient-rated reviews of this technique for the treatment of thumb CMC arthritis. The technique can be performed via an arthroscopic or open approach and, in the proper circumstance, offers the hand surgeon an additional technique that can result in accelerated recovery and return to function in relatively short order.

S. M. Jacoby, MD

Continuation of TNF blockade in patients with inflammatory rheumatic disease. An observational study on surgical site infections in 1,596 elective orthopedic and hand surgery procedures

Berthold E, Geborek P, Gülfe A (Skåne Univ Hosp, Lund, Sweden)
Acta Orthop 84:495-501, 2013

Background.—Increased infection risk in inflammatory rheumatic diseases may be due to inflammation or immunosuppressive treatment. The influence of tumor necrosis factor (TNF) inhibitors on the risk of developing surgical site infections (SSIs) is not fully known. We compared the incidence of SSI after elective orthopedic surgery or hand surgery in patients with a rheumatic disease when TNF inhibitors were continued or discontinued perioperatively.

Patients and Methods.—We included 1,551 patients admitted for elective orthopedic surgery or hand surgery between January 1, 2003 and September 30, 2009. Patient demographic data, previous and current treatment, and factors related to disease severity were collected. Surgical procedures were grouped as hand surgery, foot surgery, implant-related surgery, and other surgery. Infections were recorded and defined according to the 1992 Centers for Disease Control definitions for SSI. In 2003–2005, TNF inhibitors were discontinued perioperatively (group A) but not during 2006–2009 (group B).

Results.—In group A, there were 28 cases of infection in 870 procedures (3.2%) and in group B, there were 35 infections in 681 procedures (5.1%) (p = < 0.05). Only foot surgery had significantly more SSIs in group B, with very low rates in group A. In multivariable analysis with groups

A and B merged, only age was predictive of SSI in a statistically significant manner.

Interpretation.—Overall, the SSI rates were higher after abolishing the discontinuation of anti-TNF perioperatively, possibly due to unusually low rates in the comparator group. None of the medical treatments analyzed, e.g. methotrexate or TNF inhibitors, were significant risk factors for SSI. Continuation of TNF blockade perioperatively remains a routine at our center.

▶ The authors investigated the incidence of surgical site infection (SSI) in patients with rheumatoid arthritis. In an extensive database of almost 1600 patients, they found an increased risk for patients who continued their anti—tumor necrosis factor (TNF) medication through the surgery. Nevertheless, they report routinely continuing TNF blockade perioperatively at their institution.

Despite the impressive number of patients included in this study, its message seems ambivalent. One might assume that patient categories (hand, foot, implants, other) are too broad and collectives too heterogeneous; therefore important parameters that correlate with SSI might not have been identified.

In our practice, the incidence of surgery for patients with rheumatoid arthritis has decreased dramatically in the past decade after the introduction of new disease-modifying antirheumatic drugs. As this study beautifully demonstrates, the data on the perioperative management of these drugs are contradictory, and we tend to decide on an individual basis whether to discontinue antirheumatic medication. Apart from patient-related factors, the type and extent of the surgical intervention in particular has to be considered.

K. Megerle, MD, PhD

Silicone Arthroplasty for Nonrheumatic Metacarpophalangeal Joint Arthritis

Neral MK, Pittner DE, Spiess AM, et al (Univ of Pittsburgh Med Ctr, PA; Univ of Pittsburgh School of Medicine, Wexford, PA)
J Hand Surg Am 38:2412-2418, 2013

Purpose.—To evaluate the clinical effectiveness of metacarpophalangeal (MCP) arthroplasty for nonrheumatic arthritis. We hypothesized that MCP arthroplasty would produce significant improvement in objective measures of hand function, pain relief, and overall patient satisfaction.

Methods.—This retrospective study evaluated 30 patients with 38 MCP arthroplasties for nonrheumatic arthritis over a 12-year period. Follow-up assessment was completed at an average of 56 months after surgery. Objective measures included range of motion; grip and pinch strength; Disabilities of the Arm, Shoulder, and Hand (DASH) score; and visual analog pain score. A subjective patient questionnaire was used to assess patient satisfaction.

Results.—There was marked improvement between preoperative and follow-up range of motion, DASH, and pain. Linear regression showed strong correlations between preoperative measurements and improvement at follow-up. No difference was detected for grip or pinch strength. Results of the questionnaire showed that 73% were very satisfied, 87% would definitely do it again, and 70% experienced rare or no pain. Follow-up x-rays showed 5° mean angulation and 2-mm mean subsidence compared with immediate postoperative x-rays. Four arthroplasties (11%) required revision.

Conclusions.—This study showed improved range of motion and DASH score, excellent pain relief, and excellent patient satisfaction in patients undergoing MCP arthroplasty for nonrheumatic arthritis. Patients with more severe range of motion limitation, DASH score, and pain score experienced a greater improvement of these measures at follow-up. Strength improvement was limited although it remained comparable to the nonoperated hand. Angulation, subsidence, and complications in the study population were consistent with those reported in the literature.

Type of Study/Level of Evidence.—Therapeutic III.

▶ The authors report on Dr Imbriglia's experience with silicone arthroplasty for nonrheumatic arthritis of the metacarpophalangeal (MCP) joint. Some surgical pearls are included (maintain the collateral ligaments) in the description of the surgical technique. His postoperative regimen is included for completeness. Three different implants were used; the reasons for this are not specified.

Once the inclusion criteria were met, the cohort consisted of 38 MCP arthroplasties with minimum 8-month follow-up (mean, 56 months). Visual analog pain score and Disabilities of the Arm, Shoulder, and Hand scores were collected for most of the cohort. The results were in line with those of other studies and indicate that the procedure is effective at reducing or eliminating pain but does not significantly improve power in the hand.

The study is valuable for reporting one surgeon's experience and including the technical points he thinks are responsible for the results he is showing us. There is ample opportunity to introduce bias in such a study, but taken as it is offered, it is a valuable description of one surgeon's work.

D. J. Mastella, MD

Proximal Row Carpectomy: Minimum 20-Year Follow-Up
Wall LB, Didonna ML, Kiefhaber TR, et al (Washington Univ Orthopaedics, St Louis, MO; Indiana Univ Health Physicians, Fishers; Hand Surgery Specialists, Inc, Cincinnati, OH; et al)
J Hand Surg 38A:1498-1504, 2013

Purpose.—Proximal row carpectomy (PRC) is a motion-sparing procedure for degenerative disorders of the proximal carpal row. Reported results at a minimum 10-year follow-up consistently show maintenance of strength, motion, and satisfaction with an average conversion rate to radiocarpal arthrodesis of 12%. We hypothesized that PRC would continue to provide a high level of satisfaction and function at a minimum of 20 years.

Methods.—Seventeen wrists in 16 patients, including 7 laborers, underwent PRC for symptomatic degenerative disorders of the proximal carpal row at an average age of 36 years. Patients returned for radiographic and clinical evaluation, and the Quick Disabilities of the Arm, Shoulder and Hand (QuickDASH) questionnaire and Patient-Related Wrist Evaluation were used for subjective assessment. Follow-up was a minimum of 20 years (average, 24 y).

Results.—Eleven wrists (65%) underwent no further surgery at a minimum 20-year follow-up. The average time to failure of PRC, defined as the time from PRC to radiocarpal arthrodesis, was 11 years (range, 8 mo to 20 y). Ten of 11 patients who did not undergo radiocarpal arthrodesis continued to be satisfied, with minimal decrease in motion and grip strength compared with the uninvolved side. Average score for QuickDASH was 16 and for Patient-Related Wrist Evaluation was 26. The flexion-extension arc was 68°, and grip strength was 72% of the contralateral side. All patients returned to their original employment. There was no correlation between degenerative radiographic changes and satisfaction level. The predicted probability of failure revealed a higher risk in patients who underwent PRC at a younger age, which leveled off at age 40 years.

Conclusions.—PRC provides satisfaction at a minimum of 20 years with a survival rate of 65%. Whereas we recommend a minimum age for PRC between 35 and 40 years, young patients should not be excluded as PRC candidates; these patients should undergo appropriate preoperative counseling of their increased failure risk secondary to their young age.

Type of Study/Level of Evidence.—Therapeutic IV.

▶ Dr Stern and his colleagues present us with the longest follow-up study to date (average 24 years) on the outcomes of proximal row carpectomy (PRC). From a purely scientific standpoint, the study has many flaws (eg, roughly 25% of the original study population not followed up, no preoperative measurements or functional outcomes to compare with, small sample size); however, the article has significance in that we see this procedure can at least stand up to the test of time even in some laborers. That alone makes this a good article. Also, Dr Stern is historically highly critical of his own outcomes and quick to report failures and adverse events, so an article by him reporting favorable outcomes holds even more merit in my eyes.

I agree with the messages of this article: PRC in this series and others seems to have a conversion rate of 15% to 20%, it can be successful even in higher demand patients, and it can be successful in the long term even in some younger patients (even those younger than 40 years).

My personal approach to these conditions has been to use PRC typically in lower-demand patients or those at higher risk for nonunion while favoring scaphoid excision and midcarpal fusion (isolated capitolunate) for higher-demand and younger patients. I have always assumed the lunate articulates better with the lunate fossa than the capitate; therefore, theoretically, CL fusions will have less long-term degeneration compared with PRC. Unfortunately, we do not have the long-term data for midcarpal fusion to support this claim, and some studies have found higher rates of complications using this procedure.

Although I don't think this study will change my practice, it makes me more confident offering this procedure to higher-demand and younger patients given the results presented. This remains an unsolved problem for hand surgeons.

G. Gaston, MD

Distribution of primary osteoarthritis in the ulnar aspect of the wrist and the factors that are correlated with ulnar wrist osteoarthritis: a cross-sectional study
Katayama T, Ono H, Suzuki D, et al (Kokuho Central Hosp, Nara, Japan; et al)
Skeletal Radiol 42:1253-1258, 2013

Objective.—The purpose of this cross-sectional study was to identify the distribution of primary osteoarthritis (OA) in the ulnar aspect of the wrist, and analyze the factors correlated with OA at this site.

Materials and Methods.—A total of 1,128 cases of skeletally mature Japanese patients were collected over a 3-year period. We analyzed the posteroanterior and lateral wrist radiographs of these patients for the presence of primary OA in the ulnar aspect of the wrist, including the distal radioulnar (DRUJ), radiolunate, ulnolunate, lunotriquetral, triquetrohamate, lunohamate, and lunocapitate joints. All joints were examined for the frequency of primary OA. Multivariate logistic regression was used to investigate the factors correlated with the presence of degenerative arthritis in the ulnar aspect of the wrist joint.

Results.—Primary OA of the ulnar wrist was identified in 145 out of 1,128 cases (12.8 %). Degenerative changes were most frequently identified in the DRUJ (12.3 %), followed by the ulnolunate joint (8.1 %). Variations in radial inclination (RI), carpal height ratio (CHR), and ulnar variance (UV) correlated with OA of the ulnar aspect of the wrist, with variations in UV showing the highest correlation.

Conclusion.—Primary OA of the ulnar wrist was most frequent in the DRUJ and second most frequent in the ulnolunate joint. UV correlated most with OA in the ulnar aspect of the wrist.

▶ This is an interesting retrospective radiographic review of 1128 adult Japanese patients to quantify ulnar-sided osteoarthritis involving the distal radioulnar, radiolunate, ulnolunate, lunocapitate, lunohamate, triquetrohamate, and lunotriquetral joints. The authors specifically reviewed standard posteroanterior and lateral films in patients with no history of posttraumatic or inflammatory arthritis or congenital malformations. The authors note distal radioulnar joint arthritis to be the most common ulnar-sided site for arthritis affecting approximately 12% of the sample. They also note that the ulnar variance (positive) had the strongest correlation with the development of ulnar-sided arthritis. This is a nice study that has helped truly quantify the incidence of ulnar-sided arthritis while the authors also took great care to understand the possible influences on the development of the arthritis. This is a nice edition to the growing literature trying to define baseline incidents of conditions including basic patterns of wrist arthritis.

J. M. Froelich, MD

Number of Ruptured Tendons and Surgical Delay as Prognostic Factors for the Surgical Repair of Extensor Tendon Ruptures in the Rheumatoid Wrist
Sakuma Y, Ochi K, Iwamoto T, et al (Tokyo Women's Med Univ, Shinjuku-ku, Japan)
J Rheumatol 41:265-269, 2014

Objective.—Extensor tendon ruptures in the rheumatoid wrist are usually restored by extensor tendon reconstruction surgery. However, the factors significantly correlated with the outcomes of extensor tendon reconstruction have not been defined. We examined factors showing a statistically significant correlation with postoperative active motion after tendon reconstruction.

Methods.—Spontaneous extensor tendon ruptures of 66 wrists in patients (mean age, 52.6 yrs) with rheumatoid arthritis (RA) were evaluated. All patients underwent tendon reconstruction surgery with wrist arthroplasty or arthrodesis. Active ranges of motion of the affected fingers were evaluated at 12 weeks postsurgery. Statistical significance was determined using multiple and single regression analyses.

Results.—Forty-six (69.6%) wrists had "good" results, while 13 (19.7%) and 7 (10.6%) wrists had "fair" and "poor" results, respectively. In multiple regression analysis, an increased number of ruptured tendons and the age at operation were independent variables significantly correlated with the postoperative active motion of reconstructed tendons ($p = 0.009$). Single regression analysis also showed a significant association between the number of ruptured tendons and surgical delay ($p = 0.02$).

Conclusion.—The number of ruptured extensor tendons was significantly correlated with the results of tendon reconstruction, and the number of ruptured tendons was significantly correlated with preoperative surgical delay. Our results indicate that, in patients presenting with possible finger extensor tendon rupture, rheumatologists should consult with hand surgeons promptly to preserve hand function.

▶ The authors retrospectively analyzed outcomes of tendon reconstruction following rupture associated with rheumatoid arthritis (RA). The study is somewhat ambitious, but I applaud what the authors were trying to help us better understand: are there factors predictive of outcome following tendon rupture associated with RA?

The authors reviewed 66 hands/wrists that underwent tendon reconstruction in conjunction with treatment of distal radioulnar joint arthritis. Based on range of motion and residual extension lag, 46 cases (69.7%) had good results, 13 (19.7%) had fair results, and 7 (10.6%) had poor results. Older patients fared worse. In addition, somewhat intuitively, patients with multiple ruptures also had poorer outcomes. Finally, although it is sometimes difficult to pinpoint the precise date of rupture, the more chronic ruptures (patients who had a delay in surgery) did not do as well.

I think this study, although fairly intuitive, help us when discussing with patients their prognosis and may aid in tempering expectations for outcomes after surgery. I have also found that patients who have complete wrist fusions in association with tendon reconstruction have additional challenges secondary to the loss of tenodesis effect, which they would otherwise have if the wrist had not been fused. Interestingly, only 1 patient in the series had a complete wrist fusion, and this individual had a "good" outcome.

M. Rizzo, MD

Distribution of primary osteoarthritis in the ulnar aspect of the wrist and the factors that are correlated with ulnar wrist osteoarthritis: a cross-sectional study
Katayama T, Ono H, Suzuki D, et al (Kokuho Central Hosp, Tawaramoto, Nara, Japan)
Skeletal Radiol 42:1253-1258, 2013

Objective.—The purpose of this cross-sectional study was to identify the distribution of primary osteoarthritis (OA) in the ulnar aspect of the wrist, and analyze the factors correlated with OA at this site.

Materials and Methods.—A total of 1,128 cases of skeletally mature Japanese patients were collected over a 3-year period. We analyzed the posteroanterior and lateral wrist radiographs of these patients for the presence of primary OA in the ulnar aspect of the wrist, including the distal radioulnar (DRUJ), radiolunate, ulnolunate, lunotriquetral, triquetrohamate, lunohamate, and lunocapitate joints. All joints were examined for the frequency of primary OA. Multivariate logistic regression was used to investigate the factors correlated with the presence of degenerative arthritis in the ulnar aspect of the wrist joint.

Results.—Primary OA of the ulnar wrist was identified in 145 out of 1,128 cases (12.8 %). Degenerative changes were most frequently identified in the DRUJ (12.3 %), followed by the ulnolunate joint (8.1 %). Variations in radial inclination (RI), carpal height ratio (CHR), and ulnar variance (UV) correlated with OA of the ulnar aspect of the wrist, with variations in UV showing the highest correlation.

Conclusion.—Primary OA of the ulnar wrist was most frequent in the DRUJ and second most frequent in the ulnolunate joint. UV correlated most with OA in the ulnar aspect of the wrist.

▶ The purpose of this cross-sectional study was to identify the distribution of primary osteoarthritis (OA) affecting the ulnar side of the wrist and analyze the factors that correlated with OA at this site. The authors evaluated 1128 skeletally mature patients (mean age, 54.2; range, 19–100) with standard posteroanterior and lateral radiographs who presented to their clinic with wrist symptoms. Patients with fractures, inflammatory disease, carpal avascular necrosis, and congenital deformities were excluded. Radiographs were reviewed and included specific evaluation of the distal radioulnar joint (DRUJ), radiolunate joint (RL), ulnolunate joint (UL), lunotriquetral joint (LT), triquetrohamate joint (TH), lunatohamate joint (LH), and lunocapitate joints (LC). The authors report that of the 1128 patients, 145 (12.8%) presented with primary OA involving the ulnar side of the wrist. The DRUJ was most frequently involved (139 of 145), representing 12.3% of the total cases. Of the 139 patients, 57 exhibited ulnar positive variance. The second most frequent area involved with OA was the UL joint, seen in 91 of 1128 patients. Fifty-three of 1128 exhibited LC arthritis, 46 of 1128 exhibited RL arthritis, 40 of 1128 exhibited TH arthritis, 38 of 1128 exhibited LH arthritis, and 14 of 1128 exhibited LT arthritis. The only statistically significant radiographic finding that correlated with OA was positive ulnar variance. Based on this study, the authors propose that in the setting of symptomatic ulnar abutment, an ulnar shortening osteotomy be performed to decrease symptoms and possibly decrease the frequency of OA.

This study is interesting and notes an association between positive ulnar variance and OA about the ulnar side of the wrist. The rationale for an ulnar-shortening osteotomy in the setting of positive ulnar variance and ulnocarpal abutment is well established and is reasonably predictable. However, I do not think the study results support the notion that an ulnar-shortening osteotomy decreases the likelihood of primary OA of the DRUJ.

D. Zelouf, MD

Treatment of Little Finger Carpometacarpal Posttraumatic Arthritis With a Silicone Implant
Proubasta IR, Lamas CG, Ibañez NA, et al (Hosp Sant Pau, Barcelona, Spain; Institut Kaplan for Surgery of the Hand and Upper Extremity, Barcelona, Spain)
J Hand Surg 38A:1960-1964, 2013

Purpose.—To evaluate the short-term clinical and radiographic outcome of a flexible silicone proximal interphalangeal joint implant between the hamate and the metacarpal, to treat posttraumatic little finger carpometacarpal (CMC) osteoarthritis.

Methods.—We treated 3 men with a mean age of 30 years by means of a proximal interphalangeal silicone implant arthroplasty for CMC osteoarthritis of the little finger. Indications were disabling pain on the ulnar side of the hand, grip weakness, loss of CMC joint mobility, and disability for work and daily activities.

Results.—All patients were free of pain at a mean follow-up of 20 months. Transverse metacarpal arch mobility and grip strength were restored. The appearance was acceptable, without misalignment, malrotation, or shortening of the little finger ray. Radiographic evaluation showed no fractures or dislocations of the implant and no signs of foreign body reaction to silicone particles.

Conclusions.—This technique offers the advantages of eliminating pain, maintaining length, and restoring mobility of the transverse metacarpal arch, and results in acceptable function and grip strength.

▶ The authors present an interesting 3-case series using flexible silicone implants in treating posttraumatic little finger carpo-metacarpal (CMC) joint arthritis. These patients were reported to be pain free, with good grip strength, appearance, and metacarpal arch mobility after 20 months of follow-up. In my mind, this study provides an alternative way to treat fifth CMC arthritis but may still have limitations such as the small case number and short-term follow-up. Silicone implants act like a soft spacer and maintain good digit height for the fifth CMC joint, but arthritis may also exist in the fourth to fifth metacarpal base articulation, which may also induce pain. Silicone implants may also have problems such as related synovitis, foreign body reaction, and wear and fatigue. Currently, I have found that patients tolerate traumatic arthritis and even chronic dislocation of fifth CMC joint relatively well. For patients with disabling pain, I perform a fifth CMC joint resection arthroplasty with arthrodesis of the fourth to fifth metacarpal bases. Fifth CMC arthrodesis to the hamate may also be used.

Y.-C. Huang, MD

The Effect of Swan Neck and Boutonniere Deformities on the Outcome of Silicone Metacarpophalangeal Joint Arthroplasty in Rheumatoid Arthritis
Chetta M, Burns PB, Kim HM, et al (Univ of Michigan Health System, Ann Arbor; Univ of Michigan, Ann Arbor; Pulvertaft Hand Ctr, Derby, UK; et al)
Plast Reconstr Surg 132:597-603, 2013

Background.—Rheumatoid arthritis patients with swan neck deformities are postulated to have greater metacarpophalangeal joint arc of motion because of their need to flex the joint to make a fist, whereas the boutonniere deformity places the fingers into the flexed position, creating less demand on the joint for grip. This study analyzes the effect of these deformities on the joint's arc of motion and hand function.

Methods.—The authors measured the metacarpophalangeal joint arc of motion in 73 surgical patients. Data were allocated into groups by finger and hand deformity. Linear regression models were used to analyze the effect of the deformity on the joint's arc of motion. Functional outcomes were measured by the Michigan Hand Outcomes Questionnaire and the Jebson-Taylor Test.

Results.—Nineteen fingers had boutonniere deformity, 95 had swan neck deformities, and 178 had no deformity. The no-deformity group had the least arc of motion at baseline (16 degrees) compared with the boutonniere (26 degrees) and swan neck (26 degrees) groups. Mean arc of motion in the no-deformity group compared with the boutonniere group at baseline was statistically significant, but all groups had similar arc of motion at long-term follow-up. Only mean Jebson-Taylor Test scores at baseline between the boutonniere and no-deformity groups were significantly different.

Conclusions.—The results did not support the hypothesis that swan neck deformities have better arc of motion compared with boutonniere deformity. Boutonniere deformity has worse function at baseline, but there was no difference in function among groups at long-term follow-up.

▶ Silicone metacarpophalangeal joint arthroplasty is a well-established surgical procedure used in patients with rheumatoid arthritis. Despite this, there is limited information about patient-related outcomes and factors predicting outcomes for such procedures. The senior author in this study is at the forefront of applying rigorous scientific method in the study of the surgical treatment of rheumatoid arthritis. This multicenter report involving key hand centers in the United Kingdom and United States is an important step in the direction to fill knowledge gaps in our surgical treatment of rheumatoid arthritis.

This study suggests that the presence and type of finger deformity does not affect the outcome of silicone metacarpophalangeal joint arthroplasty. In this study, the primary outcome studied was arc of motion. This parameter provided the basis to calculate the sample size for the study. In contrast to their original stated hypothesis, apart from a lower arc of motion in the no-deformity group compared with the other 2 groups at baseline, the authors did not find any difference in the mean arc of motion between the groups at baseline or subsequent time points. Specifically, they did not find an expected increase in arc of motion of the metacarpophalangeal joint in swan neck deformity compared with boutonniere deformity. Between groups, they found that mean Jebsen-Taylor Test scores were worse for boutonniere deformity compared with the no-deformity group at baseline. There was no difference between the swan-neck group and no-deformity group at baseline. They also did not find differences in the Michigan Hand Outcomes Questionnaire (MHQ) scores between groups either at baseline or at follow-up. This may be because the sample sizes are quite small in the MHQ and Jebsen-Taylor Test because of dropouts. This is one of the limitations of the study.

In addition, as the authors note, the variety in forms and severity of deformities across the patients complicates such studies. The deformities could not be graded because evaluation was done with photographs and radiographs. This study also did not consider other factors such as the number of digits involved, and the position (radial or ulnar) of the affected digits.

The patients in this study were part of a multicenter prospective clinical trial that was reported separately.[1] That report complements this article. In that study, the patients were not randomly selected because of strong patient preference. It found that at baseline, the surgical group had worse MHQ scores compared with the nonsurgical group. At 1-year follow-up, there was a significant improvement in MHQ scores in the surgical group, although the mean Arthritis Impact Measurement Scales scores, grip, and pinch strength did not show any significant change.

A. K. S. Chong, MD

Reference

1. Chung KC, Burns PB, Wilgis EF, et al. A multicenter clinical trial in rheumatoid arthritis comparing silicone metacarpophalangeal joint arthroplasty with medical treatment. *J Hand Surg Am.* 2009;34:815-823.

2 Wrist Arthroscopy

Coexisting Intraarticular Disorders Are Unrelated To Outcomes After Arthroscopic Resection of Dorsal Wrist Ganglions
Kang HJ, Koh IH, Kim JS, et al (Yonsei Univ College of Medicine, Seodaemun-gu, Seoul, South Korea)
Clin Orthop Relat Res 471:2212-2218, 2013

Background.—Dorsal wrist ganglions are one of the most frequently encountered problems of the wrist and often are associated with intraarticular disorders. However, it is unclear whether coexisting intraarticular disorders influence persistent pain or recurrence after arthroscopic resection of dorsal wrist ganglions.

Questions/Purposes.—We investigated (1) which intraarticular disorders coexist with dorsal wrist ganglions and (2) whether they influenced pain, function, and recurrence after arthroscopic ganglion resection.

Methods.—We retrospectively reviewed 41 patients with primary dorsal wrist ganglions who underwent arthroscopic resection. We also obtained VAS pain scores and the Mayo Wrist Scores (MWS) preoperatively and at 2 weeks, 6 weeks, 3 months, 6 months, 1 year, and annually thereafter postoperatively. Minimum followup was 24 months (mean, 38.9 months; range, 24—60 months).

Results.—Twenty-one patients had other coexisting intraarticular disorders: 18 triangular fibrocartilage complex tears and nine intrinsic ligament tears. All coexisting disorders were treated simultaneously. Two years after surgery, the mean VAS pain score decreased from 2.4 to 0.6, and mean grip strength increased from 28 to 36 kg of force. The mean active flexion-extension showed no change. The mean MWS improved from 74 to 91. Three ganglions recurred. There was no difference in mean VAS pain score and MWS preoperatively and at 2 years after surgery or recurrence of ganglions between patients with or without coexisting lesions.

Conclusions.—Intraarticular disorders commonly coexist with ganglions but we found they were unrelated to pain, function, and recurrence after arthroscopic resection of the ganglion when the intraarticular disorders were treated simultaneously.

Level of Evidence.—Level IV, therapeutic study. See Guidelines for Authors for a complete description of levels of evidence.

▶ The authors discuss the utility of arthroscopic management of dorsal wrist ganglion excision as it relates to the often underappreciated recognition of concomitant intraarticular disorders of the wrist. Previous studies have reported on the incidence of intraarticular wrist pathology (including triangular fibrocartilage complex [TFCC] and intrinsic wrist ligament injuries) identified during arthroscopic ganglion excision. However, this series of 41 patients with at least 2-year follow-up shows that if properly identified and treated, additional wrist pathology was unrelated to pain, function, and recurrence of the ganglion. Interestingly, this study found that the most common concomitant condition was TFCC tear, as opposed to scapho-lunate injury as seen in multiple other case series. This may be the result of relative ulnar-positive variance among Asians. Specifically, only 21 of 41 patients were noted to have additional pathology, and in only 9 of 41 patients was the dorsal stalk identified. Finally, the presence of intraarticular pathology did not correlate with ganglion recurrence.

The central message of this case series is to report on the frequency of additional pathology observed during arthroscopic dorsal ganglion excision. The ability to identify and treat concomitant pathology from both the radiocarpal and midcarpal joints should result in greater patient satisfaction, as traditional, open surgical excision naturally precludes treatment of additional pathology. I have found the technique offered Yao and Trindade[1] particularly helpful in localizing the dorsal ganglion stalk with inert dye. This allows for complete excision of the visualized stalk, which ultimately minimizes the chance of ganglion recurrence.

S. M. Jacoby

Reference

1. Yao J, Trindade MC. Color-aided visualization of dorsal wrist ganglion stalks aids in complete arthroscopic excision. *Arthroscopy.* 2011;27(3):425-429. http://dx.doi.org/10.1016/j.arthro.2010.10.017.

Utility of Magnetic Resonance Imaging for Detection of Longitudinal Split Tear of the Ulnotriquetral Ligament

Ringler MD, Howe BM, Amrami KK, et al (Mayo Clinic, Rochester, MN)
J Hand Surg 38A:1723-1727, 2013

Purpose.—Wrist magnetic resonance imaging (MRI) has established utility in the diagnosis of wrist ligament tears, including complete tears of the ulnotriquetral ligament (UTL) and other components of the triangular fibrocartilage complex. A new type of longitudinal split tear of the UTL has recently been described with no imaging correlate. Our aims were to describe putative MRI findings associated with longitudinal UTL split tears and to assess diagnostic accuracy.

Methods.—We randomly selected 40 patients with arthroscopically proven longitudinal UTL split tears and 20 patients with intact UTLs, all of whom had preoperative 3 T MRI of the same wrist performed, from a list of operative notes spanning from January 1997 through October 2011, filtered with the terms "ulnotriquetral ligament" and "ulnar triquetral ligament." Two musculoskeletal radiologists who were blinded to surgical results and clinical information independently reviewed the exams. They recorded the degree of certainty of whether a longitudinal UTL split tear was present and whether several other hypothesized associated abnormalities were present.

Results.—Overall sensitivity for definitive longitudinal UTL split tear detection on MRI was 58% for reader 1 and 30% for reader 2. Specificity was 60% for both. There were no statistically significant discriminatory findings.

Conclusions.—Among a selected group of patients who all had wrist arthroscopy, preoperative noncontrast 3 T wrist MRI had poor sensitivity and specificity for detection of the longitudinal split type of UTL tear. To date, MRI may be more helpful to exclude potential alternative diagnoses in the patient with ulnar wrist pain.

▶ Ulnar-sided wrist pain remains one of the most difficult problems in the hand surgeon's office. As our understanding of the ulnar wrist has improved, we have been able to more clearly understand these patients' symptoms. Longitudinal ulnotriquetral ligament (UTL) tears are one of these diagnoses that have added to our understanding of these problems.

This study has 2 significant limitations, one of which they recognize. The list of cases that they mined for the diagnosis of UTL tears included cases performed before the description of UTL tears. Therefore, the presence or absence of mention of these injuries in the early years is suspect. The authors do not provide any information on the incidence of the diagnosis relative to the years of the index procedure. This they recognize.

The more significant limitation with this approach is that presumed positives based on arthroscopy may not represent what we currently think of as positive. In this group, if the magnetic resonance imaging (MRI) appropriately diagnoses the UTL as intact by current standards, but the abnormality noted at the time of arthroscopy does not meet the standard currently for a longitudinal tear, the usefulness of MRI is inappropriately minimized.

Regardless, this study shows what many clinicians see routinely in their practice: patients with foveal tenderness, normal distal radioulnar joint stability, and a normal MRI. At arthroscopy they have synovitis and an intact triangular fibrocartilage complex disc but some abnormality at the UTL. This study's demonstration of poor MRI sensitivity helps clinicians by encouraging them to rely more on physical examination and history.

T. Hughes, MD

Arthroscopic Excision of Dorsal Wrist Ganglion: Factors Related to Recurrence and Postoperative Residual Pain
Kim JP, Seo JB, Park HG, et al (Dankook Univ School of Medicine, Cheonan, Korea)
Arthroscopy 29:1019-1024, 2013

Purpose.—The purpose of this study was to assess the recurrence rate and postoperative residual pain rate after arthroscopic excision of dorsal wrist ganglia and the risk factors for recurrence and residual pain.

Methods.—A total of 115 wrists (111 patients: 57 men, 54 women; average age 34 years; range, 9 to 72 years) treated with arthroscopic excision for wrist dorsal ganglia between April 2005 and December 2009 were enrolled. The follow-up averaged 32 months (range, 12 to 67 months). Demographic data and operative details, including the presence of a ganglion stalk, were retrospectively reviewed and tested against recurrence and residual pain at final follow-up.

Results.—The recurrence rate of dorsal wrist ganglia after arthroscopic excision was 11% (13 of 115 wrists). Recurrence was on the dominant side in 12 of 13 (91%) patients, which was the most important risk factor for recurrence (odds ratio [OR], 8.0; 95% confidence interval [CI], 0.94 to 68.49), followed by female sex (OR, 4.9; 95% CI, 0.84 to 28.39) and age 24 years or younger (OR, 3.1; 95% CI, 0.75 to 12.74). Twenty-seven wrists (23%) had postoperative residual pain at final follow-up. The results of logistic regression showed that pain before surgery was the most important risk factor for residual pain after surgery (OR, 4.9; 95% CI, 1.36 to 18.3), followed by female sex (OR, 3.2; 95% CI, 1.22 to 8.53).

Conclusions.—Dominant side, female sex, and age of 24 years or younger are considered to be the most influential risk factors for recurrence after arthroscopic excision of dorsal wrist ganglia. However, the presence or absence of the cyst stalk was not a significant factor for recurrence. Female patients who have preoperative pain around the dorsal wrist ganglia were most likely to experience residual pain after surgery.

Level of Evidence.—Level IV, therapeutic case series.

▶ The authors present a retrospective study to assess the recurrence rate and postoperative residual pain rate after arthroscopic excision of dorsal wrist ganglia and the risk factors for recurrence and residual pain. In a large series of 111 patients followed up for an average of 32 months, the authors reported a recurrence rate of 11% with hand dominance, female sex, and age of 24 years or younger being the most influential risk factors for recurrence. Interestingly, the authors noted that the presence or absence of the cyst stalk was not a significant factor for recurrence. The findings of this study add little to the existing evidence of outcomes after arthroscopic excision of dorsal wrist ganglions. There are several weaknesses in this study, including the methods to determine postoperative recurrence, a retrospective study design, and absence of a control group. In addition, the authors did not routinely examine the midcarpal joint, and they were unable to determine the correlation of recurrence with scapholunate instability. The main options for the treatment of wrist ganglia are reassurance and benign neglect, aspiration, arthroscopic resection, and open excision. Variations within each option have been described, and the literature is clouded by widespread variability in the results reported. Osterman and Raphael[1] pioneered the arthroscopic resection of dorsal wrist ganglions and reported on 150 procedures with only 1 recurrence. Arthroscopic excision is a less-invasive surgical alternative to open resection with the benefits of visualizing and treating other intra-articular pathology, fewer potential complications, and earlier return to activities. Several investigators believe that the recurrence rate depends on adequate visualization and resection of the ganglion stalk.[2,3] In a recent prospective, randomized study, Kang et al[4] concluded that the rates of recurrence with arthroscopic dorsal ganglion excision are comparable with and not superior to those of open excision. Currently, I prefer arthroscopic resection for dorsal wrist ganglions. I introduce a 2-0 PDS suture through a 21-gauge hypodermic needle introduced through the ganglion cyst. This helps visualize the stalk and the redundant tissue at all times and also prevents "blue-out" caused by the injection of methylene blue. I perform a systematic examination of the radiocarpal and midcarpal joints. This helps identify any ligament injuries and presence of occult ganglions.

A. L. Wahegaonkar, MD, FACS, MCh (Orth)

References

1. Osterman AL, Raphael J. Arthroscopic resection of dorsal ganglion of the wrist. *Hand Clin.* 1995;11:7-12.
2. Gallego S, Mathoulin C. Arthroscopic resection of dorsal wrist ganglia: 114 cases with minimum follow-up of 2 years. *Arthroscopy.* 2010;26:1675-1682.
3. Yao J, Trindade MC. Color-aided visualization of dorsal wrist ganglion stalks aids in complete arthroscopic excision. *Arthroscopy.* 2011;27:425-429.
4. Kang L, Akelman E, Weiss AP. Arthroscopic versus open dorsal ganglion excision: A prospective, randomized comparison of rates of recurrence and of residual pain. *J Hand Surg.* 2008;33:471-475.

3 Carpus

In Vivo **3-Dimensional Analysis of Dorsal Intercalated Segment Instability Deformity Secondary to Scapholunate Dissociation: A Preliminary Report**
Omori S, Moritomo H, Omokawa S, et al (Osaka Univ Graduate School of Medicine, Japan; Osaka Yukioka College of Health Science, Japan; Nara Med Univ, Japan)
J Hand Surg 38A:1346-1355, 2013

Purpose.—To investigate *in vivo* 3-dimensional patterns of dorsal intercalated segment instability deformity resulting from scapholunate dissociation.

Methods.—We studied 6 patients with stage IV scapholunate dissociation in which there were complete tears of the scapholunate interosseous ligament and dorsal intercalated segment instability deformity. Of these, 3 patients had a dorsally displaced distal radius malunion, a condition known to aggravate or produce a dorsal intercalated segment instability deformity. With the wrist in neutral, we created 3-dimensional bone models of the wrists from computed tomography. We calculated centroid locations of each carpal and the rotational angle of the scaphoid and lunate relative to the radius and compared them with those of 6 normal subjects. The joint contact area was visualized to evaluate congruity of the radiocarpal and midcarpal joints.

Results.—In the scapholunate dissociated wrists, the scaphoid translated dorsally and radially with rotation in the direction of flexion and pronation. The lunate was extended and supinated. The capitate, trapezoid, and trapezium translated dorsally. Contact area of the radioscaphoid joint shifted dorsoradially owing to dorsoradial subluxation of the scaphoid proximal pole. Congruity was retained in the radiolunate, lunocapitate, and scaphotrapeziotrapezoid joints. In the malunion cases, the scaphoid and distal carpal rows translated more dorsally along dorsal angulation of the distal radius; therefore, incongruity of the radioscaphoid joint became more pronounced.

Conclusions.—Dorsoradial subluxation of the scaphoid proximal pole over the dorsal rim of the radius led to incongruity of the radioscaphoid joint. Dorsal translation of the distal carpal row occurred with maintaining congruency of the radiolunate, lunocapitate, and scaphotrapeziotrapezoid joints. These results suggest that for realignment of the carpal axis of an advanced scapholunate dissociated wrist, we should restore scapholunate rotational malalignment and reduce the dorsally translated distal carpal row back to the anatomical position.

▶ This report provides a novel 3-dimensional computed tomography (CT) analysis of dissociative and nondissociative dorsal intercalated segment instability (DISI) patterns caused by scapho-lunate ligament disruption (CID) and distal radius malunion with dorsal malalignment.

This article is significant in that it provides a detailed 3-dimensional CT surface bone model analysis, including measurements of centroid translation, carpal rotation, and joint congruency for each of the carpal bones relative to the distal radius in both dissociative and nondissociative types of DISI deformity. It is a well-designed and well-executed study that provides valuable in vivo data from patients with these types of carpal instability patterns. The joint contact and bone surface pressure figures provide pictures that add to our understanding of this problem.

The strengths of this study include its design, its execution, and a relatively clear presentation of the results and discussion; weaknesses are the small sample size and lack of matched controls. One could also argue that the patients selected for inclusion in the CID group had less than 3 months of observation, as injury and the full DISI deformity had not yet developed. However, this study provided an insightful and visual in vivo analysis of DISI patterns that has furthered my understanding of this complicated injury process.

J. L. Tueting, MD

Multiplanar reconstruction computed tomography for diagnosis of scaphoid waist fracture union: a prospective cohort analysis of accuracy and precision
Hannemann PFW, Brouwers L, van der Zee D, Stadler A, et al (Maastricht Univ Med Centre, The Netherlands)
Skeletal Radiol 42:1377-1382, 2013

Objective.—To examine reliability and validity concerning union of scaphoid fractures determined by multiplanar reconstruction computed tomography randomized at 6, 12, and 24 weeks after injury.

Materials and Methods.—We used Fleiss' kappa to measure the opinions of three observers reviewing 44 sets of computed tomographic scans of 44 conservatively treated scaphoid waist fractures. We calculated kappa for the extent of consolidation ($0-24$ %, $25-49$ %, $50-74$ %, or $75-100$ %) on the transverse, sagittal and coronal views. We also calculated kappa for no union, partial union, and union, and grouped the results for 6, 12, and 24 weeks after injury. As the reference standard for union, CT scans were performed at a minimum of 6 months after injury to determine validity.

Results.—Overall inter-observer agreement was found to be moderate ($\kappa = 0.576$). No union ($\kappa = 0.791$), partial union ($\kappa = 0.502$), and union ($\kappa = 0.683$) showed substantial, moderate, and substantial agreement, respectively. The average sensitivity of multiplanar reconstruction CT for diagnosing union of scaphoid waist fractures was 73 %. The average specificity was 80 %.

Conclusions.—Our results suggest that multiplanar reconstruction computed tomography is a reliable and accurate method for diagnosing union or nonunion of scaphoid fractures. However, inter-observer agreement was lower with respect to partial union.

▶ The authors present an interesting and well-designed prospective cohort analysis of accuracy and precision using multiplanar reconstruction computed tomography (CT) for the diagnosis of scaphoid waist fracture union. They suggest that multiplanar reconstruction CT is a reliable and accurate method for diagnosing union or nonunion of scaphoid fractures. However, interobserver agreement was lower with respect to partial union. Despite extensive literature supporting the use of CT scans in evaluating scaphoid fractures, there is no consensus on the methodology for defining and quantifying union.[1] This study might help build more evidence regarding the methodology for determining union status after scaphoid fractures using CT. However, there are serious concerns about radiation exposure and costs with the implementation of this method to assess scaphoid nonunion in most practice settings. Scaphoid fractures are particularly prone to nonunion, avascular necrosis, and other fracture complications. Although there has been long-standing debate over the optimal method of diagnosing scaphoid fractures, the best and most cost-effective methods combine clinical examination with other imaging modalities, such as plain films including stress views, CT, and magnetic resonance imaging (MRI) for particularly questionable presentations. Currently, I prefer plain radiographs and CT scanning for diagnosing scaphoid waist nonunions. However, I rely on a gadolinium-enhanced MR scan in patients with a proximal pole nonunion in which there is a questionable vascularity of the proximal pole fragment.

A. L. Wahegaonkar, MD, FACS, MCh (Orth)

Reference

1. Grewal R, Frakash U, Osman S, McMurtry RY. A quantitative definition of scaphoid union: determining the inter-rater reliability of two techniques. *J Orthop Surg Res.* 2013;8:28.

Radiographic Diagnosis of Scapholunate Dissociation Among Intraarticular Fractures of the Distal Radius: Interobserver Reliability
Gradl G, Science of Variation Group (Univ of Aachen Med Ctr, Germany; Massachusetts General Hosp, Boston; Rhön Klinikum AG, Bad Neustadt Saale, Germany; et al)
J Hand Surg 38A:1685-1690, 2013

Purpose.—To evaluate the reliability and accuracy of diagnosis of scapholunate dissociation (SLD) among AO type C (compression articular) fractures of the distal radius.

Methods.—A total of 217 surgeons evaluated 21 sets of radiographs with type C fractures of the distal radius for which the status of the scapholunate interosseous ligament was established by preoperative 3-compartment computed tomographic arthrography with direct operative visualization of diagnosed SLD (reference standard). Observers were asked whether SLD was present, and if yes, whether they would recommend operative treatment. Diagnostic performance characteristics were calculated with respect to the reference standard. We assessed interobserver reliability using the Fleiss generalized kappa.

Results.—The interobserver agreement for radiographic diagnosis of SLD was moderate ($\kappa = 0.44$). Correct diagnosis for a given set of radiographs ranged from 8% to 98% (average, 79%) of observers. Diagnostic performance characteristics were: 69% sensitivity, 84% specificity, 84% accuracy, 68% positive predictive value, and 84% negative predictive value. Based on a prevalence of 5%, Bayes adjusted positive and negative predictive values were 18% and 98%, respectively. Raters recommended operative treatment in 74% to 100% of patients diagnosed with SLD.

Conclusions.—Radiographs are moderately reliable and are better at ruling out than ruling in SLD associated with type C fracture of the distal radius.

▶ This interesting study is an example of cooperation among a large number of surgeons working all over the world called the Science of Variation Group. It assessed the sensitivity, specificity, accuracy, positive predictive value, and negative predictive value when evaluating scapholunate dissociation (SLD) in radiographs of patients with AO type C distal radius fracture. The study also supports treatment of these instabilities based on the recommendations of these surgeons. From my personal feeling, this study describes more the weakness of radiographs when diagnosing SLD than problems with interobserver reliability. It is interesting that less agreement was found among more experienced surgeons. On the other hand, precise diagnosis with suggested 3-compartment computed tomographic arthrography with direct operative visualization of diagnosed SLD is rarely possible in trauma departments treating these complicated injuries.

In my clinical practice, I evaluate radiographs looking for clear SLD symptoms, and only in these cases I perform reduction and percutaneous pinning for 6 weeks. I don't attempt to visualize the SL complex. I also suggest, based on a few irreducible SLD cases I've seen, that some of them may be old previous injuries and do not need to be treated.

P. Czarnecki, MD

An innovative orthotic design for midcarpal instability, non-dissociative: Mobility with stability
O'Brien MT (Brigham and Women's Hosp, Chestnut Hill, MA 02467)
J Hand Ther 26:363-364, 2013

Assisting carpal instability patients with regaining pain free and symptom free movement is a primary goal of therapy. This author describes her version of an orthotic device for carpal instability non-dissociative. She also describe her typical treatment plan for these patients.

▶ The author's goal of providing an orthotic device that would allow for pain-free movement in the setting of carpal instability is novel. This is a well-described classification of instability and brief history on the causation of proximal carpal instability. Providing dorsal stability of the distal ulnar is something previous designs lacked or previous designs, in effect, were too immobilizing. Orthotic fabrication that allows for improved function and patient compliance is always the goal in hand therapy. I would have liked to see comments on the compliance of splint wear and midrange strengthening in this particular program. This article provided detail and easy-to-follow instructions on the fabrication of the orthotic. It could be duplicated by practitioners, with photographs to compare and emulate, providing a design that does not promote stiffness and muscle atrophy due to immobilization, which would allow for quicker return to functional activities. Some of the variables that were included in the article were the treatment protocol of midrange strengthening exercise and some type of heat modality.

Could pain decrease be caused by therapy exercise program versus the orthotic device that allows for freedom in movement? This is certainly a topic for further study.

S. Kranz, OTR/L, CHT

Effect of Capitate Morphology on Contact Biomechanics After Proximal Row Carpectomy
Tang P, Swart E, Konopka G, et al (Allegheny Health Network, Pittsburgh, PA; Columbia Univ Med Ctr, NY; Univ of Texas, Houston; et al)
J Hand Surg 38A:1340-1345, 2013

Purpose.—Proximal row carpectomy (PRC) is used as a treatment for a variety of wrist pathologies to maintain motion and to improve strength and decrease pain. Several studies have looked at how PRC alters wrist characteristics, although they did not provide an explanation for the variability observed in outcomes. Studies have classified the capitate into 3 unique types: round, V-shaped, or flat. We hypothesized that these differences in morphology could affect the contact biomechanics between the radius and the capitate after PRC.

Methods.—A total of 14 cadaveric wrists underwent PRC. They were classified by capitate morphology and then loaded to 200 N in a neutral position, flexion, and extension. We measured contact area, contact pressure, and location using pressure-sensitive film in all 3 positions and compared their morphology types.

Results.—Nine wrists had a round-type capitate, 4 had a V-shaped capitate, and 1 had a flat capitate, which we excluded from statistical analysis. Comparing round and V-shaped types, we found no differences in contact area, pressure, or location in any wrist position For the V-shaped capitates, there was increased contact pressure in flexion and extension compared with the wrist in neutral. Center of pressure translated dorsal and radial in flexion to volar and ulnar in extension for all types.

Conclusions.—When we compared V-shaped and round-type capitates, we found no significant differences in contact characteristics of the wrist after PRC. There were some differences in contact pressure for V-shaped capitates in various wrist positions.

Clinical Relevance.—Differences between round and V-shaped capitates do not appear to affect contact biomechanics after PRC. Thus, these 2 capitate shapes may not necessarily be a factor in the decision-making process to perform PRC.

▶ Proximal row carpectomy (PRC) is a time-tested treatment for scapholunate advanced collapse wrist as well as other conditions. It has worked successfully in most patients for whom it is recommended. However, there are still concerns over its durability and long-term success. As the shape of the capitate does not completely resemble that of the lunate, it has matched the lunate facet of the radius sufficiently enough to provide good clinical outcomes. However, there is a trend to maintain the lunate (with mid-carpal fusions) in younger patients to more exactly match the lunate facet.

This study measures contact pressures and contact areas after PRC. Specifically, they looked at different capitate morphologies (flat, round, and v-shaped) to evaluate if the forces were different based on capitate shape. Presumable, if the capitate is flat, it might more closely resemble the lunate, which on the anteroposterior view is typically flat. The authors do not even propose this connection (likely because their data could not detect differences) and speak only of "the possibility that gross morphologic differences in capitate shapes cause differences in the mechanical environment."

The obvious weakness of the usefulness of this study is the inability to prove any significant differences. However, my criticism is not that they couldn't find differences but in their suggestion that a 16% difference in contact pressures would not be clinically meaningful. They use this statement to justify the low power of the study. However, given the good results of PRCs in general, it would probably take a very small difference in pressure over a significant length of time to lead to a clinical difference.

The addition of these data to the literature likely helps only to suggest the need for further study.

T. Hughes, MD

Scaphoid Overstuffing: The Effects of the Dimensions of Scaphoid Reconstruction on Scapholunate Alignment
Capito AE, Higgins JP (MedStar Union Memorial Hosp, Baltimore, MD)
J Hand Surg Am 38:2419-2425, 2013

Purpose.—Osteochondral replacement of the proximal scaphoid has been reported using a vascularized flap from the medial femoral trochlea. A concern with this technique is the loss of stability of the scapholunate relationship with resection of the scaphoid proximal pole. Overexpansion of the scaphoid dimensions (overstuffing) during scaphoid reconstruction with the osteochondral flap may play a role in maintaining scapholunate alignment. Our purpose was to determine if overstuffing the scaphoid can correct rotatory carpal instability in a cadaveric model studied radiographically.

Methods.—The radiolunate angle and scapholunate interval were measured for 5 fresh cadaver wrists. We completely incised the scapholunate interosseous ligament and performed an osteotomy to excise the proximal third of the scaphoid to simulate a proximal pole deficiency nonunion and create a dorsal intercalated segmental instability deformity. Radiographic measurements were repeated. The proximal pole of the scaphoid was replaced with its original piece of bone; radiographic measurements were repeated without scapholunate ligament repair. The osteotomy site was overstuffed with a 4-mm sawbone spacer without scapholunate ligament repair, and radiographs were obtained.

Results.—Sectioning of scapholunate ligaments and proximal pole excision successfully created carpal instability demonstrated by abnormal radiolunate angles. Without ligament repair, proximal pole replacement did not restore normal radiolunate angles. Expansion of the scaphoid dimensions corrected radiolunate angles on lateral unloaded radiographs and improved scapholunate intervals on clenched fist radiographs. These findings were statistically significant compared with the unexpanded (replaced) scaphoid.

Conclusions.—These findings suggest that scaphoid reconstruction that results in expansion of the scaphoid's normal dimensions will restore carpal alignment without scapholunate ligament reconstruction.

Clinical Relevance.—Osteochondral reconstruction of difficult proximal pole nonunions may not require any preservation or reconstruction of scapholunate integrity if the reconstruction expands the normal dimensions of the native scaphoid. Scapholunate interval and carpal alignment may be restored by scaphoid overstuffing. The effects on increased contact pressure and range of motion require further investigation.

▶ The authors hypothesized that expanding the proximo-distal dimensions of the scaphoid by inserting a nonanatomically correctly sized osteochondral graft (termed *overstuffing*) might improve the scapholunate angle in patients with necrotic nonunion of the proximal pole of the scaphoid treated with this osteochondral graft. In a small series of 5 cadaver wrists, they excised the proximal pole and divided the intrinsic and extrinsic ligaments, creating a dorsal intercalated segmental instability (DISI) pattern. They replaced the resected proximal pole and saw some improvement in metrics but much more significant improvement when they added a 4-mm wedge between the proximal pole and remaining scaphoid, presumably increasing scaphoid dimensions (overstuffing the scaphoid.) They opine that purposefully overstuffing the scaphoid would improve kinematics. Their model creates the ideal reconstruction in that the normally shaped proximal pole is replaced, with extra bone stuffing. The clinical circumstance is much removed from the ideal. The residual proximal pole may have shriveled into something resembling a dried pea. In this case, the chondral part of the osteochondral graft must be carved freehand to fit as best as possible in the scaphoid fossa of the radius. Having performed many successful rib osteocutaneous grafts for these cases, I've never seen one that looked ideal. So what works in this nice cadaver model may not yield the same result in the typical clinical setting. It is still my advice to my hand fellows to stop taking x-rays once you are sure the bony part of your graft has healed to the distal scaphoid. It is not at all clear that a mild residual DISI pattern leads to an unfavorable outcome provided that the scaphoid reconstruction prevents progressive carpal collapse. Another concern is whether too much scaphoid length may reduce wrist motion.

V. R. Hentz, MD

Reconstruction of Both Volar and Dorsal Limbs of the Scapholunate Interosseous Ligament
Henry M (Hand and Wrist Ctr of Houston, TX)
J Hand Surg 38A:1625-1634, 2013

Complete scapholunate interosseous ligament deficiency can lead to pain, reduced functional performance, and scapholunate advanced collapse arthritis. Efforts to restore carpal stability began with procedures to tether scaphoid motion. Techniques evolved to include multiple differing strategies of linking the scaphoid to the lunate dorsally in the transverse plane. Actually restoring stability has proven elusive owing to the impossibility of truly replicating the original anatomy and the multidirectional forces to which the scapholunate interface is subjected. The described surgical technique differs from others by reconstructing both the volar and dorsal limbs of the scapholunate ligament and accounting for the multiple force vectors involved in scapholunate instability.

▶ Scapholunate ligament injuries remain an unsolved problem in hand surgery. Ligament reconstructions are hampered by high-strain forces across the scapholunate gap, poor vascularity of the scaphoid and lunate, and lack of understanding of all of the structures at play. Indirect stabilization procedures that aim to prevent scaphoid flexion such as the Blatt or the Szabo capsulodeses do not address the gapping at the scapholunate interval and do not restrict proximal capitate migration. Dorsal ligament reconstructions such as the bone-tendon-bone and the modified Brunelli do not address the volar ligament, leaving the scapholunate interval gapped anteriorly and relying on the dorsal reconstruction to resist all tensile forces across the joint. Attempts at doing a circumferential reconstruction with drill holes through the proximal pole of the scaphoid have shown a high risk of avascular necrosis. The scapholunate axis method reconstruction, which I helped to develop, was an attempt to provide 2 fixation points across the scapholunate interval while limiting the insult to the proximal pole.

The volar and dorsal reconstruction detailed in this surgical technique article is promising because it takes advantage of the Brunelli scaphoid bone tunnel to reconstruct the volar scaphotrapezial-trapezoidal ligaments and the dorsal scapholunate ligament (SLIL) while also building in a volar SLIL reconstruction without further compromising the vascularity of the proximal pole of the scaphoid.

As with all reconstructions that have been devised, only time and clinical experience will tell if this reconstruction is better than any of the others before it.

D. A. Zlotolow, MD

A comparison of the rates of union after cancellous iliac crest bone graft and Kirschner-wire fixation in the treatment of stable and unstable scaphoid nonunion
Park HY, Yoon JO, Jeon IH, et al (Asan Med Ctr, Seoul, Korea)
Bone Joint J 95-B:809-814, 2013

This study was performed to determine whether pure cancellous bone graft and Kirschner (K-) wire fixation were sufficient to achieve bony union and restore alignment in scaphoid nonunion. A total of 65 patients who underwent cancellous bone graft and K-wire fixation were included in this study. The series included 61 men and four women with a mean age of 34 years (15 to 72) and mean delay to surgery of 28.7 months (3 to 240). The patients were divided into an unstable group (A) and stable group (B) depending on the pre-operative radiographs. Unstable nonunion was defined as a lateral intrascaphoid angle > 45°, or a radiolunate angle > 10°. There were 34 cases in group A and 31 cases in group B. Bony union was achieved in 30 patients (88.2%) in group A, and in 26 (83.9%) in group B (p = 0.439). Comparison of the post-operative radiographs between the two groups showed no significant differences in lateral intrascaphoid angle (p = 0.657) and scaphoid length (p = 0.670) and height (p = 0.193). The radiolunate angle was significantly different (p = 0.020) but the mean value in both groups was < 10°. Comparison of the dorsiflexion and palmar flexion of movement of the wrist and the mean Mayo wrist score at the final clinical visit in each group showed no significant difference (p = 0.190, p = 0.587 and p = 0.265, respectively). Cancellous bone graft and K-wire fixation were effective in the treatment of stable and unstable scaphoid nonunion.

▶ The authors present an interesting study comparing the rates of union after cancellous iliac crest bone graft (ICBG) and Kirschner (K-)wire fixation in the treatment of stable and unstable scaphoid nonunion. In a retrospective study, they divided 65 patients into an unstable Group A (n = 34) and stable Group B (n = 31) depending on the preoperative radiographs. Unstable nonunion was defined as a lateral intrascaphoid angle > 45° or a radiolunate angle > 10°. The study revealed that there was essentially no statistical difference between the rate, time to union, wrist range of motion, and Mayo Wrist Score between the 2 study groups. Moreover, no radiologic measurements except the radiolunate angle showed statistical difference. The authors conclude that iliac crest cancellous bone grafting and K-wire fixation provide reliable results even in unstable scaphoid nonunions. However, there are a few weaknesses in the study. It would have been interesting to compare the outcomes of K-wire fixation and cancellous ICBG with those of a more rigid fixation modality, such as a headless compression screw and cancellous ICBG in unstable scaphoid nonunions. The outcome measures would have been more reliable if cases with avascular necrosis (AVN) were excluded from the study. Lastly, of 15 patients with a preoperative dorsal intercalated segment instability (DISI), 8 had a persistent DISI postoperatively, and it puts into question the ability of cancellous bone graft alone vis-à-vis with corticocancellous ICBG in providing and maintaining structural stability in unstable scaphoid nonunions. Cancellous bone grafting combined with K-wire fixation is a relatively straightforward technique that has been shown in several studies to predictably produce healing of scaphoid nonunions. This retrospective study proves this point, albeit with some redundancy. Currently, for all established scaphoid nonunions with absence of AVN, I prefer to use a corticocancellous ICBG with a rigid headless compression screw fixation. In documented cases with AVN, I opt for vascularized bone grafts in addition to cancellous bone graft and fixation with K-wires and/or a screw, depending on the size and condition of the proximal fragment.

A. L. Wahegaonkar, MD, FACS, M.Ch(Orth)

Clinical and Radiological Outcomes of Scaphoidectomy and 4-Corner Fusion in Scapholunate Advanced Collapse at 5 and 10 Years

Cha S-M, Shin H-D, Kim K-C (Chungnam Natl Univ, Daejeon, Korea)
Ann Plast Surg 71:166-169, 2013

Summary.—This retrospective study examined clinical and radiological outcomes of scaphoidectomy and 4-corner fusion in patients with a scapholunate advanced collapse (SLAC) at 5 and 10 years.

Purpose.—Partial wrist arthrodesis is commonly performed to treat wrist arthritis because it provides pain relief without sacrificing complete wrist motion. The purposes of this retrospective study were to evaluate clinical and radiological outcomes after scaphoidectomy and 4-corner fusion after more than 10 years of follow-up and to compare the midterm and long-term results.

Methods.—Forty-two patients were enrolled. The following were evaluated annually: pain (visual analog scale); Disabilities of the Arm, Shoulder, and Hand score; range of motion; grip strength; and Modified Mayo Wrist score. Bony union and arthritic changes in the radiolunate joint were also evaluated radiologically. Midterm and long-term results were compared.

Results.—The mean (SD) follow-up period was 12.2 (1.43) years. Two patients were excluded from the study because of complications, so the final postoperative evaluation included 40 patients. Visual analog scale and Disabilities of the Arm, Shoulder, and Hand scores improved to a satisfactory level by 5 years after surgery and did not differ significantly between 5 and 10 years. Flexion, extension, and radial deviation were reduced after 5 years compared with preoperative measures, and no difference was found between 5 and 10 years. Ulnar deviation, pronation, and supination did not change significantly after surgery. Grip strength was significantly recovered from 29.7 (4.9) kg at 5 years after surgery to 32.1 (8.5) kg at 10 years. The Modified Mayo Wrist score improved significantly to 83.2 (4.1) at 5 years after surgery but did not differ significantly between 5 and 10 years. All cases showed radiological solid fusion, and the mean (SD) period of union was 9.34 (3.7) weeks. Further radiolunate arthritic change was verified in 2 patients, but Modified Mayo Wrist scores were fair. One patient experienced inexplicable pain; therefore, total wrist fusion was performed at 6 years after surgery.

Conclusions.—This retrospective cohort study of patients followed up for more than 10 years showed that the midterm and long-term results of 4-corner fusion for stage III SLAC were satisfactory, and arthritic changes in the radiolunate joint were minimal.

▶ The authors present an important study regarding clinical and radiologic outcomes of scaphoidectomy and 4-corner fusion in patients with a scapholunate advanced collapse at 5 and 10 years. The grip, Disabilities of the Arm, Shoulder, and Hand score and Visual Analog Scale score all showed much improvement after surgery and without significant difference between 5 and 10 years. Loss of some range of motion was noted after surgery, but there was no significant difference between 5 and 10 years. The radiologic follow-up showed minimal progressive arthritic change in the radiolunate joint. The results were satisfactory and durable. Currently, I perform radial styloidectomy, scaphoidectomy, and 4-corner fusion for stage II and III scapholunate advanced collapse. I have also been impressed with its durable and satisfying results. I have performed proximal row carpectomy for several patients with stage II scapholunate advanced collapse but found progressive arthritic change of the articulation between the radius and capitate and need for further surgical intervention.

Y. C. Huang, MD

4 Dupuytren's Contracture

Patterns of Recontracture After Surgical Correction of Dupuytren Disease
Dias JJ, Singh HP, Ullah A, et al (Univ of Leicester, UK)
J Hand Surg 38A:1987-1993, 2013

Purpose.—To study the evolution of deformity of the proximal interphalangeal joint over 5 years after good surgical correction of Dupuytren-induced contracture.

Methods.—We assessed 63 patients (72 fingers; 69 hands) with Dupuytren disease for the degree of contracture, its correction after surgery, and the range of movement at the proximal interphalangeal joints at 3 and 6 months, and 1, 3, and 5 years after fasciectomy with or without the use of a firebreak graft. We investigated associations between the recurrence of contracture and preoperative patient and surgical factors.

Results.—There were 4 patterns of evolution of contracture after surgical correction. A total of 31 patients (33 hands) showed good improvement that was maintained for 5 years (minimal recontracture group). Twenty patients (23 hands) showed good initial improvement, which mildly worsened (<20°) but was then maintained over 5 years (mild early recontracture group). Four patients (5 hands) worsened in first 3 months after surgery (>20°) but there was no further worsening (severe early recontracture group). Eight patients (8 hands) worsened progressively over 5 years (progressive recontracture group). Worsening of contracture more than 6 between 3 and 6 months after surgery predicted progressive recontracture at 5 years.

Conclusions.—Recurrence of contracture (not disease recurrence) could be predicted as early as 6 months after surgery for Dupuytren disease.

▶ Joint contracture after treatment for Dupuytren's disease remains a significant problem and concern. This is even more poignant in patients who undergo surgical treatment, as treatment of contractures after surgery for Dupuytren's carries greater risk and complications.

The authors attempt to provide insight into this problem, which is all too frequent after treatment for Dupuytren's contracture. Despite being a retrospective review, the article sheds interesting light on the incidence of recurrence of proximal interphalangeal (PIP) contracture after treatment. The aim was to review outcomes of PIP correction after Dupuytren's surgery to determine what, if any, information can be gleaned from these observations.

Interestingly, the authors concluded that within the first 3 to 6 months after treatment (if the patient had a greater than 6° worsening of contracture), there was an association with recurrence at 5 years.

Traditional statistical measures were not used; rather generalized estimating equations were used to assess associations between variables such as family history, bilateral involvement, diabetes, and smoking. Jonckheere-Terpstra testing was used to examine recurrence with age, degree of preoperative joint contracture, duration of disease, and operating time.

They identified 4 groups: (1) progressive contracture group, (2) severe early contracture group, (3) mild early contracture group, and (4) minimal contracture group. They measured 3 months, 6 months, 1 year, 3 years, and 5 years after surgery and found that if there was a greater than 6° worsening of contracture between 3 and 6 months, it correlated with progressive recurrence at 5 years.

Allowing for limitation of this being a retrospective observational study, I applaud the authors' attempts to help us better understand the phenomena of recurrence after surgical treatment of Dupuytren's disease. I agree that this is as much a study of joint contracture as recurrent Dupuytren's. It underscores the difficulties in managing both problems in these patients. In addition, one of the added benefits of this study includes some observations on their experience with surgery for Dupuytren's in general such as the lack of benefit with skin grafting.

M. Rizzo, MD

Dupuytren Disease: European Hand Surgeons, Hand Therapists, and Physical Medicine and Rehabilitation Physicians Agree on a Multidisciplinary Treatment Guideline: Results from the HANDGUIDE Study
Huisstede BMA, On behalf of the European HANDGUIDE Group (Erasmus MC—Univ Med Ctr Rotterdam, The Netherlands; et al)
Plast Reconstr Surg 132:964e-976e, 2013

Background.—Multidisciplinary treatment guidelines for Dupuytren disease can aid in optimizing the quality of care for patients with this disorder. Therefore, this study aimed to achieve consensus on a multidisciplinary treatment guideline for Dupuytren disease.

Methods.—A European Delphi consensus strategy was initiated. A systematic review reporting on the effectiveness of interventions was conducted and used as an evidence-based starting point for this study. In total, 39 experts (hand surgeons, hand therapists, and physical medicine and rehabilitation physicians) participated in the Delphi consensus strategy. Each Delphi round consisted of a questionnaire, an analysis, and a feedback report.

Results.—After four Delphi rounds, consensus was achieved on the description, symptoms, and diagnosis of Dupuytren disease. No nonsurgical interventions were included in the guideline. Needle and open fasciotomy, and a limited fasciectomy and dermofasciectomy, were seen as suitable surgical techniques for Dupuytren disease. Factors relevant for choosing one of these surgical techniques were identified and divided into patient-related (age, comorbidity), disease-related (palpable cord, previous surgery in the same area, skin involvement, time of recovery, recurrences), and surgeon-related (years of experience) factors. Associations of these factors with the choice of a specific surgical technique were reported in the guideline. Postsurgical rehabilitation should always include instructions and exercise therapy; postsurgical splinting should be performed on indication. Relevant details for the use of surgical and postsurgical interventions were described.

Conclusion.—This treatment guideline is likely to promote further discussion on related clinical and scientific issues and may therefore contribute to better treatment of patients with Dupuytren disease.

▶ With the multiplicity of treatments, both operative and nonoperative, now available for Dupuytren's disease, consensus is very difficult. This is because of several factors, including surgeon preference, experience, training, practice environment, and patient population. The European HANDGUIDE group used the Delphi consensus strategy to gain perspective on practice trends in Europe. This systematic review was used to gather consensus among a panel of 18 hand surgeons, 20 hand therapists, and 5 physical medicine and rehabilitation physicians on various aspect of the management of Dupuytren's disease. These individuals were considered experts in the European community. The number of experts who actually participated in the Dupuytren's portion of the HANDGUIDE study was inconsistently reported in the report. Nevertheless, the recommendations of the group were that consensus was achievable in several areas of the management of Dupuytren's disease. The group reached consensus that nonoperative management was not effective for the condition and that further data were needed on the effectiveness of collagenase therapy. There was agreement that the current array of surgical treatments (fasciotomy, limited fasciectomy, and dermofasciectomy) could be used to effectively treat the condition. Recurrent disease was identified as a factor that drove the decision on a specific surgical treatment. Agreement was reached on the importance and need for postoperative exercise therapy but agreement could not be reached on the role of postoperative splinting.

Consensus on the management of Dupuytren's disease is challenging in the United States and perhaps in other international locales given the multiplicity of viable treatment alternatives, surgical training bias, and patient population trends. The authors are to be congratulated on bringing clarity to the practice norms in the European community for Dupuytren's disease.

P. Murray, MD

Efficacy and Safety of Concurrent Collagenase Clostridium Histolyticum Injections for Multiple Dupuytren Contractures

Coleman S, Gilpin D, Kaplan FTD, et al (Brisbane Hand and Upper Limb Clinic, Queensland, Australia; Indiana Hand to Shoulder Ctr, Indianapolis; Caboolture Clinical Res Centre, Queensland, Australia; et al)

J Hand Surg Am 39:57-64, 2014

Purpose.—To assess the safety and efficacy of 2 concurrent injections of collagenase clostridium histolyticum (CCH) in the same hand to treat multiple Dupuytren flexion contractures.

Methods.—In a multicenter, open-label phase IIIb study, 60 patients received two 0.58-mg CCH doses injected into cords affecting 2 joints in the same hand during 1 visit, followed by finger extension approximately 24 hours later. Efficacy at postinjection day 30 (change in flexion contracture and active range of motion, patient satisfaction, physician-rated improvement, and rates of clinical success [flexion contracture 5° or less]) and adverse events were summarized.

Results.—The concurrent injections were most commonly administered in cords affecting metacarpophalangeal (MCP) and proximal interphalangeal (PIP) joints on the same finger (47%) or 2 MCP joints on different fingers of the same hand (37%). Mean total (sum of the 2 treated joints) flexion contracture decreased 76%, from 87° to 24° (MCP joints: 86%; PIP joints: 66%). Mean total range of motion increased from 100° to 161°. Clinical success was 76% for MCP joints and 33% for PIP joints. Most patients were very satisfied (60%) or quite satisfied (28%) with treatment. Most investigators rated treated joints as very much improved (55%) or much improved (37%). The most common treatment-related adverse events (> 75% of patients) were contusion, pain in extremity, and edema peripheral (local edema). Most adverse events were mild to moderate in severity. Serious complications included 1 pulley rupture related to study medication and 1 flexor tendon rupture (following conclusion of the study). There were no systemic complications.

Conclusions.—Results suggest that 2 affected joints can be effectively and safely treated with concurrent CCH injections. There was an increased incidence of some adverse events with concurrent treatment (pruritus, lymphadenopathy, blood blister, and skin laceration) compared with treatment of a single joint. High degrees of patient satisfaction and physician-rated improvement were reported.

▶ Most of my patients with Dupuytren contractures are currently treated with collagenase injections, a true paradigm shift in how these patients were treated just 6 years ago. Many of them require multiple injections because of the number of joints involved or the volume of pathologic tissue being treated, so clinical insight into patients receiving multiple injections is critical to defining how we use this important enzyme. It is remarkable that the rate of tendon rupture, arguably the most important local complication that can occur using this treatment modality, is as low as it is: 0.2% over 3357 procedures performed. What is also remarkable is the very high rate of tendon rupture in this cohort of patients: 1.7% (1 patient with 2 tendons in the small finger). Adding the one patient with both A2 and A4 pulley ruptures brings the complication rate to 3.3% for serious hand-related complications. Clearly, this can be a statistical glitch because of the small size of the study, but if these tendon and pulley rupture rates are verified in larger studies, administering multiple doses at the same sitting is not worth the 8-fold increase in tendon rupture.

A. Daluiski, MD

The Impact of Dupuytren Disease on Patient Activity and Quality of Life
Wilburn J, McKenna SP, Perry-Hinsley D, et al (Galen Res Ltd, Manchester, UK; Univ of Manchester, UK)
J Hand Surg 38A:1209-1214, 2013

Purpose.—To explore the impact of Dupuytren disease (DD) from the patients' perspective.

Methods.—Audio-recorded interviews were conducted for patients with Dupuytren disease (DD) attending outpatient clinics. The interviews were transcribed and subjected to content analysis. This analysis highlighted key impact areas and common themes in individuals' personal experiences. These were then allocated to categories specified by the World Health Organization International Classification of Functioning, Disability, and Health (impairments and activity limitations) and the needs-based model of quality of life (QoL).

Results.—Qualitative unstructured interviews were conducted with 34 patients (74% men; age, 41–80 y; mean [SD], 64 [13] y). The sample had a wide range of severity and duration of DD (range, 0.5–40; mean [SD], 13 [10] y). Nine hundred fifty-three statements relating to the impact of DD were identified from the interview transcripts. These statements fell into 2 major categories of impact: activity limitations (10 themes including problems with dressing, gripping, and personal care) and QoL (6 need categories: physiological, safety and security, social, affection, esteem, and cognitive needs).

Conclusions.—Findings from the interviews suggest that DD affects both performance of activities and QoL. To determine accurately the effectiveness of DD interventions from the patients' perspective, it is important to determine their impacts on both activity limitations and QoL. We intend to develop valid, reproducible, and responsive DD-specific scales for this purpose.

Clinical Relevance.—The study identifies key issues specific to DD that influence patients' functioning and QoL. The information reported will form the basis of DD-specific patient-reported outcomes measures for use in clinical practice and evaluations of interventions.

▶ This study attempts to provide patient quality-of-life data from unstructured recorded patient interviews that will contribute to a meaningful patient-reported outcomes measure (PROM) in patients with Dupuytren's disease.

Most published evaluations of patients with Dupuytren's disease focus on range of motion, overall hand function, and the complications and recurrence rates with various forms of treatment. This study provides a brief analysis of the patient's perspective on their disease with regard to the performance of simple daily activities and their quality of life. Recently, there has been a push to develop validated disease-specific PROMs, and this study makes an initial attempt at identifying some of the key features of what should be included in a PROM for Dupuytren's disease.

This study has a retrospective observational study design that provides demographic and disease information for the study population. A postinterview Disabilities of the Arm, Shoulder and Hand score was collected, but it was not used to correlate with the results of the qualitative comments collected during the interview. This report does take the first steps necessary generating items for inclusion in a Dupuytren's specific PROM, and additional investigation can and should be done in this area.

J. L. Tueting, MD

Response of Dupuytren Fibroblasts to Different Oxygen Environments

Türker T, Murphy E, Kaufman CL, et al (Christine M. Kleinert Inst for Hand and Microsurgery, Louisville, KY; Univ of Louisville School of Medicine, KY; Univ of Louisville and Jewish Hosp/St. Mary's Healthcare, KY; et al)
J Hand Surg Am 38:2365-2369, 2013

Purpose.—It is thought that local ischemia and oxygen radicals are responsible for fibroblast-to-myofibroblast cell transformation and proliferation. We hypothesized that hypoxia could differentially activate the contractility of fibroblasts from normal human palmar fascia and from fibroblasts-myofibroblasts of Dupuytren cords.

Methods.—Normal palmar fascia from 5 patients with carpal tunnel syndrome and Dupuytren cords from 5 patients were harvested. Cells were cultured from all tissue samples, and collagen lattices were prepared containing these cells. Oxygen treatment subgroups were created and incubated under hypoxic (1% O_2, 5% CO_2, and 94% N_2), normoxic (21% O_2, 5% CO_2, and 74% N_2), and hyperoxic (100% oxygen using 2.4 atm pressure twice a day for 7 d) conditions. After 7 days, each subgroup was photographed, and lattices were released from dishes. Postrelease photographs were taken immediately, 5 minutes after release, and after 1 hour. Areas of the lattices at each time point were calculated using Meta-Morph software. Actin staining and live/dead cell analysis was performed. Linear repeated measures analysis of variance was used for data analysis given that contraction levels were measured over 3 distinct time points.

Results.—We found a statistically significant difference between normal samples and Dupuytren samples in mean contraction levels over time. There was no statistically significant difference between tissue groups over the 3 time periods based on the oxygen treatment received.

Conclusions.—Our results showed a greater degree of contractility in Dupuytren disease cells than normal fibroblasts. However, the contraction in either group was not affected by oxygen level. Future *in vivo* research is needed to better understand the nature of pathophysiology of Dupuytren disease.

▶ This report evaluates the response of non-Dupuytren's and Dupuytren's fibroblasts and myofibroblasts to hypoxia in in-cell culture.

The significance of this study is that it provides a well-designed analysis of the effects of hypoxia on fibroblast and myofibroblast cells from human tissue in a controlled cell-culture environment that included a collagen lattice assay. It has been postulated in many studies that there is an association of Dupuytren's disease with tissue hypoxia and local ischemia secondary to oxygen free radical formation. This *in vitro* study seems to provide data that do not support this association.

This study has strengths that include its well-controlled design and execution; weaknesses are that it is an *in vitro* study that does not recreate the disease process and physiologic environment present in Dupuytren's disease. This study will hopefully stimulate additional well-designed *in vivo* research that contributes to our understanding of the pathophysiology and treatment of Dupuytren's disease.

J. L. Tueting, MD

A Comparison of Percutaneous Needle Fasciotomy and Collagenase Injection for Dupuytren Disease

Nydick JA, Olliff BW, Garcia MJ, et al (Florida Orthopaedic Inst and the Foundation for Orthopaedic Res and Education (FORE), Tampa)
J Hand Surg Am 38:2377-2380, 2013

Purpose.—To compare percutaneous needle fasciotomy (PNF) with collagenase injection in the treatment of Dupuytren contracture.

Methods.—A retrospective review was performed for patients with Dupuytren disease treated with PNF or collagenase. Range of motion, patient satisfaction, and complications were recorded.

Results.—There were 29 patients in the collagenase group with mean baseline contractures of 40° for 22 affected metacarpophalangeal joints and 50° for 12 affected proximal interphalangeal joints. The PNF group was composed of 30 patients with mean baseline contractures of 37° for 32 affected metacarpophalangeal joints and 41° for 18 affected proximal interphalangeal joints. All patients were observed for a minimum of 3 months. Clinical success (reduction of contracture within 0° to 5° of normal) was accomplished in 35 of 50 joints (67%) in the PNF group and in 19 of 34 joints (56%) in the collagenase group. Patient satisfaction was similar between groups. Only minor complications were observed, including skin tears, ecchymosis, edema, pruritus, and lymphadenopathy.

Conclusions.—In the short term, both PNF and collagenase have similar clinical outcomes and patient satisfaction.

Type of Study/Level of Evidence.—Therapeutic III.

▶ The authors performed a retrospective study comparing the 3-month post-treatment outcomes of collagenase or percutaneous needle fasciotomy (PNF) in patients with Dupuytren contractures. There was no statistical difference in terms of reduction of contractures or patient satisfaction between the 2 treatments. They did have more PNF patients with metacarpophalangeal (MP) joint contractures achieve full or nearly full correction. The collagenase outcomes for MP joint contractures (64% achieving full or near-full correction) is less than that achieved at this joint in the multicenter (CORD) study (77%), but some CORD subjects had more than 1 injection. However, this difference may be somewhat offset by the ability of the authors to anesthetize their patients. Local anesthesia was seldom used in the CORD trial. They state that collagenase treatment is more expensive but give no data regarding actual costs. Their 2 groups included patients with contractures of both the MP and proximal interphalangeal (PIP) joints, but they don't indicate when both joints were contracted in the same digit. This information would have been helpful because all offending cords can be treated at the same time by PNF, whereas the manufacturer of collagenase and the US Food and Drug Administration guidelines advise treating a specific cord causing a contracture of a specific joint, that is, not injecting multiple cords at the same treatment time. Clearly, an advantage of PNF is the ability to keep slicing until full correction is achieved, particularly at the MP joint when cord anatomy is simple compared with the PIP joint and, most importantly, where the flexion contracture does not result in collateral ligament shortening as is the case at the PIP joint. As a CORD trial investigator, I have first-hand experience in its use in the investigative and now clinical sphere. As the authors found, almost no collagenase patient wants a second injection to the same joint for residual contracture if they achieved any notable success with the first injection. Good enough is good enough!

V. R. Hentz, MD

The Effect of Night Extension Orthoses Following Surgical Release of Dupuytren Contracture: A Single-Center, Randomized, Controlled Trial
Collis J, Collocott S, Hing W, et al (Manukau SuperClinic, Auckland, New Zealand; AUT Univ, Auckland, New Zealand)
J Hand Surg 38A:1285-1294.e2, 2013

Purpose.—To clarify the efficacy and detrimental effects of orthoses used to maintain finger extension following surgical release of Dupuytren contracture.

Methods.—We conducted a single-center, randomized, controlled trial to investigate the effect of night extension orthoses on finger range of motion and hand function for 3 months following surgical release of Dupuytren contracture. We also wanted to determine how well finger extension was maintained in the total sample. We randomized 56 patients to receive a night extension orthosis plus hand therapy (n = 26) or hand therapy alone (n = 30). The primary outcome was total active extension of the operated fingers (°). Secondary outcomes were total active flexion of the operated fingers (°), active distal palmar crease (cm), grip strength (kg), and self-reported hand function using the Disabilities of the Arm, Shoulder, and Hand questionnaire (0–100 scale).

Results.—There were no statistically significant differences between the no-orthosis and orthosis groups for total active extension or for any of the secondary outcomes. Between the first postoperative measure and 3 months after surgery, 62% of little fingers had maintained or improved total active extension.

Conclusions.—The use of a night extension orthosis in combination with standard hand therapy has no greater effect on maintaining finger extension than hand therapy alone in the 3 months following surgical release of Dupuytren contracture. Our results indicate that the practice of providing every patient with a night extension orthosis following surgical release of Dupuytren contracture may not be justified except for cases in which extension loss occurs after surgery. Our results also challenge clinicians to research ways of maintaining finger extension in a greater number of patients.

▶ The authors randomly assigned patients undergoing surgery for Dupuytren contractures into 2 groups, those who had postoperative therapy alone or those who had therapy plus a static night splint. They determined that the addition of a night splint had no effect on outcome and question the routine prescribing of night splints. It's refreshing when a widely held, reflexive therapeutic algorithm is unseated by a proper study. Night splinting after surgical release of contracture is likely engrained in most of us because it kind of made sense. The goal of surgery was to straighten a crooked finger. During awake hours, the patient is actively opening and closing the hand. During sleep, our fingers generally rest in flexion, and this seems antithetical to the surgical goal. For years I have rationalized prescribing night splints in the belief that this is resisting surgery-generated scar contraction and is needed only for some finite period consistent with scar maturation. Now I will either have to give up this cherished belief or ignore the findings of this study. I think I will continue to prescribe night splinting in my patients who are doing their own therapy, at least until the authors answer the question, is formal therapy after this surgery uniformly necessary?

V. R. Hentz, MD

Collagenase Clostridium Histolyticum for Dupuytren Contracture: Patterns of Use and Effectiveness in Clinical Practice

Peimer CA, Skodny P, Mackowiak JI (Michigan State Univ, Lansing; Marquette General Healthcare, MI; Auxilium Pharmaceuticals, Inc, Malvern, PA)

J Hand Surg 38A:2370-2376, 2013

Purpose.—To collect data on the real-world effectiveness of collagenase clostridium histolyticum (CCH) during its first year of use following U.S. Food and Drug Administration approval and compare those results with clinical trial efficacy data.

Methods.—This retrospective chart review was conducted at 10 U.S. community and academic practice sites with major experience using CCH. Charts of patients treated with CCH between February and December 2010 were abstracted, and anonymized data were analyzed. Clinical use, including number of injections per cord and effectiveness outcomes (joint contracture and range of motion) were compared with results from 2 registration trials.

Results.—Data were collected from 501 patients (74% male; 48% employed; mean [SD] age, 65 [10] y); 463 patients had sufficient data for analysis. We found that 1.08 CCH injections were used per treated joint, compared with a mean of 1.7 injections in registration trials. Ninety-three percent of joints received only 1 injection. The mean (SD) number of visits per injection was 2.92 (1.0). Mean (SD) contracture was reduced by 75% from 49 (21) at baseline to 12 (17), similar to the 71% to 79% reduction in clinical trials. Mean (SD) range of motion was improved by 37 from 44 (20) at baseline to 81 (14), similar to the increase of 35 and 37 in the 2 clinical trials; and 67% of first injections resulted in full correction to 0 to 5, compared with the clinical trial rate of 39%.

Conclusions.—Despite a lower injection rate, correction of joint contracture and range of motion was similar to findings from clinical trials. Effectiveness reports using this kind of surveillance design could provide patients, physicians, and payers with the information needed to make better treatment and reimbursement decisions.

Type of Study/Level of Evidence.—Therapeutic III.

▶ This report is a retrospective review of the use of mixed clostridial collagenase (CCH) in 10 practices during its first year after US Food and Drug Administration (FDA) approval for treatment of Dupuytren contracture. Although the sites are not identified, it can be assumed that a high percentage of these early adopters were involved in the clinical trials leading to CCH approval. The report compares the use of CCH in real world practice with the prior published data, which is derived from use under clinical trial protocols intended for FDA submission. The results of this review are useful for practitioners considering the use of CCH in their practice who want to be able to answer patients' questions (all of which I have been asked multiple times) including:

1 How many injections will I need?
2 How many office visits will I need?
3 How much correction will I get?
4 What are the chances I will get full correction with one injection?

The answers this study provides are on average: (1) 1.08 injections per joint, (2) 2.9 visits per injection (3) 75% contracture reduction, and (4) two-thirds (67%). These numbers are different from those seen under the FDA trial protocols for the number of injections and percentage of full correction: 1.08 injections per joint in contrast to 1.7 and 67% chance of full correction in contrast to the published trial rate of 39%.

The authors point out that many interventions fall short when compared with the results seen under the rigorous protocols of a clinical trial. However, this study has results that are similar to the trial data in contracture reduction and superior in percentage of full correction and number of injections needed. An explanation suggested is that most patients were manipulated using local anesthesia, whereas that was for a minority in the FDA submission trials. Further, in clinical practice, clinicians are able to modify their protocols to maximize their results according to what works for them. As a CORD I investigator, the major changes I have made in my practice from the CORD I protocol include:

1 Distributing the dose of CCH in 3 or more areas along the cords or cords to be addressed.
2 Aggressive manipulation under local anesthesia at a longer interval than 24 hours.
3 Splinting significant proximal interphalangeal contractures according to a protocol similar to that of Skriven et al.[1]

P. Blazar, MD

Reference

1. Skirven TM, Bachoura A, Jacoby SM, Culp RW, Osterman AL. The effect of a therapy protocol for increasing correction of severely contracted proximal interphalangeal joints caused by dupuytren disease and treated with collagenase injection. *J Hand Surg Am*. 2013;38:684-689.

Patterns of Recontracture After Surgical Correction of Dupuytren Disease
Dias JJ, Singh HP, Ullah A, et al (Univ of Leicester, UK)
J Hand Surg 38A:1987-1993, 2013

Purpose.—To study the evolution of deformity of the proximal interphalangeal joint over 5 years after good surgical correction of Dupuytren-induced contracture.

Methods.—We assessed 63 patients (72 fingers; 69 hands) with Dupuytren disease for the degree of contracture, its correction after surgery, and the range of movement at the proximal interphalangeal joints at 3 and 6 months, and 1, 3, and 5 years after fasciectomy with or without the use of a firebreak graft. We investigated associations between the recurrence of contracture and preoperative patient and surgical factors.

Results.—There were 4 patterns of evolution of contracture after surgical correction. A total of 31 patients (33 hands) showed good improvement that was maintained for 5 years (minimal recontracture group). Twenty patients (23 hands) showed good initial improvement, which mildly worsened (< 20°) but was then maintained over 5 years (mild early recontracture group). Four patients (5 hands) worsened in first 3 months after surgery (>20°) but there was no further worsening (severe early recontracture group). Eight patients (8 hands) worsened progressively over 5 years (progressive recontracture group). Worsening of contracture more than 6° between 3 and 6 months after surgery predicted progressive recontracture at 5 years.

Conclusions.—Recurrence of contracture (not disease recurrence) could be predicted as early as 6 months after surgery for Dupuytren disease (Fig 1).

▶ The authors followed up with a series of patients who had undergone surgical release of proximal interphalangeal (PIP) joint contractures secondary to Dupuytren's disease to determine the pattern of recurrence of contracture. They found that patients whose contracture worsened, even a little (the authors' statistical methodology stated as little as 6°) after 3 months were likely to have progressive recontracture (Fig 1). These patients were a little younger, had developed their contracture more rapidly, and had longer operating times, indicating more extensive dissection to correct the deformity. Other studies,

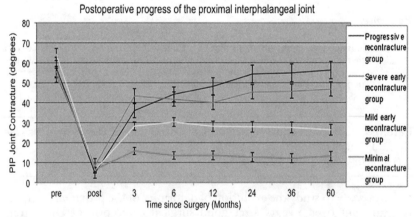

FIGURE 1.—Postoperative progress of PIP joint recontracture in the 4 groups. Error bars represent the SEM. (Reprinted from Dias JJ, Singh HP, Ullah A, et al. Patterns of recontracture after surgical correction of Dupuytren disease. *J Hand Surg*. 2013;38A:1987-1993, with permission from ASSH.)

cited by the authors, have recognized similar patterns. My reading of the article doesn't tell me whether measurements were active or passive. If these are passive measurements, then likely, active extension in these patients would be less. The authors mention several factors that may play a role in recontracture, including surgical scarring, skin tightness, and residual disease. For the commonly affected small finger (the majority in this study), I think residual contracture is frequently associated with incompetence of the extensor mechanism, a consequence of the prolonged flexed posture of the PIP joint.

V. R. Hentz, MD

5 Compressive Neuropathies

Persistence of Abnormal Electrophysiological Findings after Carpal Tunnel Release
Merolli A, Luigetti M, Modoni A, et al (The Catholic Univ School of Medicine, Rome, Italy)
J Reconstr Microsurg 29:511-516, 2013

Practitioners may refer to experienced hand surgeons to differentiate a recurrence in carpal tunnel syndrome (CTS) from a failed carpal tunnel release. The patient may complain about the reappearance of symptoms, whatever is the cause. Nerve conduction studies (NCS) are often required by the practitioner to assist the final diagnosis. We observed abnormal values in NCS in patients who were clinically healed from CTS. We evaluated the changes preoperatively and, then, at 1, 3, 6, 9, and 12 month postoperatively. At the same time, we performed a retrospective study on a group of 37 clinically healed patients. Follow-up ranged from 2 to 20 years. Surgical treatment let the electrophysiological parameters to improve toward physiological values; however, normality is hardly ever reached. This sort of "electrophysiological scar" is true for all the parameters measured. In presence of CTS, the latency difference between the radial and median sensory nerve action potentials, recorded following thumb stimulation, produces a double peak shift. The "double peak shift" best described this "electrophysiological scar," being a parameter that should measure about zero in the normal population. In conclusion, abnormal postoperative electrophysiological findings cannot substantiate the diagnosis of a poor outcome of a carpal tunnel release nor a recurrence of CTS.

▶ This study calls in to question the diagnostic value of electrophysiologic testing in the management of carpal tunnel syndrome and the value of electrophysiologic testing in differentiating carpal tunnel syndrome from other neurologic conditions. Some hand surgeons have remained reliant on electrophysiologic studies in part because most patients with carpal tunnel syndrome have already had electrodiagnostic studies before seeing them and in part because of various external pressures such as insurance payment criteria, national professional organization recommendation, and the medical legal climate.

The findings of the prospective portion of this study were that nerve conduction studies (NCS) improve for the first 3 months after carpal tunnel release;

however, they never completely return to normal. Unfortunately, the cohort of this portion of the study is small (20 patients), and the reader is not told how the patients were selected or if this was a randomly acquired group. The second portion of the study was a retrospective review of 37 patients who volunteered to be re-evaluated after carpal tunnel release surgery, again, giving the reader pause as to inclusion criteria. Also, the reader is not told what the average follow-up was, only that a range of 2 to 20 years existed. Nevertheless, the authors found that the NCS never returned to normal in this group, although the absolute numbers did improve.

Although the methods of this study are lacking, this is another study questioning the relevance of NCS in the diagnosis and management of carpal tunnel syndrome, particularly in the patient with suspected recurrent carpal tunnel syndrome. The authors conclude that electrophysiologic studies can neither substantiate outcomes after carpal tunnel release surgery nor define recurrence of carpal tunnel syndrome after surgery. These findings are in alignment with the previous work of Glowacki et al[1] and Szabo et al[2] who found that electrodiagnostic testing did not correlate with outcome after carpal tunnel release and that electrodiagnostic testing did not increase the diagnostic accuracy beyond standard clinical testing for the condition, respectively.

P. Murray, MD

References

1. Glowacki KA, Breen CJ, Sachar K, Weiss AP. Electrodiagnostic testing and carpal tunnel release outcome. *J Hand Surg Am*. 1996;21:117-121.
2. Szabo RM, Slater RR Jr, Farver TB, Stanton DB, Sharman WK. The value of diagnostic testing in carpal tunnel syndrome. *J Hand Surg Am*. 1999;24:704-714.

Sonographically Guided Percutaneous Needle Release of the Carpal Tunnel for Treatment of Carpal Tunnel Syndrome: Preliminary Report
McShane JM, Slaff S, Gold JE, et al (Sports Medicine, Villanova, PA; Temple Univ, Philadelphia, PA; et al)
J Ultrasound Med 31:1341-1349, 2012

Objectives.—The purpose of this study was to evaluate the effectiveness of a novel treatment procedure, sonographically guided percutaneous needle release of the carpal tunnel, for individuals with carpal tunnel syndrome.

Methods.—Seventeen patients (89% female; mean age, 62 years; SD, 13.6 years) with a clinical diagnosis of carpal tunnel syndrome who had undergone a sonographically guided percutaneous needle release of the carpal tunnel at least 6 months before follow-up evaluation were retrospectively reviewed. At the follow-up evaluation, to ascertain previous and current symptoms as well as functional impairment, the patients filled out a hand diagram and a questionnaire. In addition, medical records were reviewed, and patients were queried regarding complications such as infection or nerve damage. Median nerve sonographic measurements and a physical evaluation were performed on a subset of 13 patients who came to the office for evaluation.

Results.—Postprocedure sonography showed that patients had a significantly smaller ($P = .03$) cross-sectional area of the median nerve compared to pretreatment values. In addition, patients had significantly fewer symptoms ($P < .0001$), less functional impairment ($P = .0002$), and an improved hand diagram score ($P < .0001$). Postprocedure patients had grip strength that was 12 lb below average (≈ 1 SD below) compared to grip strength norms. However, most patients (84.6%) had negative clinical diagnostic test results for carpal tunnel syndrome, and 86% said they were satisfied with the procedure. There were no procedure-related infections or nerve injuries.

Conclusions.—Of the patients with carpal tunnel syndrome who agreed to participate in this study, most had favorable symptomatic and functional outcomes. Sonographically guided percutaneous needle release of the carpal tunnel may be an alternative option to traditional surgical treatment of carpal tunnel syndrome.

▶ The authors present a novel technique for percutaneous release of the transcarpal ligament for treatment of carpal tunnel syndrome. Under direct ultrasound guidance, they repeatedly fenestrate the ligament and then use hydrodissection to disrupt and stretch the ligament. They provide information regarding pre— and post—physical examination of the patient's symptoms, pain scales, and ultrasound-directed cross-sectional area of the median nerve at the wrist. Their results indicate that there is a statistical decrease in the size of the cross-sectional area of the median nerve and improvement in grip strength after the procedure. They also identified that there is less functional impairment and improved hand diagram scores.

The authors point out many weaknesses to this study. One is a very small sample size, including only 13 patients that had this novel procedure performed. Of these 13 patients, there was inconsistent pre- and postprocedure information regarding physical examination and lack of any consistent electromyography identification of median neuropathy. There was no randomization presented, and the patient's symptoms were by recall. After the procedure there was no attempt to identify that the transcarpal ligament was actually disrupted.

The conclusion of this study, that this novel technique of percutaneous needle release of carpal tunnel syndrome, is a viable alternative to surgical treatment, is a bit premature. It is difficult to draw any conclusions from this study given the small sample size and inconsistent data obtained. This is a novel procedure that does have significant potential to revolutionize the treatment of carpal tunnel syndrome, but further higher-powered studies are needed.

J. Brault, MD

Clinical Outcomes of Endoscopic Carpal Tunnel Release in Patients 65 and Over

Beck JD, Wingert NC, Rutter MR, et al (Geisinger Orthopaedics, Danville, PA)
J Hand Surg 38A:1524-1529, 2013

Purpose.—To examine outcomes of endoscopic carpal tunnel release (ECTR) in patients 65 and older. We hypothesized that this population could expect relief of pain, night pain/numbness, and numbness.

Methods.—A retrospective review was conducted of all patients 65 years of age and over who had ECTR for nerve conduction study-confirmed carpal tunnel syndrome (CTS) from October 2007 to July 2010. The charts were reviewed for demographic data, symptoms and physical findings, patient satisfaction, and 3 patient-reported outcome scores. Preoperative and postoperative results for pain, night pain/numbness, and numbness were compared. Logistic regression analysis was used to assess whether age influenced symptom resolution. Boston carpal tunnel, Short Form-36 and Disabilities of the Arm, Shoulder, and Hand scores were compared between patients with mild, moderate, or severe CTS.

Results.—A total of 78 patients had ECTR. Their ages ranged from 65 to 93 years (mean, 73 y). Before surgery 69% of patients had constant numbness. Night pain/numbness was present in 65 patients before surgery, and 61 had complete resolution. All 70 patients who presented with pain reported complete relief by the 6-month follow-up. Following ECTR, the average Boston carpal tunnel symptom severity, functional status, and Disabilities of the Arm, Shoulder, and Hand scores were 1.5, 1.5, and 13, respectively. At final evaluation, 79% of patients were very satisfied or satisfied with their outcome. A significant number of patients were found to have improvement in pain, night pain/numbness, and numbness following ECTR.

Conclusions.—This study has demonstrated relief of symptoms in a statistically significant number of patients following ECTR. We found that preoperative CTS severity, based on nerve conduction study result, did not significantly correlate with patient outcome following ECTR. Advanced symptoms at presentation do not preclude symptom resolution and should not be a contraindication to ECTR.

Type of Study/Level of Evidence.—Therapeutic III.

▶ In this report, the authors provide a single surgeon retrospective review of 78 patients with age greater than 65 years who had nerve conduction study–confirmed carpal tunnel syndrome (CTS) and all of whom had single-incision endoscopic carpal tunnel release (E-CTR) as definitive treatment.

The report is significant in that it provides meaningful new data that E-CTR is an effective treatment in mild, moderate, and severe CTS in an elderly patient population. Previous studies evaluating elderly patients with CTS have focused on open carpal tunnel release (O-CTR) and have reported that elderly patients do not respond as well to O-CTR surgery as their younger cohort. In this study, most elderly patients responded favorably to E-CTR, including many who had severe CTS by electrodiagnostic criteria. This study reports that 100% of patients had relief of pain, and 94% of patients reported improvement in pain and paresthesias.

The strengths of this study include the patient demographics, inclusion criteria, and postoperative evaluation; weaknesses included the retrospective study design, single surgeon experience, lack of preoperative functional scores, and relatively short 6-month follow-up.

When I first entered practice, I performed equal numbers of E-CTRs and O-CTRs, and I based my decisions on patient return to work status, bilateral involvement, and patient requests. As my practice has evolved, I perform many more E-CTRs relative to O-CTRs and typically perform O-CTRs in revision cases and in patients with severe wrist arthritis with very narrow or limited space in the carpal canal with which to safely place the endoscope. My patients seem to benefit from the faster short-term recovery and earlier return to work afforded by E-CTR, and this study provides confidence that elderly patients will also respond favorably to E-CTR.

J. L. Tueting, MD

Ultrasound as a First-line Test in the Diagnosis of Carpal Tunnel Syndrome: A Cost-effectiveness Analysis
Fowler JR, Maltenfort MG, Ilyas AM (Univ of Pittsburgh Med Ctr, PA; Rothman Inst, Philadelphia, PA)
Clin Orthop Relat Res 471:932-937, 2013

Background.—The American Academy of Orthopaedic Surgeons (AAOS) recommends that surgeons obtain a confirmatory test in patients for whom carpal tunnel surgery is being considered. The AAOS, however, does not specify a preferred test. Ultrasound reportedly causes less patient discomfort and takes less time to perform, while maintaining comparable sensitivity and specificity to electrodiagnostic testing (EDX).

Questions/Purposes.—We determined whether ultrasound as a first-line diagnostic test is more cost-effective than using EDX alone or using ultrasound alone: (1) when used by a general practitioner; and (2) when used by a specialist.

Methods.—A fictional population of patients was created and each patient was randomly assigned a probability of having true-positive, false-positive, true-negative, and true-positive ultrasound and EDX tests over an expected range of sensitivity and specificity values using Monte Carlo methods. Charges were assigned based on Medicare charges for diagnostic tests and estimates of missed time from work.

Results.—The average charge for the use of ultrasound as a first-line diagnostic test followed by EDX for confirmation of a negative ultrasound test was $562.90 per patient in the general practitioner scenario and $369.50 per patient in the specialist scenario, compared with $400.30 and $428.30 for EDX alone, respectively.

Conclusions.—The use of diagnostic ultrasound as a first-line test for confirmation of a clinical diagnosis of carpal tunnel syndrome is a more cost-effective strategy in the specialist population and results in improved false-negative rates in the generalist population despite increased cost.

Level of Evidence.—Level III, economic and decision analyses. See the Guidelines for Authors for a complete description of levels of evidence.

▶ This interesting study was a cost analysis of ultrasound scan (US) and electrodiagnostic testing (EDX) for the diagnosis of carpal tunnel syndrome (CTS). The conclusions from this study are that US used by a specialist, who understands CTS, is more cost effective as an adjunct test than EDX. But in the hands of a generalist, who will not be as accurate clinically diagnosing CTS, US is not as cost effective. This study uses Monte Carlo modeling, which is a statistical method to run many simulations to obtain probabilities, to assess the cost effectiveness of EDX and US in different scenarios. Although the results are interesting, there are some flaws that limit the study. First, the output of the modeling is based on what initial parameters are entered. The authors used numbers based on literature review, but some may complain that a sensitivity of 69% for EDX is too low. Second, the article does not address an important aspect of EDX, which is the role of testing to assess severity of CTS. A surgeon can temper patient expectations when they present with a nonresponsive nerve on EDX. US is not able to assess severity or prognosticate. This article is timely, as there has been increasing interest in the role of US for CTS diagnosis. US is appealing because it is nonpainful and less expensive. Some of this interest in US may be generated from the American Academy of Orthopaedic Surgeons guidelines, which suggest additional testing beyond history and physical before performing a carpal tunnel release. Some surgeons feel that classic clinical examination and history is sufficient; thus, if compelled to perform adjunct testing, a less painful option would be preferable. Overall, the article raises some interesting issues but is not likely to change practice.

C. Curtin, MD

Persistence of Abnormal Electrophysiological Findings after Carpal Tunnel Release
Merolli A, Luigetti M, Modoni A, et al (The Catholic Univ School of Medicine, Rome, Italy)
J Reconstr Microsurg 29:511-516, 2013

Practitioners may refer to experienced hand surgeons to differentiate a recurrence in carpal tunnel syndrome (CTS) from a failed carpal tunnel release. The patient may complain about the reappearance of symptoms, whatever is the cause. Nerve conduction studies (NCS) are often required by the practitioner to assist the final diagnosis. We observed abnormal values in NCS in patients who were clinically healed from CTS. We evaluated the changes preoperatively and, then, at 1, 3, 6, 9, and 12 month postoperatively. At the same time, we performed a retrospective study on a group of 37 clinically healed patients. Follow-up ranged from 2 to

20 years. Surgical treatment let the electrophysiological parameters to improve toward physiological values; however, normality is hardly ever reached. This sort of "electrophysiological scar" is true for all the parameters measured. In presence of CTS, the latency difference between the radial and median sensory nerve action potentials, recorded following thumb stimulation, produces a double peak shift. The "double peak shift" best described this "electrophysiological scar," being a parameter that should measure about zero in the normal population. In conclusion, abnormal postoperative electrophysiological findings cannot substantiate the diagnosis of a poor outcome of a carpal tunnel release nor a recurrence of CTS.

▶ This is an important study to consider when treating patients with carpal tunnel syndrome. Often decisions are based on objective testing when considering surgical care of carpal tunnel syndrome. This article is essential when considering the use of nerve conduction studies after carpal tunnel surgery. The presence of residual changes in the postsurgical electrodiagnostic study is not a presage of a good or poor outcome. The clinical presentation and examination require additional complementary evaluation with the electrical studies. Care decisions should not be based on the electrical studies without considering the whole picture. Carpal tunnel syndrome should be a clinical diagnosis, and electrical studies should be used to help make the diagnosis in unclear clinical situations.

C. Carroll, MD

Early versus Delayed Endoscopic Surgery for Carpal Tunnel Syndrome: Prospective Randomized Study
Chandra PS, Singh PK, Goyal V, et al (All India Inst of Med Sciences, New Delhi)
World Neurosurg 79:767-772, 2013

Objective.—To compare the effects of early versus delayed endoscopic surgery in patients with moderately severe carpal tunnel syndrome (CTS).

Methods.—The study included 100 patients with CTS. Investigations performed before surgery excluded secondary causes. Patients with moderately severe CTS (grade 3—4) were randomly assigned. Bland's neurophysiologic grading scale for CTS was used to assess the patients. Patients underwent an endoscopic carpal tunnel release using an indigenously designed instrument.

Results.—Following a course of conservative treatment, surgical treatment was offered in two groups: early surgery ($n = 51$; <1 week after diagnosis) and delayed surgery as per the usual waiting list ($n = 49$; >6 months after diagnosis). Improvement in both groups was significant ($P < 0.001$). When both groups were compared, improvement was better for the early surgery group ($P < 0.001$; confidence interval 6.35—9.12).

Conclusions.—On the basis of this study, early endoscopic surgery is proposed in patients with moderately severe CTS.

▶ The authors present an important study regarding early versus delayed endoscopic release for patients with moderately severe carpal tunnel syndrome (CTS). In this elegant study, they randomly assigned 51 patients to undergo early endoscopic release (after 1–2 weeks) and another 49 patients to undergo delayed endoscopic carpal tunnel release after 6 months of conservative treatment. The authors found that there was statistically better clinical and electrophysiologic improvement in the early surgery group. The return to daily activities was also complete and better in the early surgery group. This study indicates that surgical intervention in patients with moderate to severe CTS should be performed early, to possibly allow better recovery. Currently, for patients with moderately severe CTS, I prefer to give a trial of conservative treatment for 2 to 3 months. If there is no subjective improvement, I consider surgical release. I have found that patients who have a longer duration of symptoms need a longer period of recovery. This experience may be compatible with the results of this study. The reason the delayed surgery group had an inferior outcome may be explained by the delayed interval before surgery. These patients with remaining numbness after surgery showed improvement within several months.

Y.-C. Huang, MD

Transforming Growth Factor-β (TGF-β) Expression Is Increased in the Subsynovial Connective Tissues of Patients With Idiopathic Carpal Tunnel Syndrome
Chikenji T, Gingery A, Zhao C, et al (Mayo Clinic, Rochester, MN)
J Orthop Res 32:116-122, 2014

Non-inflammatory fibrosis of the subsynovial connective tissue (SSCT) is a hallmark of carpal tunnel syndrome (CTS). The etiology of this finding and its relationship to the development of CTS remain poorly understood. Recent studies have found that transforming growth factor-β (TGF-β) plays a central role in fibrosis. The purpose of this study was to investigate the expression of TGF-β and connective tissue growth factor (CTGF), a downstream mediator of TGF-β, in the pathogenesis of CTS. We compared SSCT specimens from 26 idiopathic CTS patients with specimens from 10 human cadaver controls with no previous diagnosis of CTS. Immunohistochemistry was performed to determine levels TGF-β1, CTGF, collagen 1(Col1) and collagen 3 (Col3) expression. TGF-β1 ($p < 0.01$), CTGF ($p < 0.01$), and Col3 ($p < 0.01$) were increased in SSCT of CTS patients compared with control tissue. In addition, a strong positive correlation was found between TGF-β1 and CTGF, ($R^2 = 0.80$, $p < 0.01$) and a moderate positive correlation between Col3 and TGF-β1 ($R^2 = 0.49$, $p < 0.01$). These finding suggest that there is an increased expression of TGF-β and CTGF, a TGF-β regulated protein, and that this TGF-β activation may be responsible for SSCT fibrosis in CTS patients.

▶ This study showed that transforming growth factor-β (TGF-β)—mediated fibrosis occurred in the subsynovial connective tissue (SSCT) in the carpal tunnel in patients with carpal tunnel syndrome (CTS). This finding suggests that reducing TGF-β expression in the carpal tunnel has potential as a treatment for CTS.

A weakness of this study is the lack of demographic information about the CTS patients and the normal cadaveric controls, from whom the SSCT specimens in the carpal tunnel were taken. The expression of TGF-β can be influenced by age and sex. For example, male sex hormones and female sex hormones have different effects on signaling pathways downstream from TGF-β receptors.[1] It has also been reported that the serum TGF-β1 level is significantly higher in children than in adults.[2] The authors should have compared TGF-β expression in CTS patients with those of sex- and age-matched controls. They should also have confirmed that none of the CTS patients or the normal controls was affected by any disease relating to systemic fibrosis before starting this study.

R. Kakinoki, MD

References

1. Kumar A, Ruan M, Clifton K, Syed F, Khosla S, Oursler MJ. TGF-β mediates suppression of adipogenesis by estradiol through connective tissue growth factor induction. *Endocrinology.* 2012;153:254-263.
2. Okamoto Y, Gotoh Y, Uemura O, Tanaka S, Ando T, Nishida M. Age-dependent decrease in serum transforming growth factor (TGF)-beta 1 in healthy Japanese individuals; population study of serum TGF-beta 1 level in Japanese. *Dis Markers.* 2005;21:71-74.

Pain and Carpal Tunnel Syndrome
Duckworth AD, Jenkins PJ, Roddam P, et al (Queen Margaret Hosp, Dunfermline, Fife; Wrightington Hosp, Wigan, Lancashire, UK; Massachusetts General Hosp, Boston)
J Hand Surg 38A:1540-1546, 2013

Purpose.—Pain is not a classical symptom of carpal tunnel syndrome (CTS), with the exception of numbness that is so intense that it is described by patients as painful. The primary aim of our study was to determine which factors correlated with pain for patients diagnosed with CTS.

Methods.—We prospectively assessed all patients diagnosed with CTS in our unit over a 1-year period. We recorded demographic details for all patients, including past medical history, body mass index, smoking, and occupation. The diagnosis and severity of carpal tunnel syndrome were established through a combination of history, clinical assessment, and nerve conduction studies. Of 275 patients diagnosed and treated for

CTS, 183 were women (67%), the mean age was 55 years (range, 22−87 y), and 166 cases were bilateral (60%). The mean body mass index was 29.5 kg/m² (range, 17−48 kg/m²), and 81 patients smoked (30%). Patients completed a Short Form−McGill pain questionnaire (SF-MPQ) as a measure of pain at initial presentation. We assessed outcome 1 year after intervention using the *Quick* Disabilities of the Arm, Shoulder, and Hand (*Quick*DASH) score.

Results.—We found no association between pain according to the SF-MPQ and the positive clinical signs of CTS or positive nerve conduction studies. Multivariate analysis demonstrated that smoking and bilateral disease independently correlated with the overall SF-MPQ, with similar findings on subanalysis. Independent factors associated with an increased improvement in the *Quick*DASH at 1 year were the presentation *Quick*DASH score, positive nerve conduction studies, and smoking.

Conclusions.—The only independent factors that correlated with pain at presentation of CTS were smoking and bilateral disease. Pain according to the SF-MPQ was not associated with classical clinical findings of the disease or with positive findings on nerve conduction testing.

Type of Study/Level of Evidence.—Prognostic I.

▶ This study was conducted prospectively and included a large cohort of patients with carpal tunnel syndrome (CTS), and there was a high response rate for the questionnaire to determine the pain and disability scores. CTS was diagnosed using nerve conduction studies combined with a clinical questionnaire, with a positive predictive value for diagnosing CTS of 90%.

However, I wonder if it was appropriate to assess pain induced by CTS using the Short Form−McGill Pain Questionnaire (SF-MPQ). Few patients with CTS experience such strong pain, including throbbing, shooting, stabbing pain, as described in the SF-MPQ. The SF-MPQ may not be a good tool to assess pain in CTS patients.

Abnormal sensation associated with strong discomfort may be expressed as pain and may be recognized as dysesthesia when the discomfort is not strong. The intensity of discomfort can be determined by assessing the intensity of the abnormal sensation and the patient's threshold for the sensation. Even in the same person, the threshold can change, depending on the emotional and psychological state. Therefore, the emotional and psychological state of the patients in this study might have affected the threshold and may have prevented finding any correlation between the nerve conduction studies and the SF-MPQ at the patients' presentation. Each patient's emotional and psychiatric state should have been assessed using batteries including self-rating depression scores.

It is known that CTS is often associated with other compression neuropathy (so-called double-crush syndrome) including thoracic outlet syndrome, pronator teres syndrome, and cervical spondylosis. CTS patients covered by workers' compensation insurance show worse patient-based outcomes than do those without workers' compensation. It would have been interesting if the authors would have described how they managed CTS patients with another associated compression neuropathy and those covered by workers' compensation.

R. Kakinoki, MD

Revision Carpal Tunnel Surgery: A 10-Year Review of Intraoperative Findings and Outcomes
Zieske L, Ebersole GC, Davidge K, et al (Washington Univ in Saint Louis School of Medicine, MO)
J Hand Surg 38A:1530-1539, 2013

Purpose.—To evaluate intraoperative findings and outcomes of revision carpal tunnel release (CTR) and to identify predictors of pain outcomes.

Methods.—We performed a retrospective cohort study of all adult patients undergoing revision CTR between 2001 and 2012. Patients were classified according to whether they presented with persistent, recurrent, or new symptoms. We compared study groups by baseline characteristics, intraoperative findings, and outcomes (strength and pain). Within each group, we analyzed changes in postoperative pinch strength, grip strength, and pain from baseline. Predictors of postoperative average pain were examined using both multivariable linear regression analyses and univariable logistic regression to calculate odds ratios of worsened or no change in pain.

Results.—We performed revision CTR in 97 extremities (87 patients). Symptoms were classified as persistent in 42 hands, recurrent in 19, and new in 36. The recurrent group demonstrated more diabetes and a longer interval from primary CTR, and was less likely to present with pain. Incomplete release of the flexor retinaculum and scarring of the median nerve were common intraoperative findings over all. Nerve injury was more common in the new group. Postoperative pinch strength, grip strength, and pain significantly improved from baseline in all groups, apart from strength measures in the recurrent group. Persistent symptoms and more than 1 prior CTR had higher odds of not changing or worsening postoperative pain. Higher preoperative pain, use of pain medication, and workers' compensation were significant predictors of higher postoperative average pain.

Conclusions.—Carpal tunnel release may not always be entirely successful. Most patients improve after revision CTR, but a methodical approach to diagnosis and adherence to safe surgical principles are likely to improve outcomes. Symptom classification, number of prior CTRs, baseline pain, pain medications, and workers' compensation status are important predictors of pain outcomes in this population.

▶ This study is significant in that it adds to our knowledge of the outcomes of revision carpal tunnel release (CTR) and attempts to identify predictors of pain outcomes.

Strengths of this study include the relatively high number of extremities (87 patients) in whom revision CTR was performed, the fact that one surgical technique by one surgeon was performed for all of the cases, and the methodic way in which the data were collected and presented. Weaknesses include the retrospective nature of the study, relatively short follow-up (all mean follow-ups were less than 5 months after surgery), and the high number of secondary procedures that were performed in each of the 3 categories (persistent, recurrent, or new).

This study's findings are important for the future treatment of persistent, recurrent, or new symptoms after primary CTR, mostly because we are now armed with more data to present to these subpopulations of patients who require a revision CTR and data to support revision CTR as a worthwhile procedure for pain relief.

Revision CTR, although uncommon in my practice, is certainly one that I perform but never entirely know what the patient's symptoms will be like after the surgery. Without formal data from my practice, I would also state that pain and, less commonly, numbness and paresthesias are the reasons for revision CTR, and most (but not all) improve with time. My technique for revision CTR is the same as described in this article, and I also no longer perform hypothenar fat flaps or other soft tissue coverage procedures.

S. S. Shin, MD, MMSc

Quality of Information on the Internet About Carpal Tunnel Syndrome: An Update

Lutsky K, Bernstein J, Beredjiklian P (Thomas Jefferson Univ, Philadelphia, PA; Univ of Pennsylvania, Philadelphia)
Orthopedics 36:e1038-e1041, 2013

The use of the Internet for health-related information has increased significantly. In 2000, the current authors examined the source and content of orthopedic information on the Internet. At that time, Internet information regarding carpal tunnel syndrome was found to be of limited quality and poor informational value. The purposes of the current study were to reevaluate the type and quality of information on the Internet regarding carpal tunnel syndrome and to determine whether the quality of information available has improved compared with 1 decade ago.

The phrase *carpal tunnel syndrome* was entered into the 5 most commonly used Internet search engines. The top 50 nonsponsored and the top 5 sponsored universal resource locators identified by each search engine were collected. Each unique Web site was evaluated for authorship and content, and an informational score ranging from 0 to 100 points was assigned. Approximately one-third of nonsponsored Web sites were commercial sites or selling commercial products. Seventy-six percent of sponsored sites were selling a product for the treatment of carpal tunnel syndrome. Thirty-eight percent of nonsponsored sites provided unconventional information, and 48% of sponsored sites provided misleading information. Just more than half of nonsponsored sites were authored by a physician or academic institution. The informational mean score was 53.8 points for nonsponsored sites and 14.5 points for sponsored sites.

The informational quality on the Internet on carpal tunnel syndrome has improved over the past decade. Despite this progress, significant room exists for improvement in the quality and completeness of the information available.

▶ This article evaluated the quality of information available on the Internet for carpal tunnel syndrome (CTS) and compared it with a similar study published 10 years ago. Its purpose was to see if the quality of available information online had improved compared with the prior published study. The authors searched "carpal tunnel syndrome" using the 5 most common search engines and came up with 250 sites. They then eliminated all but 65 sites for various reasons and provided each site with an informational score from 0 to 100. Interestingly, they found that approximately one-third of the nonsponsored Web sites were commercial sites or selling commercial products. Not surprisingly, the percentage was even higher for sponsored sites, with 76% selling a product for the treatment of CTS. After reviewing the sites, they concluded that 38% of the nonsponsored sites provided "unconventional information" and 48% of the sponsored sites provided "misleading information." They also reported that the informational mean score was 53.8 points for the nonsponsored sites and 14.5 points for the sponsored sites. They concluded that there has been a modest increase in informational value compared with one decade ago.

This article is interesting and supports the notion that the Internet continues to propagate misinformation, although with some improvement over the last decade. Commercially sponsored sites tout products that have no proven scientific benefit, and patients have no way of knowing this. As far as patient education goes, I continue to believe the Internet is clearly a mixed bag at best.

D. Zelouf, MD

Median Nerve Deformation and Displacement in the Carpal Tunnel During Finger Motion

Yoshii Y, Ishii T, Tung W-L, et al (Tokyo Med Univ Ibaraki Med Ctr, Ami, Inashiki, Japan; Tsukuba Med Ctr Hosp, Japan; et al)
J Orthop Res 31:1876-1880, 2013

The objective of this study was to evaluate the correlations between deformation and displacement of median nerve and flexor tendons during finger motion in the carpal tunnel for both carpal tunnel syndrome (CTS) patients and healthy controls. Sixty-two wrists of 31 asymptomatic volunteers and fifty-one wrists of 28 idiopathic CTS patients were evaluated by ultrasound. The displacement of the median nerve and the middle finger flexor digitorum superficialis (FDS) tendon, as well as area, perimeter, aspect ratio of a minimum enclosing rectangle, and circularity of the median nerve were measured in finger extension and flexion positions.

Deformation indices were defined as the ratios of indices in finger extension and flexion positions. The correlations between displacement and deformation indices were evaluated. There were significant correlations between nerve palmar–dorsal displacement and deformation indices ($p < 0.05$). The aspect ratio deformation index showed the strongest correlation to palmar–dorsal displacement of the nerve (-0.572, $p < 0.01$). This study showed that there is a relationship between median nerve deformation indices and nerve palmar–dorsal displacement in the carpal tunnel. Since the highest correlations were between palmar–dorsal nerve displacement direction and aspect ratio deformation index, these parameters may be helpful to understand the pathophysiology of CTS.

▶ The authors performed a study comparing the shape and motion of the median nerve during finger motion in patients with and without carpal tunnel syndrome. From a scientific standpoint, the authors did not perform a power analysis, so although they did find statistically significant differences in palmar displacement of the median nerve and flexor tendon displacement in a palmar direction, it is unclear whether this is due to chance, as the study could have been underpowered. The same is true for the deformation of the nerve between those patients with and without carpal tunnel syndrome.

This article does help with our understanding of what happens to the median nerve during normal use of the hand. At this point, the clinical relevance is unclear, as it will not affect treatment. With further investigation, there may eventually be a role for dynamic ultrasound scan, and it may have prognostic implications. At this time, there does not appear to be clinical indication for dynamic ultrasound scan for diagnosis or treatment of carpal tunnel syndrome.

W. C. Hammert, MD

Treatment of Ulnar Neuropathy at the Elbow: Cost-Utility Analysis
Song JW, Chung KC, Prosser LA (Univ of Michigan Health System, Ann Arbor; Univ of Michigan, School of Public Health, Ann Arbor)
J Hand Surg Am 37:1617-1629.e3, 2012

Purpose.—The choice of surgical treatment for ulnar neuropathy at the elbow (UNE) remains controversial. A cost–utility analysis was performed for 4 surgical UNE treatment options. We hypothesized that simple decompression would emerge as the most cost-effective strategy.

Methods.—A cost–utility analysis was performed from the societal perspective. A decision analytic model was designed comparing 4 strategies: (1) simple decompression followed by a salvage surgery (anterior submuscular transposition) for a poor outcome, (2) anterior subcutaneous transposition followed by a salvage surgery for a poor outcome, (3) medial epicondylectomy followed by a salvage surgery for a poor outcome, and (4) anterior submuscular transposition. A poor outcome when anterior submuscular transposition was the initial surgery was considered an end point in the model. Preference values for temporary health states for UNE, the surgical procedures, and the complications were obtained through a time trade-off survey administered to family members and friends who accompanied patients to physician visits. Probabilities of clinical outcomes were derived from a Cochrane Collaboration meta-analysis and a systematic MEDLINE and EMBASE search of the literature. Medical care costs (in 2009 U.S. dollars) were derived from Medicare reimbursement rates. The model estimated quality-adjusted life-years and costs for a 3-year time horizon. A 3% annual discount rate was applied to costs and quality-adjusted life-years. Incremental cost-effectiveness ratios were calculated, and sensitivity analyses performed.

Results.—Simple decompression as an initial procedure was the most cost-effective treatment strategy. A multi-way sensitivity analysis varying the preference values for the surgeries and a model structure sensitivity analysis varying the model assumptions did not change the conclusion. Under all evaluated scenarios, simple decompression yielded incremental cost-effectiveness ratios less than US$2,027 per quality-adjusted life-year.

Conclusions.—Simple decompression as an initial treatment option is cost-effective for UNE according to commonly used cost-effectiveness thresholds.

Type of Study/Level of Evidence.—Economic and Decision Analysis III.

▶ The purpose of this study was to determine which of 4 possible surgical treatments for cubital tunnel syndrome was the most cost-effective initial treatment, when taking into consideration both patient preference and cost of treatment. To this end, 117 people (drawn from people accompanying patients to a clinic appointment) completed a time trade-off survey. The authors found that in situ decompression was the most cost-effective initial surgical treatment.

Like any cost-utility survey of nonpatients, this study is based on myriad assumptions. The incidence of complications was gleaned from prior reports in the literature. The authors assumed that any patient who did not respond to their initial treatment underwent a salvage procedure. They tried to include some estimate of indirect cost, but limited this to just 2 days off work at the average wage. Their description of symptomatology does not account for the wide spectrum of severity experienced by an actual patient population.

The statistical analysis description in the materials and methods is very involved, so much so that the authors elected to include a 1-page appendix of terminology used in the study. The end result of this somewhat complicated study is further support that in situ decompression should be the default initial surgical procedure for cubital tunnel syndrome.

C. M. Ward, MD

The High-Resolution Ultrasonography and Electrophysiological Studies in Nerve Decompression for Ulnar Nerve Entrapment at the Elbow

Zhong W, Zhang W, Zheng X, et al (Affiliated to Shanghai Jiaotong Univ School of Medicine, China)
J Reconstr Microsurg 28:345-348, 2012

Objective.—To discuss a combination of high-resolution ultrasound and electrophysiological examination in diagnosis and evaluation of ulnar nerve entrapment at the elbow.

Method.—We retrospectively reviewed 20 healthy volunteers and 278 patients of ulnar nerve entrapment divided into three groups by McGowan grade, and we treated patients with subcutaneous or modified submuscular ulnar nerve transposition randomly. All the patients were followed for 2 years. The diagnosis and effects were confirmed by preoperative or postoperative cross-sectional area (CSA), motor conduction velocity (MCV), sensory conduction velocity, and nerve action potential (NAP).

Results.—Healthy volunteers and grade I patients had significant differences in CSA, MCV, and NAP; grade I, II, and III patients had significant differences in CSA, MCV, and NAP; all patients had significant differences in CSA, MCV, and NAP before and after operations.

Conclusion.—High-resolution ultrasound and electrophysiological examination can be used in diagnosis and evaluation of operations of ulnar nerve entrapment at the elbow.

▶ This study confirms previous reports of a correlation between electrophysiologic studies and high-resolution ultrasound scan in the diagnosis of ulnar nerve entrapment. In addition, this study suggests a correlation between changes in the cross-sectional area of the nerve (on ultrasound examination) and the severity of the patient's symptoms (McGowan grade). They also found that surgical transposition of the ulnar nerve resulted in statistically significant changes in both the electrophysiologic and ultrasound parameters measured.

Unfortunately, the authors provide limited details in the materials and methods. How was the McGowan grade determined (by chart review, before or after nerve studies were performed)? Patients were randomly assigned to submuscular or subcutaneous transposition, but there is no mention of how they were assigned. Nor is there any discussion of the demographics of the different groups. Were the providers who performed the nerve studies blinded to the patients McGowan grade or surgical technique? Also of note is that the preoperative values for all study measurements were exactly the same between the 2 groups (subcutaneous and submuscular, see Table 1 in the original article).

Ultrasound offers a potentially noninvasive and painless diagnostic tool for cubital tunnel syndrome, but further work is necessary to establish diagnostic criteria and correlation with clinical outcome.

C. M. Ward, MD

An Outcome Study for Ulnar Neuropathy at the Elbow: A Multicenter Study by the Surgery for Ulnar Nerve (SUN) Study Group

Song JW, for the Surgery for the Ulnar Nerve (SUN) Study Group (Drexel Univ College of Medicine, Philadelphia, PA; et al)

Neurosurgery 72:971-982, 2013

Background.—Many instruments have been developed to measure upper extremity disability, but few have been applied to ulnar neuropathy at the elbow (UNE).

Objective.—We measured patient outcomes following ulnar nerve decompression to (1) identify the most appropriate outcomes tools for UNE and (2) to describe outcomes following ulnar nerve decompression.

Methods.—Thirty-nine patients from 5 centers were followed prospectively after nerve decompression. Outcomes were measured preoperatively and at 6 weeks, 3 months, 6 months, and 12 months postoperatively. Each patient completed the Michigan Hand Questionnaire (MHQ), Carpal Tunnel Questionnaire (CTQ), and Disabilities of the Arm, Shoulder, and Hand (DASH) questionnaires. Grip, key-pinch strength, Semmes-Weinstein monofilament, and 2-point discrimination were measured. Construct validity was calculated by using Spearman correlation coefficients between questionnaire scores and physical and sensory measures. Responsiveness was assessed by standardized response means.

Results.—Key-pinch ($P = .008$) and Semmes-Weinstein monofilament testing of the ulnar ring ($P < .001$) and small finger (radial: $P = .004$; ulnar: $P < .001$) improved following decompression. Two-point discrimination improved significantly across the radial ($P = .009$) and ulnar ($P = .007$) small finger. Improved symptoms and function were noted by the CTQ (preoperative CTQ symptom score 2.73 vs 1.90 postoperatively, $P < .001$), DASH ($P < .001$), and MHQ: function ($P < .001$), activities of daily living ($P = .003$), work ($P = .006$), pain ($P < .001$), and satisfaction ($P < .001$). All surveys demonstrated strong construct validity, defined by correlation with functional outcomes, but MHQ and CTQ symptom instruments demonstrated the highest responsiveness.

Conclusion.—Patient-reported outcomes improve following ulnar nerve decompression, including pain, function, and satisfaction. The MHQ and CTQ are more responsive than the DASH for isolated UNE treated with decompression.

▶ Song and colleagues have strived to give surgeons a tool to evaluate their effectiveness in treating ulnar neuropathy at the elbow with in situ decompression. As noted by the authors, although recent studies have suggested no difference in treatment options for decompression of the ulnar nerve at the elbow, most of those studies did not use similar outcome measures, nor were the outcome measures previously validated for ulnar nerve decompression at the elbow. The authors evaluated physical examination outcomes as well as questionnaire outcomes including the Michigan Hand Questionnaire (MHQ), Disabilities of the Arm, Shoulder, and Hand, and Carpal Tunnel Questionnaire (CTQ). After prospective review of 39 consecutive patients (94 were originally enrolled) with isolated ulnar nerve neuropathy at the elbow at multiple centers, the authors note the ability of the CTQ and MHQ to measure improvement in patients and its correlation with physical examination findings. This article is an important first step in helping to create a necessary standard for measuring clinical outcomes for surgical treatment of ulnar nerve neuropathy at the elbow in the hope of strengthening comparison studies moving forward.

J. M. Froelich, MD

An Outcome Study for Ulnar Neuropathy at the Elbow: A Multicenter Study by the Surgery for Ulnar Nerve (SUN) Study Group
Song JW, for the Surgery for the Ulnar Nerve (SUN) Study Group (Drexel Univ College of Medicine, Philadelphia, PA; et al)
Neurosurgery 72:971-981, 2013

Background.—Many instruments have been developed to measure upper extremity disability, but few have been applied to ulnar neuropathy at the elbow (UNE).

Objective.—We measured patient outcomes following ulnar nerve decompression to (1) identify the most appropriate outcomes tools for UNE and (2) to describe outcomes following ulnar nerve decompression.

Methods.—Thirty-nine patients from 5 centers were followed prospectively after nerve decompression. Outcomes were measured preoperatively and at 6 weeks, 3 months, 6 months, and 12 months postoperatively. Each patient completed the Michigan Hand Questionnaire (MHQ), Carpal Tunnel Questionnaire (CTQ), and Disabilities of the Arm, Shoulder, and Hand (DASH) questionnaires. Grip, key-pinch strength, Semmes-Weinstein monofilament, and 2-point discrimination were measured. Construct validity was calculated by using Spearman correlation coefficients between questionnaire scores and physical and sensory measures. Responsiveness was assessed by standardized response means.

Results.—Key-pinch ($P = .008$) and Semmes-Weinstein monofilament testing of the ulnar ring ($P < .001$) and small finger (radial: $P = .004$; ulnar: $P < .001$) improved following decompression. Two-point discrimination improved significantly across the radial ($P = .009$) and ulnar ($P = .007$) small finger. Improved symptoms and function were noted by the CTQ (preoperative CTQ symptom score 2.73 vs 1.90 postoperatively, $P < .001$), DASH ($P < .001$), and MHQ: function ($P < .001$), activities of daily living ($P = .003$), work ($P = .006$), pain ($P < .001$), and satisfaction ($P < .001$). All surveys demonstrated strong construct validity, defined by correlation with functional outcomes, but MHQ and CTQ symptom instruments demonstrated the highest responsiveness.

Conclusion.—Patient-reported outcomes improve following ulnar nerve decompression, including pain, function, and satisfaction. The MHQ and

CTQ are more responsive than the DASH for isolated UNE treated with decompression.

▶ The authors from this multicenter study sought to validate existing patient-reported outcome measures when applied specifically for ulnar neuropathy at the elbow (UNE) using a comparison to functional data, given that no gold standard exists. They found that the Michigan Hand Questionnaire, Disabilities of the Arm, Shoulder, and Hand questionnaire scores, and Carpal Tunnel Questionnaire all had strong construct validity and responsiveness over time. No surgical treatment for UNE has proven superior, and with these validated outcome measures, surgeons can now meaningfully combine studies from multiple sources to guide proper treatment. Prospectively collecting these data on all patients with UNE may ultimately help differentiate which surgical intervention may best benefit a particular subset of patients. The authors are commended on establishing a valid baseline for which we can measure surgical quality for UNE.

R. Endress, MD

Surgical management of cubital tunnel syndrome: a comparative analysis of outcome using four different techniques

Saint-Cyr M, Lakhiani C, Tsai T-M (Mayo Clinic, Rochester MN; Univ of Texas Southwestern Med Ctr, Dallas; Christine M. Kleinert Inst for Hand and Microsurgery, Louisville KY)

Eur J Plast Surg 36:693-700, 2013

Background.—Various options exist for the surgical management of cubital tunnel syndrome. The goals of this study were to compare the outcome of four different surgical techniques: (1) simple decompression, (2) endoscopic decompression, (3) anterior subcutaneous transposition, and (4) anterior sub-muscular transposition for the treatment of cubital tunnel syndrome.

Methods.—One hundred ten patients (117 cases) with cubital tunnel syndrome were reviewed from 1986 to 2000. Parameters measured included signs and symptoms, medical comorbidity, other nerve compressions, and anatomical pathology. Severity was evaluated using the Dellon classification and the symptom severity score (SSS). SSS included evaluation of pain, clawing, the Froment sign, and the Wartenberg sign. Bishop's rating was measured at final follow-up. Statistical analysis included ANOVA, Kruskal—Wallis tests, and Spearman's Rho for correlation.

Results.—Correlation between severity of nerve compression and symptom duration was not statistically significant. A significant weak positive correlation existed between Dellon score and SSS. Bishop's rating was 46.5 % excellent, 39.5 % good, 7.9 % fair, and 6.1 % poor overall. A significant weak negative correlation existed between the Dellon score and Bishop's rating. The average Bishop score was 1.74 ± 0.85, and no significant difference existed when comparing each surgical technique to one another. No significant association was found between the severity of compression (Dellon) and the surgery type performed. A weak negative correlation existed between severity of ulnar nerve compression and clinical outcome. No significant differences were found between the type of surgeries performed in regard to outcome and Dellon score.

Conclusions.—We found patients with the most severe compressive symptoms benefited the least from operative intervention regardless of surgical technique used. However, for mild to moderate disease, performing any of the purposed surgical techniques in accordance with the physician's experience and comfort level is adequate in treating ulnar nerve compression at the elbow joint.

▶ The authors studied cubital tunnel syndrome and the clinical outcomes of 4 surgical paradigms. One should consider that patients with severe compressive symptoms benefit the least from surgical care regardless of the technique used. As surgeons we should consider selecting the least traumatic procedure we can perform for patients with severe disease. In mild to moderate disease, surgeons should select the procedure they are most comfortable performing based on training and experience. The outcomes are similar among all the procedures studied. I believe this article offers further clarity on the dilemma of which surgical procedure one should perform for the surgical treatment of cubital tunnel syndrome.

C. Carroll, MD

Validity and Responsiveness of the DASH Questionnaire as an Outcome Measure following Ulnar Nerve Transposition for Cubital Tunnel Syndrome
Ebersole GC, Davidge K, Damiano M, et al (Washington Univ School of Medicine, St Louis, MO)
Plast Reconstr Surg 132:81e-90e, 2013

Background.—This study sought to determine the validity and responsiveness of the Disabilities of the Arm, Shoulder, and Hand (DASH) questionnaire in cubital tunnel syndrome.

Methods.—Consecutive patients with cubital tunnel syndrome treated by anterior ulnar nerve transposition between September of 2009 and December of 2011 were reviewed retrospectively. Questionnaires were completed preoperatively and 1.5, 3, 6, and 12 months postoperatively. The relationship of the questionnaire to measures of pain, health status (Short Form-8), and pinch and grip strength was evaluated using Spearman's correlation coefficients. Responsiveness of the questionnaire was analyzed using Cohen's effect size, and was compared with responsiveness of the physical examination, pain, and Short Form-8 measures.

Results.—The final cohort included 69 patients with isolated cubital tunnel syndrome and 39 with concurrent cubital and carpal tunnel syndrome. Questionnaire scores correlated as expected with other measures. Moderate to strong correlations were observed with pain visual analogue scale and Short Form-8 scores, and weak to moderate correlations were observed with pinch and grip strength. Effect sizes for the DASH questionnaire were small (<0.3) at 6 weeks and moderate (0.35 to 0.57) at 3, 6, and 12 months postoperatively in both groups. Pain visual analogue scale scores demonstrated large effect sizes (>0.8) at all postoperative time points, whereas Short Form-8 and pinch and grip strength were poorly responsive.

Conclusion.—The Disabilities of the Arm, Shoulder, and Hand questionnaire is a valid measure in cubital tunnel syndrome, and is moderately responsive to change beyond 3-month follow-up.

Clinical Question/Level of Evidence.—Diagnostic, II.

▶ This retrospective review assessed the validity and responsiveness of the Disabilities of the Arm, Shoulder, and Hand (DASH) questionnaire in cubital tunnel syndrome. A cohort of 69 patients with cubital tunnel and a separate subgroup of cubital tunnel with concomitant carpal tunnel were identified and completed a postoperative assessment of a pinch and grip assessment, DASH, visual analogue, and Short Form—8. The pinch and grip assessment and Short Form-8 showed poor responsiveness. The DASH showed moderate to moderately strong responsiveness between 3 and 12 months, whereas the visual analogue was more responsive up to 6 weeks postoperatively. The DASH and visual analogue also showed strong correlation. The DASH was equally predictive in isolated cubital tunnel and concomitant cubital as carpal tunnel.

I agree with the authors that the surgical treatment of cubital tunnel has yet to reach a consensus. This article provides support for the use of the DASH score in future studies to further elucidate the surgical management of cubital tunnel.

C. Heinrich, MD

6 Nerve

Limitations of nerve repair of segmental defects using acellular conduits
Berrocal YA, Almeida VW, Levi AD (Univ of Miami Miller School of Medicine, FL)
J Neurosurg 119:733-738, 2013

The authors present the case of a 20-year-old man who, 3 months after his initial injury, underwent repair of a 1.7-cm defect of the ulnar nerve at the wrist; repair was performed with an acellular nerve allograft. Given the absence of clinical or electrophysiological recovery at 8 months postrepair, the patient underwent reexploration, excision of the "regenerated cable," and rerepair of the ulnar nerve with sural nerve autografts. Histology of the cable demonstrated minimal axonal regeneration at the midpoint of the repair. At the 6- and 12-month follow-ups of the sural nerve graft repair, clinical and electrophysiological evidence of both sensory and motor reinnervation of the ulnar nerve and associated hand muscles was demonstrated. In this report, the authors describe a single case of failed acellular nerve allograft and correlate the results with basic science and human studies reporting length and diameter limitations in human nerve repair utilizing grafts or conduits devoid of viable Schwann cells.

▶ The authors present a concise case report of a failed ulnar nerve reconstruction using an acellular nerve allograft followed by a literature review of case reports describing nonautograft peripheral nerve reconstruction.

This is a well-written and referenced study that collates many case series looking at acellular conduits in different scenarios: sensory, motor, and mixed nerves. It should be clear that the referenced cases are a heterogeneous population—acellular allografts and conduits are inherently different in their architecture. Compared with native nerve autograft, acellular allografts still retain endoneurial tubes as part of their internal microarchitecture but lack Schwann cells. Nerve conduits lack both Schwann cells and any internal microarchitecture, rendering them a more inferior reconstructive option.[1]

Acellular conduits do have the advantage of being readily available, in an off-the-shelf fashion, and, as referenced by the authors, can result in satisfactory sensory and motor restoration. Autograft nerve grafts, such as sural nerve or median antebrachial cutaneous nerve, have the inherent risks of donor site morbidity and painful neuroma, which are eliminated with acellular conduit utilization.

Although further basic science and clinical studies are needed to fully delineate the limitations of acellular allografts and conduits, it is clear that there exists a clinical place for their utilization. However, to avoid clinical failures, I favor autologous nerve reconstruction for motor reconstruction, critical sensory reconstruction, or any large-diameter peripheral nerve.[2]

M. Nicoson, MD

References

1. Whitlock EL, Tuffaha SH, Luciano JP, et al. Processed allografts and type I collagen conduits for repair of peripheral nerve gaps. *Muscle Nerve.* 2009;39:787-799.
2. Mackinnon SE. Technical use of synthetic conduits for nerve repair. *J Hand Surg Am.* 2011;36:183.

The Middle Finger Flexion Test to Locate the Thenar Motor Branch of the Median Nerve

Rodriguez R, Strauch RJ (Columbia Univ Med Ctr, NY)
J Hand Surg 38A:1547-1550, 2013

Purpose.—To assess the accuracy of a physical examination maneuver, the middle finger flexion test, in locating the thenar branch of the median nerve (TBMN).

Methods.—Forty-one cadaveric hands were studied. The TBMN was dissected and identified as it emerged from the median nerve. The middle finger was then passively flexed to 90° at both the metacarpophalangeal and the proximal interphalangeal joints with the distal interphalangeal joint at neutral, which allowed the fingertip to contact the thenar eminence. The distance of the TBMN in millimeters with respect to the position of the center of the tip of the middle finger was measured. Two measurements were obtained from each specimen: the distance from the origin of the TBMN to the tip of the finger (+ distal to fingertip, − proximal to fingertip), and the radioulnar distance from the center of the middle fingertip (+ radial, − ulnar).

Results.—The average location of the TBMN was 1.9 mm ulnar and 0.9 mm proximal to the tip of the flexed middle finger. There were 2 transligamentous median nerve thenar branches.

Conclusions.—This physical examination method accurately located the TBMN. This method is simple to perform, does not require secondary landmarks to derive vectors, and may more closely approximate the position of the TBMN than the previously described methods.

Clinical Relevance.—Understanding the location of the TBMN in the palm will aid in accurate identification of this structure and prevent damage to it during surgery.

▶ The authors present a new, simple method to estimate the position of the motor branch of the median nerve. Although the study is well performed, is well presented, and gives the reader a handy rule of thumb to localize the position of the nerve branch, I feel that its practical use is probably limited. It is well known that the motor branch has a remarkable variability, and even in the data presented, 2 of the specimens show a branch far from the expected position. Therefore, careful dissection of the median nerve is always mandatory. Especially in open injuries in the thenar region, the nerve has to be exposed completely anyway. I also like to visualize the branch in all open carpal tunnel releases to make sure there is no further compression of the branch.

K. Megerle, MD, PhD

Collagen Conduit Versus Microsurgical Neurorrhaphy: 2-Year Follow-Up of a Prospective, Blinded Clinical and Electrophysiological Multicenter Randomized, Controlled Trial
Boeckstyns MEH, Sørensen AI, Viñeta JF, et al (Univ of Copenhagen, Denmark; et al)
J Hand Surg 38A:2405-2411, 2013

Purpose.—To compare repair of acute lacerations of mixed sensory-motor nerves in humans using a collagen tube versus conventional repair.

Methods.—In a prospective randomized trial, we repaired the ulnar or the median nerve with a collagen nerve conduit or with conventional microsurgical techniques. We enrolled 43 patients with 44 nerve lacerations. We performed electrophysiological tests and hand function using a standardized clinical evaluation instrument, the Rosen scoring system, after 12 and 24 months.

Results.—Operation time using the collagen conduit was significantly shorter than for conventional neurorrhaphy. There were no complications in terms of infection, extrusion of the conduit, or other local adverse reaction. Thirty-one patients with 32 nerve lesions, repaired with collagen conduits or direct suture, attended the 24-month follow-up. There was no difference between sensory function, discomfort, or total Rosen scores. Motor scores were significantly better for the direct suture group after 12 months, but after 24 months, there were no differences between the treatment groups. There was a general further recovery of both motor and sensory conduction parameters at 24 months compared with 12 months. There were no statistically significant differences in amplitudes, latencies, or conduction velocities between the groups.

Conclusions.—Use of a collagen conduit produced recovery of sensory and motor functions that were equivalent to direct suture 24 months after repair when the nerve gap inside the tube was 6 mm or less, and the collagen conduit proved to be safe for these nerve lacerations in the forearm.

Type of Study/Level of Evidence.—Therapeutic II.

▶ The study present results from a randomized trial comparing direct suture repair with repair with a nerve conduit for lacerations of the median or ulnar nerves in the forearm. In 32 patients with nerve lacerations, the authors found similar functional outcomes and similar motor and sensory nerve recovery in both groups. The authors tackled a complex subject in a difficult subset of patients. As such, the patient population is heterogeneous with several associated injuries. This, combined with variations in surgical technique, make conclusions difficult to draw. A relatively large number of patients were also lost to follow-up. Despite these inherent limitations, the authors were able to document the timeline for nerve recovery in these difficult injuries, noting that nerve recovery continues after 12 months into 2 years after nerve repair.

The study is also valuable in that it documents the expected outcome from nerve lacerations in the forearm. Indeed, the authors found that outcomes from ulnar nerve injuries are worse than for median nerve injuries and motor and sensory latencies, and conduction velocities after injury recover to less than 50% of the contralateral hand. These data allow treating surgeons to counsel patients and set appropriate expectations for nerve recovery after laceration repair. Inclusion of a patient-reported outcome score would have added further strength to the study.

T. D. Rozental, MD

Type I Collagen Nerve Conduits for Median Nerve Repairs in the Forearm

Dienstknecht T, Klein S, Vykoukal J, et al (Univ Med Ctr Aachen; Univ Hosp Regensburg, Germany; Univ of Texas MD Anderson Cancer Ctr, Houston)
J Hand Surg Am 38:1119-1124, 2013

Purpose.—To evaluate patients with median nerve damage in the distal forearm treated with type 1 collagen nerve conduits.

Methods.—Nine patients with damage to the median nerve in the distal forearm underwent treatment with a type 1 collagen nerve conduit. The nerve gaps ranged between 1 and 2 cm. An independent observer reexamined patients after treatment at a minimal follow-up of 14 months and a mean follow-up of 21 months. Residual pain was evaluated using a visual analog scale. Functional outcome was quantified by assessing static 2-point discrimination, nerve conduction velocity relative to the uninjured limb, and Disabilities of the Arm, Shoulder, and Hand outcome measure scoring. We also recorded quality of life measures including patients' perceived satisfaction with the results and return to work latency.

Results.—We observed no implant-related complications. Of 9 patients, 7 were free of pain, and the mean visual analog scale was 0.6. The mean Disabilities of the Arm, Shoulder, and Hand score was 6. The static 2-point discrimination was less than 6 mm in 3 patients, between 6 and 10 mm in 4 patients, and over 10 mm in 2 patients. Six patients reached a status of M4 or higher. Eight patients were satisfied with the procedure and would undergo surgery again.

Conclusions.—This study indicates that purified type 1 bovine collagen conduits are a practical and efficacious method for the repair of median nerves in the distal forearm.

Type of Study/Level of Evidence.—Therapeutic IV.

▶ The authors have provided a retrospective review of their experience reconstructing mixed median nerve lacerations in the forearm. As a retrospective study, this lacks a cohort for comparison, but the authors used both subjective and objective outcomes. Their results are better than I would anticipate based on animal data for mixed nerves.[1] Both synthetic conduits and acellular allograft nerves have been reported to provide good results for sensory nerves, but the literature at this time is not compelling for mixed nerves. There are several commercially available synthetic conduits. The collagen conduits are flexible enough that extrusion does not seem to be an issue compared with the polyglycolic acid conduits, which have less flexibility and more prone to extrude, especially when soft tissue is compromised or positioned around joints in the fingers.

This is a challenging problem, and the use of an off-the-shelf replacement, which will decrease operating time and donor site morbidity associated with the use of autograft nerves, is appealing. Currently, there is not sufficient evidence for me to use synthetic conduits for critical mixed nerves, but additional studies such as this and the use of acellular allograft nerve will set the stage for a prospective study comparing the reconstructive options.

W. C. Hammert, MD

Reference

1. Lee JY, Giusti G, Friedrich PF, et al. The effect of collagen nerve conduits filled with collagen-glycosaminoglycan matrix on peripheral motor nerve regeneration in a rat model. *J Bone Joint Surg Am.* 2012;94:2084-2091.

Split Flexor Pollicis Longus Tendon Transfer to A1 Pulley for Correction of Paralytic Z Deformity of the Thumb
Rath S (Hitech Med College, Orissa, India)
J Hand Surg 38A:1172-1180, 2013

Purpose.—To test the hypothesis that split flexor pollicis longus (FPL) transfer to the A1 pulley will correct a thumb paralytic Z deformity and that the transfer can be subjected to early postoperative active mobilization protocol.

Methods.—In a prospective trial, 19 consecutive thumbs with ulnar or combined ulnar and median nerve paralysis received split FPL transfer to the thumb A1 pulley and active mobilization of transfer after 48 hours. Outcomes were assessed by correction of Z deformity during pinch, tendon transfer insertion pullout during early active mobilization, range of motion at the thumb metacarpophalangeal and interphalangeal joints, and postoperative treatment time. Data from historical records of 20 thumbs with split FPL to extensor pollicis longus (EPL) and 3 weeks' immobilization, treated before the prospective trial in the same institution, were used for comparison.

Results.—All 19 thumbs with split FPL to A1 pulley achieved Z deformity correction at discharge from rehabilitation. There was no incidence of transfer insertion pullout during active mobilization, and patients were discharged 22 days earlier than the controls who received transfer of

FPL to EPL insertion. Seventeen thumbs were available for follow-up more than 1 year after the index procedure. Fifteen thumbs retained deformity correction, and 2 had recurrence of Z deformity. The interphalangeal joint had considerably greater active motion following split FPL to A1 pulley compared with transfer of split FPL to EPL insertion.

Conclusions.—This study supports the hypothesis. Split FPL tendon transfer to thumb A1 pulley can correct paralytic thumb Z deformities and be mobilized early for transfer re-education. Improved interphalangeal joint active motion and reduced treatment time are added advantages over FPL transfer to the EPL insertion.

Type of Study/Level of Evidence.—Therapeutic III.

▶ This report describes a novel way to treat Z deformity of the thumb; that is metacarpophalangeal (MCP) joint hyperextension and interphalangeal (IP) joint flexion in the presence of ulnar nerve and, more commonly, mixed median and ulnar nerve paralysis. The point is made in the introduction that this Z deformity often coexists with the lack of thumb opposition, and, yet, thumb opposition transfers do not directly treat this. Often, thumb opposition transfers are combined with a second transfer to treat this Z deformity. The authors make a case for a preliminary surgery to provide the MCP joint flexion that will render a later opposition transfer successful in this preliminary surgery. Therefore, the patients presented underwent this procedure as a preliminary surgery in advance of a thumb opposition transfer. The goals of designing this procedure are to have a surgery from which the patient recovers quickly, has a minimal rehabilitation to achieve full range of motion, and a successful restoration of the normal position of the thumb in advance of opposition transfer. Opposition transfers are offered after successful claw deformity correction, usually at the second or third postoperative visit. As such, the outcomes of this procedure are measured while simulating opposition by actually physically holding the thumb in abduction, because this procedure occurs before opposition transfer. Only one thumb in the cohort of 20 thumbs had recurrence of the Z deformity. The authors conclude that split flexor pollicis longus (FPL) to extensor pollicis longus tenodesis is a simple technique for Z deformity correction in the flexor pollicis brevis deficient thumb.

This novel technique for stabilizing a thumb with hyperextension at the MCP joint caused by flexor pollicis brevis deficiency stands out among other transfers because it disobeys the rule that posits one tendon should have only one function. Nonetheless, it seems simple to accomplish, and it may be applicable along a wider array of indications. The question left unanswered by the report is whether this can be used in patients who do not have nerve palsies but have a lax MCP volar plate for other reasons such as primary soft-tissue laxity or secondary to basal joint arthritis. If, indeed, this simple transfer can be done in conjunction with surgeries used to realign the base of the thumb, then the results of this limited cohort may be applied to a very large group of patients that confound surgeons for an easy treatment as it is.

One final thought involves patients who have Charcot-Marie-Tooth disease. Those patients develop a stocking glove denervation of their upper and lower extremities and can develop weakness of thenar musculature that results in the Z deformity. Could this split flexor pollicis longus transfer be appropriate treatment for them or for other patients who suffer from primary arthritic causes of Z deformity? This issue remains unexplored, and, yet, the availability of a simple transfer in the split FPL as presented in this report leaves the door open for further investigation.

J. Elfar, MD

Multiple schwannomas of the upper limb related exclusively to the ulnar nerve in a patient with segmental schwannomatosis
Molina AR, Chatterton BD, Kalson NS, et al (Queen Victoria Hosp, East Grinstead, UK)
J Plast Reconstr Aesthet Surg 66:e376-e379, 2013

Schwannomas are benign encapsulated tumours arising from the sheaths of peripheral nerves. They present as slowly enlarging solitary lumps, which may cause neurological defects. Multiple lesions are rare, but occur in patients with neurofibromatosis type 2 or schwannomatosis. Positive outcomes have been reported for surgical excision in solitary schwannomas. However, the role of surgery in patients with multiple lesions is less clear. The risk of complications such as iatrogenic nerve injury and the high likelihood of disease recurrence mean that surgical intervention should be limited to the prevention of progressive neurological deficit.

We report a case of a 45 year old male who presented with multiple enlarging masses in the upper limb and sensory deficit in the distribution of the ulnar nerve. The tumours were found to be related exclusively to the ulnar nerve during surgical exploration and excision, a rare phenomenon. The masses were diagnosed as schwannomas following histopathological analysis, allowing our patient to be diagnosed with the rare entity segmental schwannomatosis. One year post-operatively motor function was normal, but intermittent numbness still occurred. Two further asymptomatic schwannomas developed subsequently and were managed conservatively.

▶ This article presents a case report of segmental schwannomatosis as well as a review and the differential diagnosis of schwannomatosis and how it differs from neurofibromatosis. Most patients with neurofibromatosis will have a diagnosis before seeing a surgeon. However, isolated schwannomas are less likely to have been diagnosed.

Schwannomas should be considered in the differential diagnosis when evaluating patients with masses around nerves. The differential diagnosis includes schwannomas (neurilemmomas), neurofibromas, and perineuriomas. Pathologic evaluation can be consumed with malignant peripheral nerve sheath tumors. Clinical examination with a tinels over a mass in association with neurologic deficit should trigger the clinician to be suspicious. Further evaluation with magnetic resonance imaging including low T1 signal with high T2 signal and enhancement can aid in surgical planning and diagnosis. This article reviews the authors' surgical technique for resection with tips to facilitate the excision, including use of the microscope and hydrodissection. In addition, this patient did have 2 recurrent schwannomas that were asymptomatic and managed conservatively, which aids in patient counseling.

C. Heinrich, MD

Approach to radial nerve palsy caused by humerus shaft fracture: Is primary exploration necessary?
Korompilias AV, Lykissas MG, Kostas-Agnantis IP, et al (Univ of Ioannina School of Medicine, Greece; Hosp for Special Surgery, NY)
Injury 44:323-326, 2013

Introduction.—While recommendations for early exploration and nerve repair in cases of open fractures of the humeral shaft associated with radial nerve palsy are clear, the therapeutic algorithm for the management of closed humeral shaft fractures complicated by radial nerve palsy is still uncertain. The purpose of this study was to determine whether patients with complete sensory and motor radial nerve palsy following a closed fracture of the humeral shaft should be surgically explored.

Patients and Methods.—Twenty-five patients with closed humeral shaft fractures complicated by complete radial nerve palsy were retrospectively reviewed during a 12-year period. Surgical intervention was indicated if functional recovery of the radial nerve was not present after 16 weeks of expectant management.

Results.—Surgical exploration was performed in 12 patients (48%) after a mean period of expectant management of 16.8 weeks (range: 16—18 weeks). In 2 of them (10%) total nerve transection was found. In the rest 10 patients underwent surgical exploration the radial nerve was found to be macroscopically intact. All intact nerves were fully recovered after a mean time of 21.6 weeks (range: 20—24 weeks) post-injury. In 13 patients (52%) in whom surgical exploration was not performed the mean time to full nerve recovery was 12 weeks (range: 7—14 weeks) post-injury.

Conclusions.—We proposed immediate exploration of the radial nerve in case of open fractures of the humeral shaft, irreducible fractures or unacceptable reduction, associated vascular injuries, radial nerve palsy after manipulation or intractable neurogenic pain. Due to high rate of spontaneous recovery of the radial nerve after closed humeral shaft fractures we recommend 16—18 weeks of expectant management followed by surgical intervention.

▶ The goal of this study was to determine whether patients with complete sensory and motor radial nerve palsy after closed fracture of the humeral shaft should be surgically explored. This retrospective review of 25 patients treated by a specific algorithm was performed to determine the ultimate outcome of patients treated using these guidelines. Twenty-three of 25 patients had complete nerve recovery. Eight of these patients underwent exploration or neurolysis because there was no recovery at 16 weeks. The 2 patients in the study who underwent exploration and repair of a completely lacerated radial nerve 16 weeks after injury had no recovery of nerve function. This study provides additional information regarding the natural history of these injuries and provides a treatment scheme that resulted in nerve recovery in 23 of 25 patients. Nonetheless, it is still not clear how to best detect complete nerve injuries early so that repair can be performed as soon as possible.

T. J. Payne, MD

Collagen Conduit Versus Microsurgical Neurorrhaphy: 2-Year Follow-Up of a Prospective, Blinded Clinical and Electrophysiological Multicenter Randomized, Controlled Trial
Boeckstyns MEH, Sørensen AI, Viñeta JF, et al (Univ of Copenhagen, Denmark; et al)
J Hand Surg Am 38:2405-2411, 2013

Purpose.—To compare repair of acute lacerations of mixed sensory-motor nerves in humans using a collagen tube versus conventional repair.

Methods.—In a prospective randomized trial, we repaired the ulnar or the median nerve with a collagen nerve conduit or with conventional microsurgical techniques. We enrolled 43 patients with 44 nerve lacerations. We performed electrophysiological tests and hand function using a standardized clinical evaluation instrument, the Rosen scoring system, after 12 and 24 months.

Results.—Operation time using the collagen conduit was significantly shorter than for conventional neurorrhaphy. There were no complications in terms of infection, extrusion of the conduit, or other local adverse reaction. Thirty-one patients with 32 nerve lesions, repaired with collagen conduits or direct suture, attended the 24-month follow-up. There was no difference between sensory function, discomfort, or total Rosen scores. Motor scores were significantly better for the direct suture group after 12 months, but after 24 months, there were no differences between the treatment groups. There was a general further recovery of both motor and sensory conduction parameters at 24 months compared with 12 months. There were no statistically significant differences in amplitudes, latencies, or conduction velocities between the groups.

Conclusions.—Use of a collagen conduit produced recovery of sensory and motor functions that were equivalent to direct suture 24 months after repair when the nerve gap inside the tube was 6 mm or less, and the collagen conduit proved to be safe for these nerve lacerations in the forearm.

Type of Study/Level of Evidence.—Therapeutic II.

▶ The authors performed a multicenter prospective trial comparing the use of a collagen conduit versus primary neurorrhaphy (direct repair or nerve grafting) with a 2-year follow-up analysis. A relatively equal distribution between median and ulnar nerves were treated, and gapping no greater than 2 cm was acceptable for inclusion in the study. The surgeons aimed to leave a gap no greater than 6 mm in the conduit group.

Results demonstrated that the conduit group had a significantly shorter operative time, and outcomes of conduits fared equally to those of primary neurorrhaphy. The median nerve repairs generally did better than ulnar nerve injuries in both groups. In addition, at final follow-up, there was significantly poorer function of the injured side compared with the uninjured extremity.

I think the authors had a solid study model, and the conclusions of this investigation are well founded. Although more research and study is required, this article provides valuable information to the science of nerve tubes and their use in nerve injuries.

M. Rizzo, MD

Early posttraumatic psychological stress following peripheral nerve injury: A prospective study
Ultee J, Hundepool CA, Nijhuis THJ, et al (Univ Med Ctr, Rotterdam, The Netherlands; et al)
J Plast Reconstr Aesthet Surg 66:1316-1321, 2013

Background.—Psychological symptoms frequently accompany severe injuries of the upper extremities and are described to influence functional outcome. As yet, little knowledge is available about the occurrence of posttraumatic psychological stress and the predictive characteristics of peripheral nerve injuries of the upper extremity for such psychological symptoms. In this prospective study, the incidence of different aspects of early posttraumatic stress in patients with peripheral nerve injury of the forearm is studied as well as the risk factors for the occurrence of early psychological stress.

Methods.—In a prospective study design, patients with a median, ulnar or combined median—ulnar nerve injury were monitored for posttraumatic psychological stress symptoms with the Impact of Event Scale (IES) questionnaire up to 3 months postoperatively.

Results.—Psychological stress within the first month after surgery occurred in 91.8% of the population (IES mean = 22.0, standard deviation (SD) = 17.3). Three months postoperatively, 83.3% (IES mean = 13.3, SD = 14.1) experienced psychological stress. One month postoperatively 24.6% and 3 months postoperatively 13.3% of the patients had IES scores indicating for the need for psychological treatment. Female gender, adult age and combined nerve injuries were related to the occurrence of psychological stress symptoms 1 month postoperatively.

Conclusions.—In the majority of these patients, peripheral nerve injury of the forearm is accompanied by early posttraumatic psychological stress, especially in female adults who suffered from combined nerve injuries.

▶ The article deals with the evaluation of posttraumatic psychological stress after reconstruction of peripheral nerve lesions. The primary concern of surgeons after a reconstructive procedure has always been functional outcome. Even though there have been a few studies dealing with posttraumatic stress disorder (PTSD) after hand surgery in general, the article provides insight into an aspect that has not been investigated so far, as this report is focused on the prospective investigation of patients with peripheral nerve lesions.

The authors observed a high incidence of PTSD in patients after nerve surgery (91.8% in the first month and 83.3% in the third month). Female gender, adult age, and combined nerve injury were identified as predisposing factors for PTSD. These findings are interesting when compared with the incidence of PTSD in other populations. A study on burn patients indicates that PTSD is more likely to occur in males, whereas other investigators did not find any difference between males and females. Another interesting finding is that adults with peripheral nerve surgery had a higher risk of PTSD development. Investigations on trauma patients in general indicated that children were more likely to develop psychological stress.

The report points out that the importance of prevention and therapy of PTSD has been underestimated in the rehabilitation of patients after peripheral nerve surgery. This is clinically important, as stress is known to have a negative impact on wound healing, which in turn could impede functional recovery of patients with peripheral nerve injuries.

M. Choi, MD

Allograft Reconstruction for Digital Nerve Loss

Taras JS, Amin N, Patel N, et al (Thomas Jefferson Univ, Philadelphia, PA; Drexel Univ College of Medicine/Hahnemann Univ Hosp, Philadelphia, PA; Philadelphia Hand Ctr, PA)
J Hand Surg 38A:1965-1971, 2013

Purpose.—To investigate the outcomes of digital nerve repairs using processed nerve allograft for defects measuring 30 mm or less.

Methods.—Seventeen patients with 21 digital nerve lacerations in the hand underwent reconstruction with processed nerve allograft. Outcome data for 14 patients with 18 digital nerve lacerations were available for analysis. Postoperative outcome data were recorded at a minimum of 12 months and an average of 15 months. The average nerve gap measured 11 mm (range, 5—30 mm). Outcome measures included postoperative sensory examination as assessed by Semmes-Weinstein monofilaments and static and moving 2-point discrimination. Pain was graded using a visual analog scale throughout the recovery period. In addition, patients completed the

Quick Disabilities of the Arm, Shoulder, and Hand survey before and after surgery.

Results.—Using Taras outcome criteria, 7 of 18 (39%) digits had excellent results, 8 of 18 (44%) had good results, 3 of 18 (17%) digits had fair results, and none had poor results. At final follow-up, Semmes-Weinstein monofilament testing results ranged from 0.08 g to 279 g. Quick Disabilities of the Arm, Shoulder, and Hand scores recorded at the patient's first postoperative visit averaged 45 (range, 2–80), and final scores averaged 26 (range, 2–43). There were no signs of infection, extrusion, or graft reaction.

Conclusions.—The data suggest that processed nerve allograft provides a safe and effective alternative for the reconstruction of peripheral digital nerve deficits measuring up to 30 mm.

▶ The authors present an important retrospective study that investigates the outcomes of digital nerve repairs using processed nerve allograft for defects measuring 30 mm or less with objective outcomes measures in 14 patients with 18 digital nerve lacerations. Nerve repairs and grafting techniques have been around for many years. Autogenous nerve grafts have worked reasonably well in the right circumstances but are associated with difficulties in achieving a proper donor-host match and with postsurgical sequelae at the donor site. Despite their inferiority to nerve autografts, clinical alternatives are commonly used for reconstruction of peripheral nerve injuries. Processed nerve allografts offer a promising alternative to nerve autografts in the surgical management of peripheral nerve injuries in which short deficits exist because they lead to no donor site morbidity. The data from this study add more evidence to suggest that processed nerve allografts provide a safe and effective alternative for the reconstruction of sensory nerve defects measuring up to 30 mm. There are, however, a few weaknesses in the study. These include a small sample size, a retrospective design, and absence of a control group. In addition, the average nerve defect was only 11 mm, and processed nerve allografts usually result in favorable results in such small defects. A recent multicentric study by Brooks et al[1] showed that processed nerve allografts performed well and were found to be safe and effective in sensory, mixed, and motor nerve defects between 5 and 50 mm. However, more prospective, randomized studies for large nerve defects 30 mm or more would help add evidence about the role of processed nerve allografts in bridging long nerve gaps, especially in motor or mixed nerves. Currently, in my practice, I use nerve autografts, and I have no experience with the use of processed nerve allografts, largely because of their unavailability in the region where I practice.

A. L. Wahegaonkar, MD

Reference

1. Brooks DN, Weber RV, Chao JD, et al. Processed nerve allografts for peripheral nerve reconstruction: a multicenter study of utilization and outcomes in sensory, mixed, and motor nerve reconstructions. *Microsurgery.* 2012;32:1-14.

Long-term outcomes after endothoracic sympathetic block at the T4 ganglion for upper limb hyperhidrosis
Panhofer P, Gleiss A, Eilenberg WH, et al (Med Univ of Vienna, Austria; et al)
Br J Surg 100:1471-1477, 2013

Background.—The aim of this study was to evaluate long-term results, quality of life, satisfaction and compensatory sweating after endothoracic sympathetic block at T4 (ESB4).

Methods.—Patients who underwent an ESB4 procedure for palmar or palmoaxillary hyperhidrosis between 2001 and 2008 were included in a prospective study at a university hospital. Questionnaires devised by Keller and Milanez de Campos were applied to evaluate disease-specific quality of life.

Results.—A total of 189 patients underwent 374 ESB4 procedures. Of 174 evaluated patients, 54 ($31 \cdot 0$ per cent) had palmar and 120 ($69 \cdot 0$ per cent) had palmoaxillary hyperhidrosis. Median follow-up was 92 months. In both groups, treatment successfully reduced hyperhidrosis ($P < 0 \cdot 001$) and quality of life increased significantly after ESB4 ($P < 0 \cdot 001$), remaining stable after 5 years. Overall satisfaction rates decreased owing to the development of compensatory sweating and recurrence during follow-up. Compensatory sweating affected 41 patients ($23 \cdot 6$ per cent), and was severe in 11 ($6 \cdot 7$ per cent) of 163 patients at 5-year follow-up; eight of these 11 patients had been treated for palmoaxillary sweating. The severity of compensatory sweating did not deteriorate with time. The severe recurrence rate increased to $11 \cdot 0$ per cent during follow-up, and was twice as common in patients treated for palmoaxillary sweating as in those treated for palmar sweating ($13 \cdot 2$ *versus* $6 \cdot 1$ per cent respectively). Nine reoperations ($5 \cdot 2$ per cent) were performed for persistent sweating, recurrence or compensatory sweating.

Conclusion.—T4 endothoracic sympathetic clip application is safe and effective in patients with upper limb hyperhidrosis, with stable long-term improvements in quality of life.

▶ The authors present an interesting study presenting their experience with treating palmar and palmoaxillary hyperhidrosis with an endothoracic T4 sympathetic block. This prospective study has a long follow-up average of 92 months and large cohort of 174 patients and keenly divided the groups into pure palmar and combined palmoaxillary hyperhidrosis. This article is beneficial to the literature because of its clean and concise design and data. The authors used one treatment method, endothoracic sympathetic block at T4 (ESB4), thus, allowing this large data set to be more powerful. Because of the prospective nature, the authors add strength to their findings of improved quality of life after ESB4, with isolated palmar symptoms more resilient to reoccurrence versus palmoaxillary patients. The strong design and concise presentation of data by the authors makes this an important article for anyone treating palmar or palmoaxillary hyperhidrosis.

J. M. Froelich, MD

The elbow flex-ex: a new sign to detect unilateral upper extremity non-organic paresis

Lombardi TL, Barton E, Wang J, et al (Cedars-Sinai Med Ctr, Los Angeles, CA)
J Neurol Neurosurg Psychiatry 85:165-167, 2014

Objective.—To examine a new neurological sign that uses synergistic oppositional movements of the arms to evaluate for non-organic upper extremity weakness.

Methods.—Patients with unilateral arm weakness were tested in a standing or sitting position with the elbows flexed at 30°. The examiner held both forearms near the wrists while asking the patient to flex or extend the normal arm at the elbow and simultaneously feeling for flexion or extension of the contralateral (paretic) arm. In patients with organic paresis, there was not a significant detectable force of contralateral opposition of the paretic limb. Patients with non-organic arm weakness had detectable strength of contralateral opposition in the paretic arm when the normal arm was tested.

Results.—The test was first performed on 23 patients with no complaint of arm weakness. Then, 31 patients with unilateral arm weakness were tested (10 with non-organic weakness and 21 with organic weakness). The elbow flex-ex sign correctly identified the cause of weakness in all cases.

Conclusions.—The elbow flex-ex sign is useful in differentiating between functional and organic arm paresis.

▶ This article presents an interesting way to help the examiner differentiate between organic and nonorganic weakness of the arm. It is sometimes a challenge when examining the patient with weakness to differentiate between lack of effort or true muscular weakness. This test takes advantage of the reflex synergistic activation of muscles on the contralateral side. If the patient was asked to fire muscles on the normal arm and force was detected on the contralateral (paretic limb), it pointed toward a functional rather than organic etiology. This highlights another tool that the hand surgeon might use to help identify functional versus organic pathology.

J. E. Adams, MD

Complex Regional Pain Syndrome Type I: Incidence and Risk Factors in Patients With Fracture of the Distal Radius

Jellad A, Salah S, Ben Salah Frih Z (Univ of Monastir, Tunisia)
Arch Phys Med Rehabil 95:487-492, 2014

Objective.—To examine the incidence and predictors of complex regional pain syndrome type I (CRPS I) after fracture of the distal radius.

Design.—Prospective study.

Setting.—University hospital.

Participants.—A consecutive sample of patients (N = 90) with fracture of the distal radius treated by closed reduction and casting.

Interventions.—Not applicable.

Main Outcome Measures.—Occurrence of CRPS I, occurrence of pain, wrist and hand range of motion, radiographic measures, Patient-Rated Wrist Evaluation, Hospital Anxiety and Depression Scale, and Medical Outcomes Study 36-Item Short-Form Health Survey at baseline and 1, 3, 6, and 9 months follow-up.

Results.—CRPS I occurred in 29 patients (32.2%) with a mean delay ± SD of 21.7 ± 23.7 days from cast removal. Univariate analyses found significant differences between patients with CRPS I and patients without CRPS I at baseline for sex ($P = .021$), socioeconomic level ($P = .023$), type of trauma ($P = .05$), pain at rest and activity ($P = .006$ and $P < .001$, respectively), wrist dorsiflexion and pronation ($P = .002$ and $P = .001$, respectively), finger flexion ($P = .047$), thumb opposition ($P = .002$), function of the hand ($P < .001$), and physical quality of life (QOL) ($P = .013$). Logistic regression showed that risk for CRPS I was higher in cases of women (odds ratio [OR] = 5.774; 95% confidence interval [CI], 1.391–23.966), medium and low energy trauma patients (OR = 7.718; 95% CI, 1.136–52.44), patients with a Medical Outcomes Study 36-Item Short-Form Health Survey physical functioning score <40 (OR = 4.931; 95% CI, 1.428–17.025), and patients with Patient-Rated Wrist Evaluation pain subscale score >16 (OR = 12.192; 95% CI, 4.484–43.478).

Conclusions.—CRPS I occurs frequently during the third and fourth week after cast removal, especially in women who report severe pain and impairment of physical QOL. Additional prospective studies are required to verify these findings in comminuted and operated fractures of the distal radius.

▶ The authors provide a report examining the incidence of complex regional pain syndrome (CRPS) type I associated with distal radius fractures. A second aim of the study was to identify risk factors associated with the development of complex regional pain syndrome. They analyzed prospectively persons with a distal radius fracture treated nonoperatively over a 2-year period.

A total of 121 fractures were identified, of which 90 fit the inclusion criteria for study. If the patient exhibited 4 of 5 of the Veldman characteristic signs for CRPS (diffuse pain, diffuse swelling, limited range of motion, abnormal skin color, and temperature relative to the other limb), they were diagnosed with the condition.

Nearly one-third of the patients were diagnosed with CRPS, which is far more than what I have seen in my experience. Most patients presented at the third or fourth week after cast removal. Women were more commonly affected. In addition, clinical data were obtained and included pain, range of motion, function of the hand, anxiodepressive profile, and quality of life (QOL). The authors found that impairment of the QOL score was predictive of developing CRPS.

M. Rizzo, MD

Anatomical Relationships and Branching Patterns of the Dorsal Cutaneous Branch of the Ulnar Nerve
Root CG, London DA, Schroeder NS, et al (Washington Univ School of Medicine, St Louis, MO)
J Hand Surg 38A:1131-1136, 2013

Purpose.—To describe the variable branching patterns of the dorsal cutaneous branch of the ulnar nerve (DCBUN) relative to identifiable anatomical landmarks on the ulnar side of the wrist.

Methods.—We dissected the ulnar nerve in 28 unmatched fresh-frozen cadavers to identify the DCBUN and its branches from its origin to the level of the metacarpophalangeal joints. The number and location of branches of the DCBUN were recorded relative to the distal ulnar articular surface. Relationships to the subcutaneous border of the ulna, the pisotriquetral joint, and the extensor carpi ulnaris tendon were defined in the pronated wrist.

Results.—On average, 2 branches of the DCBUN were present at the level of the distal ulnar articular surface (range, 1—4). On average, 2.2 branches were present 2 cm distal to the ulnar articular surface (range, 1—4). At least 1 longitudinal branch crossed dorsal to the extensor carpi ulnaris tendon prior to its insertion at the base of the fifth metacarpal in 23 of 28 specimens (82%). In 27 of 28 specimens (96%), all longitudinal branches of the DCBUN coursed between the dorsal-volar midpoint of the subcutaneous border of the ulna and the pisotriquetral joint. In 20 of 28 specimens (71%), a transverse branch of the DCBUN to the distal radioulnar joint was present.

Conclusions.—During exposure of the dorsal and ulnar areas of the wrist, identification and protection of just a single branch of the DCBUN are unlikely to ensure safe dissection because multiple branches normally are present. The 6U, 6R, and ulnar midcarpal arthroscopy portals may place these branches at risk. In the pronated forearm, the area between the DCBUN and the pisotriquetral joint contained all longitudinal branches of the DCBUN in 96% of specimens.

Clinical Relevance.—During surgery involving the dorsal and ulnar areas of the wrist, multiple longitudinal branches and a transverse branch of the DCBUN are normally present and must be respected.

▶ This study was performed to determine the branching patterns of the dorsal cutaneous branch of the ulnar nerve (DCBUN). Twenty-eight fresh-frozen cadavers were dissected. The ulnar nerve was identified proximally and traced distally. Measurements were taken of the origin of the DCBUN. The first branch of the DCBUN was found to originate a mean 5.1 cm from the distal ulna articular surface. In 96% of specimens, the DCBUN was identified between the subcutaneous border of the ulna and the pisotriquetral joint. The 3 most common distal branching patterns accounting for 87% of specimens are described. Although this nerve has been evaluated previously by cadaver dissections, the unique element of this study is related to evaluation of the variable branching patterns of the nerve. Because multiple branches may be encountered, the surgeon should exercise caution when approaching the dorsal ulnar aspect of the wrist. Based on this study, it is important to realize that identification and protection of a single nerve branch does not ensure that injury to other branches of this nerve will be avoided.

T. J. Payne, MD

Dosage of Local Anesthesia in Wide Awake Hand Surgery
Lalonde DH, Wong A (Dalhousie Univ, Saint John, New Brunswick, Canada; Dalhousie Univ, Halifax, Nova Scotia, Canada)
J Hand Surg 38A:2025-2028, 2013

Background.—Minimal pain injection tumescent local anesthesia avoids the need for preoperative testing, does not cause tourniquet pain, means less hospital time, allows patients to speak to the surgeon during surgery, and avoids the "cloudy head" resulting from sedation. The technique was described.

Technique.—Lidocaine with epinephrine is injected subcutaneously where the surgeon will be dissecting, moving fractures, or inserting K-wires. The epinephrine provides hemostasis and is well established as safe for use in the finger.

With a 27-gauge needle the incision is less painful and the injector is reminded to proceed slowly. A 2-ml dose is injected slowly just under the skin, avoiding small subcutaneous veins by collapsing them with antegrade injection. A small amount of inadvertent intravascular (IV) lidocaine is usually well tolerated. To avoid causing pain, the injector should ensure 1 ml of visible or palpable local anesthesia is ahead of the sharp needle tip. For reinsertion to cover a large area, the site of reinsertion is within 1 cm of visible palpable local anesthesia. The surgeon can hone skills by having patients score the number of times they feel pain. At least 1 cm of adrenalized skin should appear beyond all borders of incision and dissection.

Lidocaine with epinephrine is generally given in a maximal dose of 7 mg/kg, with an average 70-kg individual safely receiving 50 ml 1% lidocaine with epinephrine. It can be effective if diluted with as much as 150 ml saline solution to 1/4% lidocaine with 1:400,000 epinephrine. The injector should be generous with the volume so augmentation is not needed. One percent lidocaine with 1:100,000 epinephrine is used if less than 50 ml volume is needed, 1/2% lidocaine with 1:200,000 epinephrine for 50 to 100 ml volume, and 1/4% lidocaine with 1:400,000 epinephrine for 100 to 200 ml volume. The preferred ratio of lidocaine to bicarbonate for reducing pain is 10 ml lidocaine to 1 ml 8.4% bicarbonate.

Bupivacine is often chosen for its longer duration of action, but lidocaine offers some advantages. IV bupivacaine can be cardiotoxic and cause death, but IV lidocaine has proved safe. Lidocaine and epinephrine have a long history of safe use in dental offices with no patient monitoring required. Bupivacaine's pain-relieving effect lasts half as long as its annoying touch and pressure numbness, both of which are objectionable to patients. However, 10 ml 0.5% bupivacaine with 1:200,000 epinephrine can be added to the injectate for cases that will exceed 2.5 hours to avoid pain occurring with lidocaine's diminished effect.

Additional Considerations.—The injection of local anesthesia should be done with the patient lying on the stretcher outside the operating room. This allows more time for the epinephrine to reach maximal optimal vasoconstriction time (26 minutes), avoid the vasovagal reaction that accompanies having the patient sit up for the injection, and not waste valuable operating room time.

For spaghetti wrist and ulnar nerve decompression at the elbow, the injection of 50 to 100 ml 0.5% lidocaine with 1:200,000 epinephrine is done from proximal to distal if dissection is planned. Forearm transfers are covered using up to 200 ml 1/4% lidocaine with 1:400,000 epinephrine, with bupivacaine added to extend the pain suppression. Sensory nerves need to be bathed in local anesthesia for wrist or forearm surgery, but the forearm motor nerves should be free of anesthetic to observe active motion after repair.

Conclusions.—Tourniquet-free injections of local anesthetics allow coverage of areas where the surgeon will be performing possibly painful manipulations. This achieves relatively pain-free injection over a large area if done slowly, and improves patient convenience and satisfaction.

▶ One of the most intriguing advances in hand and upper extremity surgery has been the development of the aptly described "wide-awake hand surgery." Critical to wide-awake hand surgery is patient comfort and active participation during hand and upper extremity surgery. In this article, the authors efficiently describe the anesthesia required to minimize the unpleasant sensory experience known as pain. This brief report reflects the authors' motivation to use a combination of lidocaine with epinephrine mixed with bicarbonate to create an effective anesthetic that also precludes the use of tourniquet control. The authors further opine that this anesthetic experience improves patient convenience and satisfaction while allowing the surgeon to operate in a controlled field and, when necessary, to engage the patient in conversation during surgical repair/fixation to educate and discuss the findings.

The authors are to be credited for scientifically refuting the age-old dogma that epinephrine should not be injected in fingers and digits. Although not an absolute requisite for wide awake hand surgery, the technique described in this article allows the surgeon to anesthetize the patient in such way that minimizes tourniquet pain and the associated postanesthetic sequelae often encountered with general sedation. It should be noted that in the rare, but potentially real, event of digital ischemia, phentolamine should be available to the surgeon as a reversal agent. Furthermore, when attempting this technique for the first time, a full complement of anesthesia personnel should be available in the event that the patient requires additional sedation or anesthesia. As one becomes comfortable with this technique, the indications for the use of tourniquet-free local anesthesia will expand quickly, as they have in my practice.

S. M. Jacoby, MD

The "Double Wrist Flexor" Tendon Transfer for Radial Nerve Palsy

Al-Qattan M (King Saud Univ, Riyadh, Saudi Arabia)
Ann Plast Surg 71:34-36, 2013

In isolated high radial nerve palsy, it is traditionally taught that one should not use both wrist flexors for tendon transfers. Over the last 17 years, the author has encountered 4 unusual cases of high radial nerve palsy with concurrent direct injury to the pronator teres, flexor digitorum superficialis, and the palmaris longus in the proximal forearm. In these cases, the author used both wrist flexors, namely, the flexor carpi radialis to restore wrist extension and the flexor carpi ulnaris to restore finger/thumb extension as well as thumb radial abduction. Despite the major loss of wrist flexion, all patients had a good overall function as per the modified Bincaz scale. It was concluded that this "double wrist flexor" transfer remains to be an acceptable option for high radial nerve palsy when the pronator teres, flexor digitorum superficialis, and the palmaris longus tendons are not available.

▶ This article presents a useful alternative to wrist fusion in crush injury cases in which the traditional median nerve innervated muscles used for transfers (pronator teres, flexor digitorum superficialis, and the palmaris longus) are not available because of direct injury to these muscles. The authors' results show that, contrary to traditional teaching, their procedure is able to create a useful degree of wrist extension and good overall wrist function, despite the loss of a significant degree of wrist flexion.

J. Toto, MD

The effectiveness of early mobilization after tendon transfers in the hand: a systematic review

Sultana SS, MacDermid JC, Grewal R, et al (Univ of Western Ontario, London, Ontario, Canada; et al)
J Hand Ther 26:1-21, 2013

Study Design.—Systematic review.
Introduction.—Over the past decade, early mobilization (initiated within a week) has become an increasing trend in postoperative rehabilitation after tendon transfer surgery in the hand. However, there are no published reviews summarizing the effectiveness of early mobilization protocols in comparison with conventional immobilization in tendon transfer rehabilitation.
Purpose.—To systematically review available evidence on the effectiveness of early mobilization protocols to conventional immobilization protocol after tendon transfers in the hand.
Methods.—A literature search of the Cochrane Library, PubMed, PEDro, EMBASE, and CINAHL databases was conducted (1980 to date).

Randomized controlled trials (RCTs), case—control, and other study designs were included. Six articles were eligible for inclusion in the analysis (five RCTs and one retrospective study) and 260 articles that did not meet inclusion criteria were excluded. Level of evidence (Center for Evidence-based Medicine) and methodological quality (Structured Effectiveness Quality Evaluation Scale [SEQES] score) of each study were assessed by two independent reviewers.

Results.—This review found three high quality trials (SEQES score: 35—43 of 48), with level 1b and 2b evidence, supporting early mobilization of tendon transfers. The literature reports reduced total cost, total rehabilitation time, and demonstrates that early mobilization is a safe approach with no incidence of tendon ruptures or insertion pull out. In the initial phase of rehabilitation, outcomes like range of motion, grip strength, pinch strength, total active motion of digits, deformity correction, and tendon transfer integration were significantly superior with early mobilization compared with immobilization. However, in the long term, these outcomes were similar in both the groups, suggesting that early mobilization protocol improves hand function in the initial phase of rehabilitation (four weeks) and the long-term results (two months to one year) are equivalent to immobilization.

Conclusions.—Based on a limited number of small studies, there is evidence of short-term benefit for early mobilization, but inconclusive findings for longer-term outcomes. Until the body of evidence increases, clinicians should consider the clinical context, their experience in optimizing patient outcomes after surgery, and the patient's preferences when selecting between early and late mobilization after tendon transfer.

Level of Evidence.—2a.

▶ The authors did an excellent job on the systematic review and summarize evidence-based studies and protocols. The topic is relevant because early motion in postoperative rehabilitation translates to earlier return to function or work activities of daily living. The purpose of the review was determining the effectiveness of early mobilization protocols for tendon transfers compared with those in standard immobilization. The strong aspects of this article were the authors' search of databases and selection for inclusion. Unfortunately, after an extensive search, only 6 of 266 possible studies could be acceptable for comparison. It does give direction that future research should focus on these testing validities, interrater reliability, and stronger defined protocols for each type of neuromuscular tendon transfers. Even after review of the current evidence, the authors found that the final data were insufficient to draw the conclusion that early mobilization is the best protocol to follow after a hand tendon transfer. Despite the findings, they continued to assert that clinicians should consider the use of early mobilization as a treatment option because of the fewer complications and no incidence of ruptures. It also proposed that clinicians should perform high-quality random control trials for the future tendon transfer research.

S. Kranz, OTR/L, CHT

Approach to radial nerve palsy caused by humerus shaft fracture: Is primary exploration necessary?
Korompilias AV, Lykissas MG, Kostas-Agnantis IP, et al (Univ of Ioannina School of Medicine, Greece; Hosp for Special Surgery, NY; et al)
Injury 44:323-326, 2013

Introduction.—While recommendations for early exploration and nerve repair in cases of open fractures of the humeral shaft associated with radial nerve palsy are clear, the therapeutic algorithm for the management of closed humeral shaft fractures complicated by radial nerve palsy is still uncertain. The purpose of this study was to determine whether patients with complete sensory and motor radial nerve palsy following a closed fracture of the humeral shaft should be surgically explored.

Patients and Methods.—Twenty-five patients with closed humeral shaft fractures complicated by complete radial nerve palsy were retrospectively reviewed during a 12-year period. Surgical intervention was indicated if functional recovery of the radial nerve was not present after 16 weeks of expectant management.

Results.—Surgical exploration was performed in 12 patients (48%) after a mean period of expectant management of 16.8 weeks (range: 16—18 weeks). In 2 of them (10%) total nerve transection was found. In the rest 10 patients underwent surgical exploration the radial nerve was found to be macroscopically intact. All intact nerves were fully recovered after a mean time of 21.6 weeks (range: 20—24 weeks) post-injury. In 13 patients (52%) in whom surgical exploration was not performed the mean time to full nerve recovery was 12 weeks (range: 7—14 weeks) post-injury.

Conclusions.—We proposed immediate exploration of the radial nerve in case of open fractures of the humeral shaft, irreducible fractures or unacceptable reduction, associated vascular injuries, radial nerve palsy after manipulation or intractable neurogenic pain. Due to high rate of spontaneous recovery of the radial nerve after closed humeral shaft fractures we recommend 16—18 weeks of expectant management followed by surgical intervention.

▶ There is no consensus yet on how to treat closed nerve palsies, whether in the context of a humeral fracture or in any other setting. Diagnostic tools are limited to the clinical examination, electrodiagnostic testing, and imaging studies such as magnetic resonance imaging and ultrasound scan. There is no reliable diagnostic tool to differentiate an axonometric injury that has a good chance of recovery from a neurometric injury that will not recover. Neuropraxic injures are easier to diagnose because the nerve will conduct both proximal and distal to the lesion, and almost all resolve by about 12 weeks after injury.

Radial nerve palsies associated with humeral fractures are quite common and, therefore, have received much attention in the literature. Recommendations vary from early exploration of all complete palsies to prolonged observation. Most experts agree that a nerve that is compromised by a closed reduction should be explored, because there is a risk of nerve entrapment in the fracture.

In this study, 12 of their 25 patients with radial nerve palsies and humeral fractures did not recover spontaneously by 16 weeks and, therefore, underwent nerve exploration. Two patients required nerve grafting for complete transections, and 2 patients required extrication of the intact nerve from between the bone ends. Both patients who underwent grafting did not make any recovery of the radial nerve even after 4 years of follow-up but were able to function well with tendon transfers. All other patients who had an intact nerve at the time of exploration recovered fully by 6 months after the injury.

The results of this study do little to help answer the question at hand: Should I explore a radial nerve injury in the setting of a humeral shaft fracture? If 4 of 25 patients would have benefited from early exploration, but only 2 of those had long-term consequences from waiting to repair the nerve injury, and of those 2 it is unclear if their poor results would have been improved by earlier intervention, what does this teach us? The debate rages on.

D. A. Zlotolow, MD

7 Brachial Plexus

Comparative study of phrenic nerve transfers with and without nerve graft for elbow flexion after global brachial plexus injury
Liu Y, Lao J, Gao K, et al (Shanghai Huashan Hosp, China)
Injury 45:227-231, 2014

Background.—Nerve transfer is a valuable surgical technique in peripheral nerve reconstruction, especially in brachial plexus injuries. Phrenic nerve transfer for elbow flexion was proved to be one of the optimal procedures in the treatment of brachial plexus injuries in the study of Gu et al.

Objective.—The aim of this study was to compare phrenic nerve transfers with and without nerve graft for elbow flexion after brachial plexus injury.

Methods.—A retrospective review of 33 patients treated with phrenic nerve transfer for elbow flexion in posttraumatic global root avulsion brachial plexus injury was carried out. All the 33 patients were confirmed to have global root avulsion brachial plexus injury by preoperative and intraoperative electromyography (EMG), physical examination and especially by intraoperative exploration. There were two types of phrenic nerve transfers: type1 — the phrenic nerve to anterolateral bundle of anterior division of upper trunk (14 patients); type 2 — the phrenic nerve via nerve graft to anterolateral bundle of musculocutaneous nerve (19 patients). Motor function and EMG evaluation were performed at least 3 years after surgery.

Results.—The efficiency of motor function in type 1 was 86%, while it was 84% in type 2. The two groups were not statistically different in terms of Medical Research Council (MRC) grade ($p = 1.000$) and EMG results ($p = 1.000$). There were seven patients with more than 4 month's delay of surgery, among whom only three patients regained biceps power to M3 strength or above (43%). A total of 26 patients had reconstruction done within 4 months, among whom 25 patients recovered to M3 strength or above (96%). There was a statistically significant difference of motor function between the delay of surgery within 4 months and more than 4 months ($p = 0.008$).

Conclusion.—Phrenic nerve transfers with and without nerve graft for elbow flexion after brachial plexus injury had no significant difference for biceps reinnervation according to MRC grading and EMG. A delay of the surgery after the 4 months might imply a bad prognosis for the recovery of the function.

▶ This is a retrospective review of 33 brachial plexus patients who had phrenic nerve transfers with and without nerve graft for elbow flexion. One group had direct grafting of phrenic to the anterior division of the upper trunk and the other group had phrenic via nerve graft connected to the musculocutaneous nerve. The groups had no differences in final elbow flexion strength with roughly 64% obtaining M4 strength. The other important finding of the study was that those who had reconstruction later than 4 months had significantly less elbow flexion strength.

This article provides the nerve surgeon with information useful for practice. First, currently when trying to reconstruct the plexus using the phrenic nerve, the surgeon may struggle and perhaps use a less-than-ideal distal target in the hopes of eliminating the need for a graft. This article's findings lessen that concern about lost axons in the nerve graft, allowing the surgeon to use the repair with the best-quality nerve (even though it might require a graft).

Second, this article highlights the need to operate early on these patients. The patient presenting with a flail arm should have an expedited course to the surgery. Waiting even 4 months can result in significantly poorer results.

C. Curtin, MD

Dynamic Sonographic Evaluation of Posterior Shoulder Dislocation Secondary to Brachial Plexus Birth Palsy Injury

Sanchez TRS, Chang J, Bauer A, et al (Univ of California, Davis Children's Hosp, Sacramento)
J Ultrasound Med 32:1531-1534, 2013

Background.—Rotator cuff muscle imbalance can produce posterior subluxation of the humeral head and deformity of the glenohumeral joint. Neonatal and infantile hip stability can be assessed and monitored using sonographic evaluation, and the same technology is able to perform glenohumeral joint evaluations. Clinicians tend to rely on computed tomography (CT) and magnetic resonance imaging (MRI) scans, but concerns have been raised over radiation exposure, cost, and the use of sedation or anesthesia associated with CT and MRI. Sonography offers a dynamic and real-time evaluation of shoulder congruency that can alter treatment and is simple and safe. Because radiologists and orthopedic surgeons are often unaware of the procedure, a description of the technique was provided.

Technique.—A linear 12-MHz transducer is used to scan both shoulders posteriorly on the transverse plane. For infants less than age 3 months, placement on a bed on their side is appropriate for assessment of the nondependent shoulder, then the child can be turned to the other side. It is advisable to assess the normal shoulder first to note the normal anatomy and avoid manipulating the involved shoulder, which can cause anxiety and discomfort and compromise the ability to perform the examination. These young children may also be held on the parent's shoulder, with children over age 6 months usually placed on the adult's lap. Shoulders are scanned with the arm adducted against the torso and positioned in maximal internal rotation and the elbow flexed at 90 degrees. The α angle is formed where a line drawn along the posterior margin of the scapula intersects a line tangential to the humeral head from the posterior edge of the glenoid labrum. This angle is normally 30 degrees or less. The abnormal shoulder is also scanned in maximal external rotation. This reveals the dynamic movement of the glenohumeral joint from internal to external rotation and shows whether the humeral head can be returned to the joint or remains dislocated or subluxed.

Results.—It can be challenging to diagnose posterior dislocation caused by a displaced humeral head clinically, and an adjunct imaging modality that is both sensitive and accurate is needed. Sonography offers the ability to assess the shoulder accurately and safely.

Conclusions.—Sonography is accessible, less costly, and lacking in radiation exposure compared to CT and MRI studies. It also provides a dynamic and real-time examination of the nonossified humeral head and can identify persistent dislocation or relocation when the shoulder is externally rotated. It appears to be the most logical and safest imaging modality for the initial diagnosis and subsequent monitoring of infants with brachial plexus birth palsy shoulder instability who do not recover fully in the first year of life.

▶ In this article, the authors discuss the utility of sonography in evaluating the shoulder in brachial plexus birth palsy (BPBP). Dynamic sonography has many advantages over other imaging modalities, such as computed tomography (CT), radiographs, and magnetic resonance imaging (MRI). There is no radiation exposure to the child, no sedation required, and it can visualize the unossified humeral head in infants. The technique described positions the child on a bed in the lateral position or on the lap of the accompanying adult. Both the affected and unaffected shoulder are scanned posteriorly with the arm adducted against the torso in maximum internal rotation, and the α angle is measured. The affected shoulder is also evaluated in maximal external rotation to verify if the joint is reducible. Ultrasound scan presents an excellent alternative to CT and MRI as a monitoring tool for glenohumeral dysplasia in young patients. Although this article clearly shows the utility of dynamic sonography, it is important to remember that ultrasound scan is not readily available in every hospital or clinic and requires both a technician and a physician comfortable with obtaining and interpreting ultrasound images of the infant shoulder.

F. G. Fishman, MD

Deficits in Elbow Position Sense in Neonatal Brachial Plexus Palsy
Brown SH, Noble BC, Yang LJ-S, et al (Univ of Michigan, Ann Arbor; Univ of Michigan Health System, Ann Arbor)
Pediatr Neurol 49:324-328, 2013

Background.—In neonatal brachial plexus palsy, sensory recovery is thought to exceed motor recovery with little attention paid to long-term assessment of proprioceptive ability. However, there is growing evidence that reduced somatosensory function frequently accompanies motor deficits as a result of activity-dependent changes in the central nervous system. Given the importance of proprioception in everyday motor activities, this study was designed to investigate position sense about the elbow joint in neonatal brachial plexus palsy.

Methods.—A convenience sample of seven individuals with neonatal brachial plexus palsy aged 9-17 years and in seven control individuals aged 10-16 years were recruited for the study. An elbow position matching task was used in which passive displacement of the forearm (reference arm) was reproduced with the same or opposite arm. In both conditions, matching was performed in the absence of vision and required utilization of position-related proprioceptive feedback.

Results.—Position-matching errors were significantly greater for the affected versus the unaffected arm when reproducing a reference position with the same arm. When matching was performed using the opposite arm, errors were dependent upon which arm served as the reference arm. When the unaffected arm served as the reference position, affected arm matching errors were not significantly different from control values. However, in the reverse situation, in which the unaffected arm relied on reference feedback from the affected arm, matching errors doubled compared with control values.

Conclusions.—These results provide evidence that position sense is impaired in neonatal brachial plexus palsy and illustrate the importance of assessing proprioception in this population.

▶ The authors of this study sought to investigate possible residual deficits in position sense about the elbow in children with brachial plexus birth palsy (BPBP). A small sample of patients with unilateral BPBP, who had not undergone microsurgical or secondary reconstructive procedures, was tested. The mean age of the 7 patients was 12 years. Grip strength, functional ability, and elbow position matching ability were tested. They showed significant declines in grip strength and hand dexterity of the affected side. Additionally, the authors showed that proprioceptive errors in position matching were greater when performed by the affected arm compared with the unaffected arm. Although proprioceptive deficits have been described in adults after stroke and children with cerebral palsy, this is an understudied aspect of BPBP and certainly not typically addressed during a routine clinical assessment. Although this study evaluates a very small sample (7 individuals), it is an important reminder that proprioceptive deficits likely contribute to the overall function of the affected arm in patients with BPBP and that their function is not solely related to muscle strength and passive motion of the their joints.

F. G. Fishman, MD

Meta-analysis of Function After Secondary Shoulder Surgery in Neonatal Brachial Plexus Palsy

Louden EJ, Broering CA, Mehlman CT, et al (Cincinnati Children's Hosp Med Ctr, OH; Univ of Cincinnati College of Medicine; et al)
J Pediatr Orthop 33:656-663, 2013

Background.—Shoulder internal rotation contracture, active abduction, and external rotation deficits are common secondary problems in neonatal brachial plexus palsy (NBPP). Soft tissue shoulder operations are often utilized for treatment. The objective was to conduct a meta-analysis and systematic review analyzing the clinical outcomes of NBPP treated with a secondary soft-tissue shoulder operation.

Methods.—A literature search identified studies of NBPP treated with a soft-tissue shoulder operation. A meta-analysis evaluated success rates for the aggregate Mallet score (≥ 4 point increase), global abduction score (≥ 1 point increase), and external rotation score (≥ 1 point increase) using the Mallet scale. Subgroup analysis was performed to assess these success rates when the author chose arthroscopic release technique versus open release technique with or without tendon transfer.

Results.—Data from 17 studies and 405 patients were pooled for meta-analysis. The success rate for the global abduction score was significantly higher for the open technique (67.4%) relative to the arthroscopic technique (27.7%, $P < 0.0001$). The success rates for the global abduction score were significantly different among sexes ($P = 0.01$). The success rate for external rotation was not significantly different between the open (71.4%) and arthroscopic techniques (74.1%, $P = 0.86$). No other variable was found to have significant impact on the external rotation outcomes. The success rate for the aggregate Mallet score was 57.9% for the open technique, a nonsignificant increase relative to the arthroscopic technique (53.5%, $P = 0.63$). Data suggest a correlation between increasing age at the time of surgery and a decreasing likelihood of success with regards to aggregate Mallet with an odds ratio of 0.98 ($P = 0.04$).

Conclusion.—Overall, the secondary soft-tissue shoulder operation is an effective treatment for improving shoulder function in NBPP in appropriately selected patients. The open technique had significantly higher success rates in improving global abduction. There were no significant differences in the success rates for improvement in the external rotation or aggregate Mallet score among these surgical techniques (Fig 1).

▶ The meta-analysis reviews retrospective studies performed between 1950 and 2012 that evaluated the effect of soft tissue surgery on shoulder function in neonatal brachial plexus palsy (NBPP). Studies evaluating medical conditions with a low incidence often are inadequately powered to detect significant differences in patient outcomes. Meta-analysis has grown in popularity in an effort to answer these research questions that have been difficult to answer. However, when evaluating the conclusion, one must remember the inherent biases of meta-analysis, including heterogeneity of the combined studies and type II

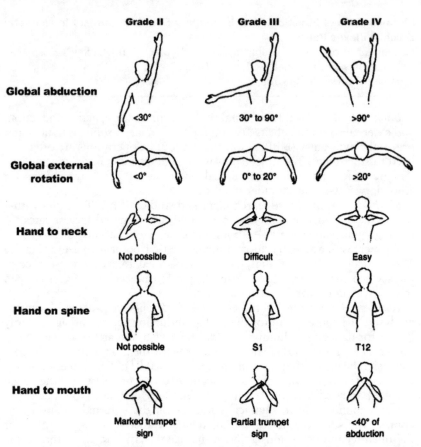

FIGURE 1.—Mallet classification system assesses brachial plexus function of the upper extremity. Each movement is evaluated from grade I indicating no function incremented up to grade V indicating normal function. Individual scores can be summed to an aggregate score where the lowest possible is a 5 and the highest possible is 25. (Reprinted from Louden EJ, Broering CA, Mehlman CT, et al. Meta-analysis of function after secondary shoulder surgery in neonatal brachial plexus palsy. *J Pediatr Orthop.* 2013;33:656-663, with permission from Lippincott Williams & Wilkins.)

error. The current analysis evaluated 3 different outcomes, including the aggregate mallet score, active shoulder abduction, and active shoulder external rotation in adduction, with study heterogeneity of 89%, 93%, and 0%, respectively. Although the authors have compiled several subjects in this review, the heterogeneity may have led to inaccurate assessment of the success of surgery. For example, the aggregate mallet score categorizes continuous variables (Fig 1), and the success of shoulder surgery was dichotomized. Thus, in a patient with global abduction of 35° that improved to 75° after soft tissue shoulder reconstruction, surgery was classified as unsuccessful because the grade remained the same. Despite these limitations, the authors have shown success rates of 58% to 71% for open soft tissue shoulder reconstruction surgery in NBPP.

A. Moeller, MD

8 Microsurgery

Toe-to-Hand Transfer: Evolving Indications and Relevant Outcomes
Waljee JF, Chung KC (Univ of Michigan Health System, Ann Arbor)
J Hand Surg 38A:1431-1434, 2013

Toe-to-hand transfer is indicated for many types of congenital and traumatic thumb absences. This review will highlight the applications of toe-to-hand transfer and their functional, aesthetic, and psychosocial

TABLE 1.—Indications for Toe-to-Hand Transfer

Adults
    Traumatic thumb amputation
    Traumatic digital amputation distal to the flexor digitorum superficialis insertion
    Multiple traumatic digital amputation
Children
    Congenital thumb absence
    Constriction ring syndrome
    Transverse arrest
    Longitudinal deficiency
    Symbrachydactyly

TABLE 2.—Advantages and Disadvantages of Toe-to-Hand Transfer Techniques

Technique	Advantages	Drawbacks
Great toe transfer	Excellent thumb stability and IP joint motion	Donor site aesthetics Larger size and contour differences compared with the contralateral toe Must preserve metatarsal head to prevent gait deficit
Second toe transfer	Donor site less apparent Can include the metatarsal joint without impeding function, and varying degrees of the metatarsal can be harvested for length	Bulbous thumb tip and smaller nail Claw deformity Less stability and motion
Wraparound toe transfer	Better size and contour match with contralateral thumb Ideal for patients with degloving injuries and intact skeletal elements and distal amputations	Requires conventional bone graft (eg, iliac crest) for support, which may resorb over time IP joint cannot be reconstructed Pulp instability
Trimmed great toe transfer	Better size and contour match with contralateral thumb Includes the IP joint	Reduced IP motion

IP, interphalangeal.

outcomes. Despite its technical complexity, toe to hand reconstruction techniques can provide an elegant option to restore function for patients with difficult hand disabilities (Tables 1 and 2).

▶ Waljee and Chung review the indications and outcomes for toe-to-hand transfer. Indications for both adults and children are summarized in Table 1. A study comparing early and delayed toe-to-hand transfer did not find a difference in survival or complications. Excellent functional and aesthetic outcomes can be achieved. However, the surgical technique used was not shown to affect outcomes. Advantages and disadvantages of different surgical techniques are summarized in Table 2. Toe-to-hand transfer has also been shown to have a profound effect on quality of life, psychosocial function, and the ability to return to work.

This report serves as a concise review of the complex topic of toe-to-hand transfer and is a useful resource summarizing the topic.

H. Chim, MD

Release of hand burn contracture: Comparing the ALT perforator flap with the gracilis free flap with split skin graft

Misani M, Zirak C, Hau LTT, et al (Brugmann ULB Univ Hosp, Brussels, Belgium)
Burns 39:965-971, 2013

Background.—The use of microsurgery in the management of burn sequelae is not a new idea. According to the properties of various types of free flaps different goals can be achieved or various additional procedures have to be combined. We report the comparison of two different free flaps on a single patient for reconstruction of both upper extremities for burn sequelae.

> *Case Report.*—A 1-year-old child sustained severe burns on both hands, arms and thorax and was initially only treated conservatively. This resulted in severe contractures. At the age of 4-years a free gracilis flap was selected for reconstruction of his left hand and a free anterolateral thigh flap for the right hand.

Results.—We noticed a better functional and esthetic result for the gracilis flap associated with a shorter operative time and a minor donor site morbidity. The intraoperative technique and time, postoperative complications, functional and esthetic results and donor site morbidities were studied in the two types of flaps chosen. A review of literature was also performed.

Conclusion.—Our experience reported a better success of the gracilis muscle flap covered with a split skin graft compared to the anterolateral

thigh flap in the reconstruction of hand function after severe burn sequelae
(Figs 3 and 8).

▶ Misani and colleagues present the results of resurfacing of bilateral hand
burns after contracture release in a 4-year-old child. On one side a gracilis
free flap with skin graft was used, whereas on the other side an anterolateral
thigh (ALT) flap was used. The authors conclude that the gracilis flap, and
other muscle flaps by extrapolation, is superior to the ALT flap because of
decreased bulk and improved versatility. In addition, they conclude that from
their experience, the ALT flap can result in circumferential scarring and subsequent bulging of the flap.

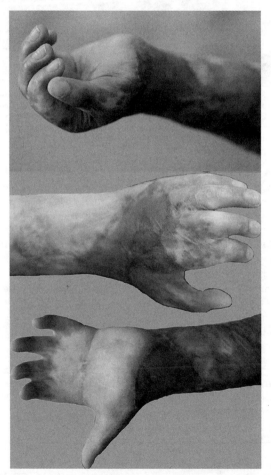

FIGURE 3.—Left hand post-op gracilis free flap: extension and flexion, dorsal and palmar view.
(Reprinted from Misani M, Zirak C, Hau LTT, et al. Release of hand burn contracture: comparing the
ALT perforator flap with the gracilis free flap with split skin graft. *Burns.* 2013;39:965-971, Copyright
2013, with permission from International Society for Burn Injuries.)

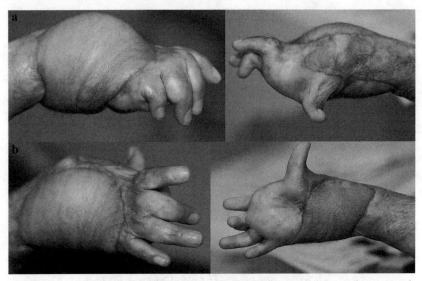

FIGURE 8.—(a) Post-op right hand with ALT free flap, lateral ulnar and radial view. (b) Post-op right hand with ALT flap, dorsal and palmar view. Extra bulck and recurrent MCP retraction at six months. (Reprinted from Misani M, Zirak C, Hau LTT, et al. Release of hand burn contracture: comparing the ALT perforator flap with the gracilis free flap with split skin graft. *Burns*. 2013;39:965-971, Copyright 2013, with permission from International Society for Burn Injuries.)

The authors are to be commended on their very nice results (Figs 3 and 8). However, it is not possible to make the broad conclusions the authors have based on the results of a single case. In addition, the authors have not presented any objective outcomes, such as range of motion at different joints. A major concern with the use of the gracilis flap, and other muscle flaps in the hand, is the possibility of tendon adhesion to the muscle flap, inhibiting tendon gliding, and limiting range of motion. In contrast, a skin or fascial flap allows better tendon gliding and has been the flap type of choice for hand resurfacing for many practitioners. A skin flap, such as the ALT, can and often is debulked at a second stage for a more aesthetically pleasing result, but the authors have not mentioned this in this report.

H. Chim, MD

Innovations in Prosthetic Interfaces for the Upper Extremity

Kung TA, Bueno RA, Alkhalefah GK, et al (Univ of Michigan Health System, Ann Arbor; Southern Illinois Univ, Carbondale, IL)
Plast Reconstr Surg 132:1515-1523, 2013

Advancements in modern robotic technology have led to the development of highly sophisticated upper extremity prosthetic limbs. High-fidelity volitional control of these devices is dependent on the critical interface between the patient and the mechanical prosthesis. Recent innovations in prosthetic interfaces have focused on several control strategies. Targeted muscle rein-nervation is currently the most immediately applicable prosthetic control strategy and is particularly indicated in proximal upper extremity amputa-tions. Investigation into various brain interfaces has allowed acquisition of neuroelectric signals directly or indirectly from the central nervous system for prosthetic control. Peripheral nerve interfaces permit signal transduc-tion from both motor and sensory nerves with a higher degree of selectivity. This article reviews the current developments in each of these interface sys-tems and discusses the potential of these approaches to facilitate motor con-trol and sensory feedback in upper extremity neuroprosthetic devices.

▶ This is a comprehensive update on the current state of myoelectric upper-extremity prostheses. In their discussion of the limitations of these devices, the authors present their novel, and elegant, approach to solving the problem of directly interfacing with the peripheral nervous system. Although the reported data were from studies performed on an animal model, this approach seems to hold great promise, and I look forward to seeing results from human clinical trials in the future.

J. Toto, MD

The Pedicled Reverse-Flow Lateral Arm Flap for Coverage of Complex Traumatic Elbow Injuries
Morrison CS, Sullivan SR, Bhatt RA, et al (The Warren Alpert School of Medicine of Brown Univ, Providence, RI; Rhode Island Hosp, Providence, RI)
Ann Plast Surg 71:37-39, 2013

Purpose.—The pedicled reverse-flow lateral arm flap has been described primarily for the reconstruction of nontraumatic elbow wounds. We describe our experience using this flap in staged operations for soft tissue coverage after elbow trauma, including acute coverage of open fractures and salvage of infected hardware.

Methods.—Review of patients who underwent staged pedicled reverse-flow lateral arm flap transfer for coverage of traumatic elbow defects.

Results.—Three patients were identified; all underwent 2-stage repair with flap delay for coverage of traumatic elbow injuries. Each patient had stable wound coverage with this flap. The only complication was 5% distal flap necrosis in 1 patient.

Conclusions.—The pedicled reverse-flow lateral arm flap provides reli-able soft tissue coverage of traumatic elbow defects with minimal donor-site morbidity.

▶ This article presents 3 cases of pedicled reverse-flow lateral arm flap for recon-struction of traumatic wounds. All patients had a preoperative angiography imag-ing showing a patent recurrent radial artery. Each patient underwent a delay procedure with full elevation of the flap, and the second stage was performed

15 days or more later. The maximum widths of the flaps were up to 7.5 cm and the donor sites were closed primarily.

The authors report that one of the patients did have a 5% superficial necrosis. They suggest assessment with a woods lamp. Another tool that is very effective in demonstrating flap perfusion is intraoperative angiography with indocyanine green. This provides a quick assessment and can be repeated after inset to determine if the flap has been pulled to tightly. A delay procedure is well documented to decrease venous congestion and partial flap necrosis. Several studies in TRAM flaps have shown that 7 days is adequate time for a delay procedure.

This article gives support to use of delayed reverse-flow lateral arm flaps in traumatic injuries but cautions that a preoperative angiogram is essential to assess for the recurrent radial artery.

C. Heinrich, MD

Vascularized Groin Lymph Node Flap Transfer for Postmastectomy Upper Limb Lymphedema: Flap Anatomy, Recipient Sites, and Outcomes
Cheng M-H, Chen S-C, Henry SL, et al (Chang Gung Univ, Taoyuan, Taiwan; Singapore General Hosp)
Plast Reconstr Surg 131:1286-1298, 2013

Background.—Vascularized groin lymph node flap transfer is an emerging approach to the treatment of postmastectomy upper limb lymphedema. The authors describe the pertinent flap anatomy, surgical technique including different recipient sites, and outcome of this technique.

Methods.—Ten cadaveric dissections were performed to clarify the vascular supply of the superficial groin lymph nodes. Ten patients underwent vascularized groin lymph node flap transfer for postmastectomy upper limb lymphedema using the wrist ($n = 8$) or elbow ($n = 2$) as a recipient site. Ten patients who chose to undergo physical therapy were used as controls. Intraoperatively, indocyanine green was injected subcutaneously on the flap margin to observe the lymph drainage. Outcomes were assessed using improvement of circumferential differentiation, reduction rate, and decreased number of episodes of cellulitis.

Results.—A mean 6.2 ± 1.3 groin lymph nodes with consistent pedicles were identified in the cadaveric dissections. After indocyanine injection, the fluorescence was drained from the flap edge into the donor vein, followed by the recipient vein. At a mean follow-up of 39.1 ± 15.7 months, the mean improvement of circumferential differentiation was 7.3 ± 2.7 percent and the reduction rate was 40.4 ± 16.1 percent in the vascularized groin lymph node group, which were statistically greater than those of the physical therapy group (1.7 ± 4.6 percent and 8.3 ± 34.7 percent, respectively; $p < 0.01$ and $p = 0.02$, respectively).

Conclusions.—The superficial groin lymph nodes were confirmed as vascularized with reliable arterial perfusion. Vascularized groin lymph node flap transfer using the wrist or elbow as a recipient site is an efficacious approach to treating postmastectomy upper limb lymphedema.

Clinical Question/Level of Evidence.—Therapeutic, III.

▶ Postmastectomy lymphedema continues to be a challenging problem for many survivors of breast cancer. The authors have shown that lymph fluid can be redirected to the venous system at a site remote from the upper extremity lymphadenectomy site by creating a lymphatic "pump"; through transfer of superficial groin lymph nodes to the upper limb. This has resulted in a significant improvement in the quality of life of some patients.

J. Toto, MD

Timing of Traumatic Upper Extremity Free Flap Reconstruction: A Systematic Review and Progress Report
Harrison BL, Lakhiani C, Lee MR, et al (Univ of Texas Southwestern Med Ctr Dallas; Mayo Clinic, Rochester, MN)
Plast Reconstr Surg 132:591-596, 2013

Background.—The recommendations on the timing of microsurgical extremity reconstruction are as variable and numerous as the flaps described for such reconstruction. Original articles suggested that reconstruction should take place within 72 hours of injury. However, significant changes in perioperative and intraoperative management have occurred in this field, which may allow for more flexibility in the timing of reconstruction. This article aims to review current literature on timing of upper extremity reconstruction to provide the microsurgeon with up-to-date recommendations.

Methods.—A structured literature search including Spanish and English language articles published between January of 1995 and December of 2011 was performed using the MEDLINE and Scopus databases. The search strategy was conducted using groups of key words, and articles were subsequently reviewed for relevance. Bibliographies of selected articles were further reviewed for additional relevant publications. Rates of total flap loss, infection, hospital stay, and bony nonunion were recorded and analyzed according to emergent (<24 hours), early (<5 days), primary (6 to 21 days), or delayed (>21 days) reconstruction.

Results.—Fifteen articles met inclusion criteria. There was no significant association between timing of reconstruction and rates of flap loss, infection, or bony nonunion. Linear regression analysis displayed a significant association between length of hospital stay and timing of reconstruction.

Conclusions.—No conclusive evidence exists to suggest that emergent, early, primary, or delayed reconstruction will eliminate or decrease complications associated with posttraumatic upper extremity reconstruction. Earlier reconstruction may decrease length of hospital stay and limit associated medical costs.

▶ The results of this study suggest that it is important to consider the patient as a whole when deciding on timing for free-flap reconstruction of an upper extremity traumatic defect. Optimizing both the patient and the recipient bed is important to good outcomes and supersedes the notion of a "one size fits all" timeframe for reconstruction.

J. Toto, MD

Upper Extremity Replantation: Current Concepts

Prucz RB, Friedrich JB (Univ of Washington, Seattle)
Plast Reconstr Surg 133:333-342, 2014

Background.—Upper extremity replantation is a procedure that has revolutionized hand surgery. Since its introduction, a rapid evolution has occurred with a shifting focus from implant survival to optimization of functional outcomes and surgical efficiency. In this review, the current concepts surrounding the indications for replantation, variations in surgical technique, the factors affecting outcomes, and future directions of the specialty are analyzed.

Methods.—A literature review was performed of all recent articles pertaining to digit, hand, and upper extremity replantation surgery. Particular emphasis was placed on comparative studies and recent meta-analyses.

Results.—The indications and contraindications for replantation surgery are largely unchanged, with mechanism of injury remaining one of the most important determinants of implant survival. With advances in surgical technique, improved outcomes have been observed with avulsion injuries. Distal tip replantations appear to be more common with improved microsurgical techniques, and for these distal injuries, digital nerve and vein repair may not be necessary. Cold ischemia time for a digit amputation should not preclude transfer to a replantation facility or significantly affect the decision to perform a replantation. However, transferring physicians should thoroughly review the options with patients to prevent unnecessary transfers, which is an area where telemedicine may be useful.

Conclusion.—This review provides an update on the current concepts of the practice of replantation and the treatment and management of patients with upper extremity amputations.

▶ The authors provide a current summary of the state of the art in replantation surgery. Unfortunately, some of the accepted indications, ideal perioperative management, and risk factors are not scientifically conclusive. Much of what we do after replantations is based on surgeon experience and personal preference.

Younger age appears to be clearly a good prognostic factor, despite the lack of comparison outcomes between children and adults. The older population is more likely to have atherosclerotic vessels and have less potential for nerve regeneration; however, decisions about treating (or not replanting) should not be based on age alone. A more appropriate variable to consider would be to assess their comorbidities and risk of anesthesia (ASA score).

The negative effects of smoking on survival after digit reattachment are somewhat intuitive and should be a consideration in determining whether to attempt replantation at all. However, although the vasoconstrictive effects of smoking are well known, a careful look at the literature shows that it is unclear how smoking affects outcomes. Nevertheless, counseling patients of the negative effects of smoking both in terms of prognosis and in general is a sound practice.

The ideal use of anticoagulation after surgery also is somewhat unclear. Aspirin is the most commonly used, and, although heparin is also quite common, its benefit over aspirin is not conclusive. The benefit of other anticoagulation medications, such as dextran and persantine, are also somewhat unclear. Additional measures such as a warm room after surgery and avoidance of caffeine and chocolate appear to be without scientific merit.

The amount of ischemia time should be a factor in more proximal amputations (ie, forearm) than in the digits. A warm ischemia time of 2 to 4 hours, and cold ischemia time of 6 to 8 hours, can result in muscle death. However, there are no muscles in the digits and, therefore, they can withstand a longer delay to treatment.

M. Rizzo, MD

Ciprofloxacin-Resistant *Aeromonas* Infection Following Leech Therapy for Digit Replantation: Report of 2 Cases
van Alphen NA, Gonzalez A, McKenna MC, et al (Mayo Clinic, Rochester, MN)
J Hand Surg Am 39:499-502, 2014

Medicinal leeches are commonly used after finger replantation to treat surgically unsalvageable venous congestion. Infection from *Aeromonas hydrophila* is a recognized complication of leech therapy that can be underestimated by the medical community. Ciprofloxacin and trimethoprim-sulfamethoxazole are the most commonly recommended prophylactic antibiotics used to prevent *A. hydrophila* infections during leech therapy. Here, we report 2 cases of ciprofloxacin-resistant *Aeromonas* infections, occurring within 4 months of each other. Both cases developed after leech therapy for unsuccessful digital replantation. These infections were successfully treated with ceftriaxone. Ciprofloxacin-resistant *Aeromonas* should be recognized when determining prophylactic antibiotic protocols for replant centers when leech therapy is used for finger replantation.

▶ The authors report a rare finding of ciprofloxacin-resistant *Aeromonas* infection associated with leech therapy after digital replantation in 2 cases. The consequences of infection were significant and resulted in amputation of the replanted digits. They concluded that ceftriaxone would be a reasonable first-line treatment for leech infection prophylaxis and has a lower reported incidence of *Aeromonas* resistance.

M. Rizzo, MD

9   Tendon

Open Versus Percutaneous Release for the Treatment of Trigger Thumb
Guler F, Kose O, Ercan EC, et al (Antalya Education and Res Hosp Orthopaedics and Traumatology Clinic, Turkey; Haydarpasa Numune Education and Res Hosp Orthopaedics and Traumatology Clinic, Istanbul, Turkey)
Orthopedics 36:e1290-e1294, 2013

The purpose of this retrospective study was to compare the outcomes and complications of conventional open surgical release and percutaneous needle release in the treatment of trigger thumb. The study comprised 87 patients with trigger thumb who were treated with either open pulley (n = 52) or percutaneous (n = 32) release between 2008 and 2011. All patients were reevaluated at a mean follow-up of 22.7 ± 9.6 months (range, 9-44 months).

Main outcome measures were the rate of recurrence, pain on movement or tenderness over the pulley, infection rate, digital nerve injury, tendon bowstringing, joint stiffness or loss of thumb range of motion, and patient satisfaction. The groups were statistically similar regarding age, sex, laterality, dominant side involvement, and trigger thumb grade on initial admission. At final follow-up, no patient had recurrence, tendon bowstringing, joint stiffness, or loss of thumb range of motion. No patients in the open pulley release group and 2 (5.7%) patients in the percutaneous release group had a digital nerve injury ($P = .159$). No statistical difference was found in the infection rate between groups ($P = .354$). A total of 98.1% of patients in the open pulley release group and 97.1% of patients in the percutaneous release group were satisfied with treatment ($P = .646$). Both techniques resulted in similar therapeutic efficacy, and the rate of potential complications was also statistically similar in each group.

Although statistically insignificant, the authors believe that the 5.7% rate of iatrogenic digital nerve injury seen in the percutaneous release group is clinically significant and serious. Therefore, they advocate using open surgical release of trigger thumb.

▶ This is a retrospective review of 87 patients who underwent open or percutaneous trigger release. The study is limited by its retrospective study design but still provides important and useful information. Overall, the results of patient satisfaction and recurrence were similar in the 2 groups. However, the complication profiles were different with the open group having 2 superficial infections and the percutaneous group having 2 digital nerve injuries (1 of which resolved at 3 months). Given the 6% rate of digital nerve injuries, the authors recommend the open approach to trigger thumbs.

This study provides important information. Percutaneous trigger finger release is increasing in prominence, and there have been several recent reports including randomized controlled trials on the efficacy and safety of this technique.[1] Yet there continues to be debate on the role of percutaneous trigger release for this thumb. This article reviews the literature on the close proximity of the nerve to the A1 pulley in the thumb and provides a clear warning for the risks of the percutaneous thumb trigger release. Digital nerve injury is a serious complication, and these data will likely outweigh appeal of the ease and potential cost savings of percutaneous trigger thumb release.

C. Curtin, MD

Reference

1. Sato ES, Gomes Dos Santos JB, Belloti JC, Albertoni WM, Faloppa F. Treatment of trigger finger: randomized clinical trial comparing the methods of corticosteroid injection, percutaneous release and open surgery. *Rheumatology (Oxford).* 2012; 51:93-99.

Systematic Review and Meta-Analysis on the Work-Related Cause of de Quervain Tenosynovitis: A Critical Appraisal of Its Recognition as an Occupational Disease

Stahl S, Vida D, Meisner C, et al (Karl Univ of Tübingen, Germany; Marienhospital Stuttgart, Germany)
Plast Reconstr Surg 132:1479-1491, 2013

Background.—The authors systematically reviewed all of the etiopathologic factors discussed in the literature to verify the classification of de Quervain tenosynovitis on the list of occupational diseases.

Methods.—The authors searched Ovid MEDLINE, EMBASE, and the Cochrane Library for articles discussing the cause of de Quervain tenosynovitis. The literature was classified by the level of evidence presented, the etiopathologic hypothesis discussed, the authors' conclusion about the role of the etiopathologic hypothesis, and the first author's professional background. The quality of reporting of the observational studies was evaluated by an extended Strengthening the Reporting of Observational Studies in Epidemiology statement checklist. A meta-analysis of all controlled cohort studies was performed. The Bradford Hill criteria were used to evaluate a causal relationship between de Quervain tenosynovitis and occupational risk factors.

Results.—A total of 179 references were found, and 80 articles were included. On average, only 35 percent (median, 35 percent; range, 16 to 60 percent) of all items on the extended Strengthening the Reporting of Observational Studies in Epidemiology checklist were addressed per article. The meta-analysis to evaluate the strength of the association between de Quervain tenosynovitis and (1) repetitive, (2) forceful, or (3) ergonomically stressful manual work suggested an odds ratio of 2.89 (95 percent CI, 1.4 to

5.97; $p = 0.004$). No evidence was found to support the Bradford Hill criteria for a causal relationship between de Quervain tenosynovitis and occupational risk factors.

Conclusion.—No sufficient scientific evidence was provided to confirm a causal relationship between de Quervain tenosynovitis and occupational risk factors.

Clinical Question/Level of Evidence.—Risk, III.

▶ This work selected 5 studies to assess the causal relationship between de Quervain tenosynovitis and occupational risk factors; it concluded there is insufficient scientific evidence for a causal relationship between tenosynovitis and these risk factors. Even if a statistically significant difference is not found in a single study with a small sample size, a significant difference may be found if the sample size is increased by combining several studies into a meta-analysis.

A meta-analysis may have several biases, which can lead one to draw a wrong conclusion; these include selection bias, publication bias, location biases (eg, English-language bias, citation bias, and multiple publication biases), and so on. To avoid these biases, we usually test the symmetry of the funnel plots. Because this meta-analysis included only 5 studies, the sample size was too small to apply the test for the symmetry of the funnel plots.

I believe that there are some patients whose de Quervain tenosynovitis appears to be work related. Because of the small number of controlled studies dealing with the relationship between causality of de Quervain tenosynovitis and occupational risks, it remains difficult to find statistically significant results and, thus, draw conclusions.

R. Kakinoki, MD

Experimental Model of Trigger Finger Through A1 Pulley Constriction in a Human Cadaveric Hand: A Pilot Study
Liu KJ, Thomson JG (Yale Univ School of Medicine, New Haven, CT)
J Hand Surg 38A:1933-1940, 2013

Purpose.—Although it can be reasonably assumed that trigger digits occur as the result of a size mismatch in the pulley-tendon system, it is unclear whether locking, histological changes, and nodule formation occur owing to an intrinsically too small pulley or an enlarged digital flexor tendon. Our purposes in this feasibility study were to (1) create a model of trigger digit by pulley constriction in nonpreserved human tissue, (2) measure the change in work of flexion as the force of pulley constriction increased, (3) compare the work of flexion between nontriggering and triggering conditions, and (4) determine whether triggering can occur at the A2, A3, and A4 pulleys under similar conditions.

Methods.—Using a tensiometer, we studied the work of flexion in 4 fingers (thumb, index, middle, and ring) in a human cadaveric hand. The load of flexion was measured as the A1 to A4 pulleys were incrementally constricted in order to induce triggering. Work of flexion was analyzed for differences among trial conditions.

Results.—Triggering was successfully induced in all 4 digits through constriction of the A1 pulley. No triggering occurred in any of the A2, A3, or A4 pulley systems in this model.

Conclusions.—We successfully created a trigger model in a human cadaveric hand. Our results demonstrate that the A1 pulley can cause triggering from manual constriction of the pulley alone.

Clinical Relevance.—A trigger model such as this may allow investigations of pathophysiology, and this may result in novel treatment strategies and modalities.

▶ In this study, the authors used a cable tie to measure the tension normalized by circumference, which is proportional to the radial constriction force. They identified the occurrence of the triggering by drawing a graph depicting the load—excursion curve of the flexor digitorum profundus (FDP) tendon. Despite constriction of both the flexor digitorum superficialis (FDS) and FDP tendons, only the FDP tendon was distracted to elicit triggering in this experimental model. Both the FDP and FDS tendons should be distracted to simulate normal flexion of the fingers. The load to produce the finger flexion was unphysiologic in this model.

The authors reported that the triggering of fingers was elicited by the constriction at the A1 pulley and that constriction of the other pulleys did not elicit the triggering. The constriction at the A1 and A3 pulleys included the volar plates and flexor tendons. However, at the A2 pulley, both the flexor tendons and the proximal phalangeal bone are constricted. At the A4 pulley, the extensor tendons were also included in the constriction. Because the constriction included different tissue structures at each pulley and the unphysiologic finger flexion model, it is unclear that this cable tie constriction system can really simulate the size mismatch of the tendon and pulley system, which elicits the triggering of digits. I believe that one of the causes of the triggering is the size mismatch between the pulleys and the flexor tendons, in which intratendinous inflammation caused by the friction at each pulley makes the circumference of the flexor tendons greater than that of the pulley.

R. Kakinoki, MD

Transcription factor EGR1 directs tendon differentiation and promotes tendon repair
Guerquin M-J, Charvet B, Nourissat G, et al (UPMC, Paris, France; et al)
J Clin Invest 123:3564-3576, 2013

Tendon formation and repair rely on specific combinations of transcription factors, growth factors, and mechanical parameters that regulate the production and spatial organization of type I collagen. Here, we investigated the function of the zinc finger transcription factor EGR1 in tendon formation, healing, and repair using rodent animal models and mesenchymal stem cells (MSCs). Adult tendons of $Egr1^{-/-}$ mice displayed a deficiency in the expression of tendon genes, including *Scx*, *Col1a1*, and *Col1a2*, and were mechanically weaker compared with their WT littermates. EGR1 was recruited to the *Col1a1* and *Col2a1* promoters in postnatal mouse tendons in vivo. *Egr1* was required for the normal gene response following tendon injury in a mouse model of Achilles tendon healing. Forced *Egr1* expression programmed MSCs toward the tendon lineage and promoted the formation of in vitro—engineered tendons from MSCs. The application of EGR1-producing MSCs increased the formation of tendon-like tissues in a rat model of Achilles tendon injury. We provide evidence that the ability of EGR1 to promote tendon differentiation is partially mediated by TGF-β2. This study demonstrates EGR1 involvement in adult tendon formation, healing, and repair and identifies *Egr1* as a putative target in tendon repair strategies.

▶ The authors investigated the function of the zinc finger transcription factor EGR1 in tendon formation, healing, and repair using genetically modified mice and mesenchymal stem cells (MSCs). They provide evidence that EGR1 promotes tendon differentiation, involvement of transforming growth factor-β, and a potential treatment target (the *Egr1*). This is a very basic scientific study using mice modified to be deficient in some genes critical to tendon formation. It may serve as a basis for future basic science investigations of tendon growth and formations, but I see no immediate applications or relevance to the clinical setting.

Other basic science investigations more directly applicable to future clinical applications have been seen in recent years, including modification of tendon sutures with MSCs or growth factors, growth factor-related gene therapy, and cell therapy using a variety of stem cells. Work by our team is focused on growth factor gene therapy. More recently, we worked on nanoparticle-based controlled-release vehicles to deliver engineered miRNA plasmids to decrease adhesion formation. The growth factor-related gene therapy has allowed us to improve healing strength in chicken models. The adhesion-limiting nanoparticle-miRNA complex has decreased adhesions at the cost of significantly weakening the repair. Clearly, the journey toward the identified goals is arduous, and further animal experimentation is required.

Biological modulation of tendon healing remains an important area of future investigations. Along with advancements in biotechnology, we expect to see future developments and clinical applications. The biological tendon healing process is complex. With each investigation, we advance our understanding.

J. Bo Tang, MD

The Effect of Surface Modification on Gliding Ability of Decellularized Flexor Tendon in a Canine Model *In Vitro*

Ozasa Y, Amadio PC, Thoreson AR, et al (Mayo Clinic, Rochester, MN)
J Hand Surg 38A:1698-1704, 2013

Purpose.—To investigate the gliding ability and mechanical properties of decellularized intrasynovial tendons with and without surface modification designed to reduce gliding resistance.

Methods.—We randomly assigned 33 canine flexor digitorum profundus tendons to 1 of 3 groups: untreated fresh tendons, to serve as a control; tendons decellularized with trypsin and Triton X-100; and tendons decellularized as in group 2 with surface modification using carbodiimide-derivatized hyaluronic acid and gelatin (cd-HA-gelatin). Tendons were subjected to cyclic friction testing for 1,000 cycles with subsequent tensile stiffness testing. We qualitatively evaluated the surface roughness after 1,000 cycles using scanning electron microscopy.

Results.—The gliding resistance of the decellularized group was significantly higher than that of both the control and cd-HA-gelatin tendons (0.20, 0.09, and 0.11 N after the first cycle; and 0.41, 0.09, and 0.14 N after 1,000 cycles, respectively). Gliding resistance between the control and cd-HA-gelatin groups was not significantly different. The Young modulus was not significantly different between groups. The surfaces of the control and cd-HA—gelatin-treated tendons appeared smooth after 1,000 cycles, whereas those of the decellularized tendons appeared roughened under scanning electron microscopy observation.

Conclusions.—Decellularization with trypsin and Triton X-100 did not change tendon stiffness. However, although this treatment was effective in removing cells, it adversely altered the tendon surface in both appearance and gliding resistance. Surface modification with cd-HA-gelatin improved the tendon surface smoothness and significantly decreased the gliding resistance.

Clinical Relevance.—The combination of decellularization and surface modification may improve the function of tendon allografts when used clinically.

▶ This well-designed study found that surface modification improves smoothness (and decreases gliding resistance) after decellularization. This is an extension of a series of studies by the authors on improvement of the gliding surface of the decellularized tendon allograft. I found this modification valuable and believe it may have clinical applications. Smoother gliding always benefits a tendon graft.

Clinically, when I have to use an allograft, I use preserved tendon allografts without decellularization. We have carefully proceeded with the allograft for 8 years with postoperative follow-up of the patients for 2 to 5 years. With these lengths of follow-up in 40 patients, all showed no problems with the preserved allografts; adhesions were not increased.

Experimental findings make surface modification after decellularization attractive. However, questions remain regarding whether surface treatment is significantly beneficial when used clinically and whether untreated and treated allografts are functionally similar. I look forward to seeing how surface modification and decellularization work when translated into clinical practice.

J. Bo Tang, MD

Distal Attachment of Flexor Tendon Allograft: A Biomechanical Study of Different Reconstruction Techniques in Human Cadaver Hands
Wei Z, Thoreson AR, Amadio PC, et al (Mayo Clinic, Rochester, MN)
J Orthop Res 31:1720-1724, 2013

We compared the mechanical force of tendon-to-bone repair techniques for flexor tendon reconstruction. Thirty-six flexor digitorum profundus (FDP) tendons were divided into three groups based upon the repair technique: (1) suture/button repair using FDP tendon (Pullout button group), (2) suture bony anchor using FDP tendon (Suture anchor group), and (3) suture/button repair using FDP tendon with its bony attachment preserved (Bony attachment group). The repair failure force and stiffness were measured. The mean load to failure and stiffness in the bony attachment group were significantly higher than that in the pullout button and suture anchor groups. No significant difference was found in failure force and stiffness between the pullout button and suture anchor groups. An intrasynovial flexor tendon graft with its bony attachment has significantly improved tensile properties at the distal repair site when compared with a typical tendon-to-bone attachment with a button or suture anchor. The improvement in the tensile properties at the repair site may facilitate postoperative rehabilitation and reduce the risk of graft rupture.

▶ This mechanical study nicely shows that a tendon graft with a piece of its inserting bone provides greater tensile strength than conventional pullout suture or micro-anchor suture using cadaveric tendons. The test setup is valid, and the results are reasonable. The authors clearly indicate the potential for future applications.

Clinically, the major problem associated with pullout suture is damage to the nail; micro-anchors may present problems with bulkiness. Distal insertion of the graft using these 2 methods is strong, and, thus, the strength is not a major concern. Harvesting bone and grafting it to the insertion site would involve the bone healing process and present additional problems with nonhealing of the bone graft. I doubt that many surgeons would adopt this method clinically; it is a more complicated surgery involving a small bone fragment that presents the possibility of nonunion. In addition, added strength is not a concern, given these methods. I wonder whether I will adopt this more complex method.

This is a pure mechanical study that does not involve tendon healing. Most hand surgeons would agree that the currently available tendon-bone junction methods, such as a pullout repair, are strong but still present the problems of complications and damage to the distal phalanx. In my practice, if there is a small remnant of the distal flexor digitorum profundus tendon, I cut that stump in half and strongly suture the graft to it using multiple reinforced suture repairs. Roughness of the repair site is a secondary concern, as this part does not glide very much. Such repairs are durable enough to withstand early active motion. I use a micro-anchor for repair if no distal tendon is available. I no longer use pull-out suture because of concerns with nail damage. Some surgeons prefer to drill a transverse tunnel at the middle part of the distal phalanx and thread a strong suture through it that is then tied to the distal graft end.

J. Bo Tang, MD

Fibrin Glue Augmentation for Flexor Tendon Repair Increases Friction Compared With Epitendinous Suture
Xu NM, Brown PJ, Plate JF, et al (Virginia Tech-Wake Forest Univ School of Biomedical Engineering and Sciences, Winston-Salem, NC)
J Hand Surg Am 38:2329-2334, 2013

Purpose.—To compare the gliding resistance, repair gapping, and ultimate strength of a common suture construct with a modified construct with fibrin glue augmentation.

Methods.—Twelve human cadaveric flexor digitorum profundus tendons were transected and repaired with a 4-strand core suture. Specimens were divided into 2 groups and augmented with epitendinous suture (n = 6) or fibrin glue (n = 6). We compared gliding resistance, 2-mm gapping, and ultimate strength of the repaired tendon between groups.

Results.—The linear stiffness, force to produce a 2-mm gap, and ultimate failure were similar in both repair methods. However, the 4-strand suture repair with fibrin glue augmentation displayed significantly higher gliding resistance compared with the 4-strand suture with a running epitendinous suture.

Conclusions.—The significantly increased gliding resistance associated with fibrin glue raises questions regarding the use of this material for flexor tendon repair augmentation.

Clinical Relevance.—In a human cadaveric study, fibrin glue augmentation to zone II flexor tendon repairs significantly increased friction in the tendon sheath compared with an epitendinous suture.

▶ The authors have evaluated the intriguing idea of using fibrin glue to augment zone II flexor tendon repairs in a cadaver model compared with the traditional method of utilizing epitendinous sutures. Fibrin glue has been used in other specialties and is used clinically in hand surgery for augmentation of peripheral nerve repair.

The study was well designed and adequately powered to detect a difference. Although the results are not what the authors anticipated (increased gliding resistance), the findings are important and may help guide future research. Zone II flexor tendon repair remains a challenge, and in spite of research regarding suturing techniques and rehabilitation variables, consistently good outcomes remain elusive.

Gliding resistance is one of the more important, but often overlooked, variables in flexor tendon repair. Techniques such as excision of one slip of the flexor digitorum superficialis (FDS) have been shown to decrease gliding resistance toward preinjury levels. In addition, there are commercially available materials that are reported to improve tendon gliding, but clinical data confirming this have not been published.

My personal approach to zone II flexor tendon repairs include a four strand core suture and epitendinous repair of the flexor digitorum profundus with excision of one slip of the FDS and repair of the remaining slip with 2 or 4 strands depending on the location of the laceration and size of the tendon. I have used fibrin glue for augmentation of peripheral nerve repairs and feel it has an important role in hand surgery. The specific indications in tendon surgery are yet to be defined.

W. C. Hammert, MD

Flexor Tendon Repair Rehabilitation Protocols: A Systematic Review
Starr HM, Snoddy M, Hammond KE, et al (Emory Univ, Atlanta, GA)
J Hand Surg 38A:1712-1717.e14, 2013

Purpose.—To systematically review various flexor tendon rehabilitation protocols and to contrast those using early passive versus early active range of motion.

Methods.—We searched PubMed and Cochrane Library databases to identify articles involving flexor tendon injury, repair, and rehabilitation protocols. All zones of injury were included. Articles were classified based on the protocol used during early rehabilitation. We analyzed clinical outcomes, focusing on incidence of tendon rupture and postoperative functional range of motion. We also analyzed the chronological incidence of published tendon rupture with respect to the protocol used.

Results.—We identified 170 articles, and 34 met our criteria, with evidence ranging from level I to level IV. Early passive motion, including both Duran and Kleinert type protocols, results included 57 ruptures (4%) and 149 fingers (9%) with decreased range of motion of 1598 tendon repairs. Early active motion results included 75 ruptures (5%) and 80 fingers (6%) with decreased range of motion of 1412 tendon repairs. Early passive range of motion protocols had a statistically significantly decreased risk for tendon rupture but an increased risk for postoperative decreased range of motion compared to early active motion protocols. When analyzing published articles chronologically, we found a statistically significant trend that overall (passive and active rehabilitation) rupture rates have decreased over time.

Conclusions.—Analyzing all flexor tendon zones and literature of all levels of evidence, our data show a higher risk of complication involving decreased postoperative digit range of motion in the passive protocols and a higher risk of rupture in early active motion protocols. However, modern improvements in surgical technique, materials, and rehabilitation may now allow for early active motion rehabilitation that can provide better postoperative motion while maintaining low rupture rates.

▶ This is an extremely detailed systematic review of the reported rehabilitation protocols after primary flexor tendon repair. I also recommend its online appendix, which is a comprehensive overview of past rehabilitation methods. However, because systematic reviews are always difficult to interpret, and because there are many variations in these reports, comparisons are more likely to identify general trends than direct and final conclusions. The outcomes, disruption rates, and ranges of motion arrived at in the conclusions of this review generally echo what I see clinically.

There have been major advances toward limited-range early active motion. Surgeons in the United Kingdom, China, and Canada have moved ahead of those in the United States where many still perform early passive motion (with or without place and hold). Briefly, the limited-range early active motion starts from 4 to 5 days after primary repair surgery, with active motion of the repaired digits over one-third to two-thirds of their total range of flexion in the first 3 weeks. From week 4, the goal of a full range of active digital flexion is achieved gradually. Active digital extension is always urged in these weeks. From week 6, the digit is moved through the full range without resistance. The rationale behind this protocol is that in the initial one-third to two-thirds of the flexion arc, the resistance to tendon motion is minimal to mild. The final third of digital flexion produces great resistance, which should be avoided in the first few weeks when healing is weak. In each session, passive finger motion starts first to decrease joint stiffness before active digital motion.

I use the limited-range early active motion and began advocating it in 2007.[1] Protocols in several countries have incorporated these elements, and we see that more surgeons are updating their protocols with these exercises. We apply the limited-range active motion in clean-cut and complex cases, with the active-motion elements modified according to trauma severity and edema. I encourage readers to consult recent publications[2,3] on motion protocols while making their way through this systematic review. Most of the updated protocols have not been included in the review, and many practitioners now use protocols very different from those published in the past decades.

J. Bo Tang, MD

References

1. Tang JB. Indications, methods, postoperative motion and outcome evaluation of primary flexor tendon repairs in Zone 2. *J Hand Surg Eur Vol.* 2007;32:118-129.
2. Elliot D, Giesen T. Primary flexor tendon surgery: the search for a perfect result. *Hand Clin.* 2013;29:191-206.
3. Lalonde DH, Martin AL. Wide-awake flexor tendon repair and early tendon mobilization in zones 1 and 2. *Hand Clin.* 2013;29:207-213.

Decellularized Human Tendon–Bone Grafts for Composite Flexor Tendon Reconstruction: A Cadaveric Model of Initial Mechanical Properties

Fox PM, Farnebo S, Lindsey D, et al (Stanford Univ Med Ctr, CA; VA Palo Alto Health Care System, Stanford, CA)
J Hand Surg Am 38A:2323-2328, 2013

Purpose.—After complex hand trauma, restoration of tendon strength is challenging. Tendon insertion tears typically heal as fibrous scars after surgical reconstruction and create a weak point at the tendon–bone interface. In addition, major tendon loss may overwhelm the amount of available autograft for reconstruction. An off-the-shelf product may help address these challenges. We hypothesized that decellularized human flexor digitorum profundus and distal phalanx tendon–bone composite grafts were a feasible option for flexor tendon reconstruction after complex hand trauma. By replacing the entire injured composite segment, the need for tendon repair within the tendon sheath, reconstruction of the tendon–bone interface, and use of limited autograft could be eliminated.

Methods.—Paired human cadaver forearms were dissected to obtain the flexor digitorum profundus tendon with an attached block of distal phalanx. Tendon–bone grafts were pair-matched and divided into 2 groups: decellularized grafts (n = 12) and untreated (control) grafts (n = 11). Grafts in the decellularized group were subjected to physiochemical decellularization. Pair-matched tendon–bone grafts (decellularized and untreated) were placed back into the flexor tendon sheath and secured distally using a tie-over button and proximally by weaving the graft into the flexor digitorum superficialis tendon in the distal forearm. The ultimate load, location of failure, and excursion were determined.

Results.—Decellularized tendon–bone composite grafts demonstrated no significant difference in ultimate failure load or stiffness compared with untreated grafts. Both groups eventually failed in varied locations along the repair. The most common site of failure in both groups was the tie-over button. The decellularized group failed at the tendon–bone insertion in 3 specimens (25%) compared with none in the untreated group. Both groups demonstrated an average tendon excursion of approximately 82 mm before failure.

Conclusions.—Decellularization of human flexor tendon–distal phalanx tendon–bone constructs did not compromise initial strength despite chemical and mechanical decellularization in a cadaveric model. At the time of repair, decellularized flexor tendon–bone grafts can exceed the strength and excursion needed for hand therapy immediately after reconstruction.

Clinical Relevance.—These tendon–bone grafts may become an option for complex hand reconstruction at or near tendon–bone insertions and throughout the tendon sheath. Further work is required to assess the role of reseeding in an *in vivo* model.

▶ The use of allogeneic intrasynovial tendon grafts for flexor tendon reconstruction is an enticing idea. Such ready-made grafts would obviate the need to harvest tendons from the patient, removing a potential source of added morbidity. It would also enable the use of intrasynovial grafts for reconstruction of flexor tendons. The use of such intrasynovial tendon grafts is still not common in clinical practice, despite a body of research evidence that intrasynovial tendons are superior to extrasynovial ones for flexor tendon grafting. This resistance is largely because of the ease of harvest and perceived reduced morbidity of harvesting extrasynovial grafts like the palmaris longus.

The senior author's group has been working to decellularize tendons for use as scaffolds for tendon tissue engineering. Their work has found that the decellularization process can successfully reduce the immunogenicity of the tissue while maintaining its biomechanical properties.

The work covered in this report extends their previous work to explore the use of an allogeneic composite bone-tendon graft for use in tendon reconstruction. Their findings suggest that it is biomechanically and surgically feasible to apply this concept to clinical practice. This contribution is important, as the bone-tendon interface, or enthesis, heals with inferior properties after injury and is a potential site for graft failure or reinjury. Using a bone-tendon composite graft would bypass the region, allowing bone-bone healing, which is stronger and more reliable.

This work does not investigate the effect of biological processes on the graft. The group intends to perform further experiments on a large animal model, which will help provide more information about the effect of healing processes in vivo on their construct and its integration. This is an important and necessary next step to see if this concept will be successful in clinical practice.

A. K. S. Chong, MD

Rehabilitation Following Extensor Tendon Repair
Canham CD, Hammert WC (Univ of Rochester Med Ctr, NY)
J Hand Surg 38A:1615-1617, 2013

Background.—Extensor tendon lacerations are repaired and then often splinted for a month before motion exercises are begun. Several approaches are available for rehabilitating the patient after repair of extensor tendon lacerations, and the evidence was weighed to determine the best choice for a specific patient.

> *Case Report.*—Man, 29, suffered a laceration of the dorsum of the middle finger metacarpal of the right hand and was unable to extend his middle finger. No skeletal injury or foreign body was detected radiographically, so the wound was irrigated and sutured, then tendon repair using a braided core suture was done 3 days later. The rehabilitation protocol chosen was early active motion.

Assessment of Evidence.—Static splints have been used with some good but several poor outcomes for extensor tendon repairs in zones 5 to 7.

Among the exercise protocols for dynamic or active motion after extensor tendon repair are dynamic extension splinting (DES), controlled early active motion, and relative motion splinting. Usually all splinting is discontinued after 6 to 8 weeks, with activity allowed with few restrictions. DES has achieved good to excellent extension and flexion and is associated with significantly greater grip strength development compared to static methods. Active motion with a volar blocking splint has also produced excellent or good results in a majority of patients. Relative motion splinting offers another good option, with the average time to return to work of 18 days. However, no comparative studies have been done between relative motion splinting and DES or early active motion with volar blocking splints.

Complicating the results of the various studies is the lack of standards for assessing outcomes after extension tendon repair. Rather than patient-based outcome measures, clinician-based assessments are generally used, which are often biased and inaccurate. In addition, the prognosis for recovery is associated with the zone of injury, with more distal lacerations evidencing poorer outcomes. It is difficult to conduct studies based on zone of injury because there are too few cases to collect a sample large enough to make meaningful conclusions.

Conclusions.—The best results after extensor tendon laceration repair appear to be associated with early active motion, whether through DES or a relative motion splint. Heavy work or manual labor should be avoided for 6 weeks, which is when the splint is discontinued. When more than three tendons are involved, use of a volar blocking splint is advised. For pediatric patients or adults whose behavior is unreliable, static splinting may minimize the risk of tendon rupture after repair, then a therapy program can be started after 3 weeks. DES may require a more expensive, more complex splint and more extensive hand therapist involvement compared to the other options, but the trade-off in terms of benefit has yet to be studied.

▶ This article confirms the need to develop treatment guidelines that are evidence based and for the consistent use of patient-based outcome measures to allow us to critically assess the efficacy of current rehabilitative protocols. This is a valuable summary of success percentages with typical extensor tendon protocols that are currently being followed. The authors quote "good or excellent" results; however, from a therapist's perspective, a definition of these terms would have been appreciated to better understand the success of a given protocol.

In our clinic, which is a hospital outpatient-based setting, we generally fabricate a static splint and use an early active motion protocol for tendon repairs. In the long term, we have experienced fairly good success with regard to range of motion (ROM), tendon excursion, avoidance of extensor lag, and ultimately functional restoration of the injured extremity.

In some situations, one must critically assess the feasibility of fabricating dynamic extension splints (DES), which require skill to ensure proper alignment, tension, pull, and a compliant patient, when less expensive, and possibly a more effective splint choice with proven successful outcomes can be considered instead.

Although I have fabricated relative motion splints for other kinds of injuries, I have not utilized it for extensor tendon repairs. I will certainly consider this splint approach among my repertoire of extensor tendon protocols. It is simple to fabricate, the patient is allowed to begin ROM immediately within the confines of the splint, and the patient can participate in light activities. Certainly, with the more complicated injuries, a DES or static splint is likely still the gold standard for extensor tendon repairs.

The authors suggest that further research with the inclusion of a multicenter database would be of great benefit to assist clinicians with choosing appropriate treatment protocols, compare data, anticipate prognosis, and implement appropriate exercise regimes for specific zones of injury.

In this age of health care reform, we must all be cognizant of cost and value of the services we provide to our patients and ensure that the treatment we provide is skilled and based on solid research and efficacy.

L. Brooke, OTR, CHT

Hand Surface Landmarks and Measurements in the Treatment of Trigger Thumb

Patel RM, Chilelli BJ, Ivy AD, et al (Northwestern Univ Feinberg School of Medicine, Chicago, IL)
J Hand Surg 38A:1166-1171, 2013

Purpose.—To determine hand surface landmarks and measurements that may be useful in localizing the A1 pulley and digital neurovascular structures in the treatment of trigger thumb.

Methods.—We highlighted 4 surface landmarks in 20 adult cadaveric hands: the radial border of the index finger, the ulnar border of the thumb, the thumb interphalangeal joint flexion creases, and the thumb metacarpophalangeal joint creases. We injected the radial arteries with red latex and dissected the thumbs.

Results.—The proximal margin of the A1 pulley was located an average of 0.3 mm proximal (range, 3.2 mm proximal to 2.3 mm distal) to the most proximal metacarpophalangeal joint flexion crease. The ratio of measurements from the thumb tip to the midpoint of the interphalangeal joint flexion creases and from this point to the proximal margin of the A1 pulley averaged 1.1:1. The radial digital nerve crossed obliquely over the flexor pollicis longus tendon and approached the proximal margin of the A1 pulley at a mean distance of 2.7 mm (range, 0—12.9 mm). The ulnar digital nerve was located deep to intersecting lines drawn along the radial border of the index finger and the ulnar border of the thumb and coursed parallel to the A1 pulley at a mean distance of 5.4 mm (range, 0—11.1 mm). At the level of the A1 pulley, the digital arteries were positioned dorsal to the digital nerves, and both nerves were located 1.0 to 4.2 mm from the skin surface.

Conclusions.—The findings from our study clarify hand surface landmarks in localizing the thumb A1 pulley and digital neurovascular structures.

Clinical Relevance.—Awareness of topographical landmarks in localizing the A1 pulley and digital neurovascular structures and the relationships between the digital neurovascular structures and the A1 pulley may improve the safety and efficacy of trigger thumb treatment.

▶ The authors present a study of cadaver dissection of hand surface landmarks and measurement of the A1 pulley of thumbs. They highlighted 4 surface landmarks in 20 adult cadaveric hands: the radial border of the index finger, the ulnar border of the thumb, the thumb interphalangeal joint flexion creases, and the thumb metacarpophalangeal joint creases. They measured the location and margin of the A1 pulley and its distance to vital digital neurovascular structures that might be injured during percutaneous needle release. The results showed compatible findings to those of previous studies and provided helpful information to circumvent iatrogenic injuries with injection and percutaneous release. However, the authors point out the limitation of this study affecting and leading to variable results, including a small number of specimens from different body builds and genders. In addition, the methods of incision and dissection may alter the native structures. In my clinical practice, I perform injection with the needle entrance point over the tendon at the proximal third of proximal phalanx aiming toward the A1 pulley to avoid iatrogenic injury. I prefer open release for patients with recalcitrant trigger finger. I have found the injected local anesthetic will distend the soft tissue over the A1 pulley, which may create more of a safe zone to avoid iatrogenic injuries to neurovascular structures.

Y.-C. Huang, MD

Effectiveness of cast immobilization in comparison to the gold-standard self-removal orthotic intervention for closed mallet fingers: A randomized clinical trial

Tocco S, Boccolari P, Landi A, et al (Studio Terapico Kaiser, Via Trento, Parma, Italy; Policlinico of Modena, Italy; et al)
J Hand Ther 26:191-201, 2013

Study Design.—Randomized clinical trial.

Introduction.—Although orthotic immobilization has become the preferable treatment choice for closed mallet injuries, it is unclear whether orthosis self-removal has an impact on the final outcome.

Purpose.—To evaluate the treatment efficacy of cast immobilization of closed mallet fingers using Quickcast® (QC) compared to a removable, lever-type thermoplastic orthosis (LTTP).

Methods.—57 subjects were randomized in 2 groups. DIPj extensor lag and the Gaberman success scale were used as primary outcomes.

Results.—LTTP subjects resulted in greater extensor lag than QC subjects ($x = 5°$; $p = 0.05$) at 12 weeks from baseline, and high edema and older age negatively affected DIPj extensor lag. No other differences were found between groups.

Conclusion.—Cast immobilization seems to be slightly more effective than the traditional approach probably for its greater capacity to reduce edema.

Level of Evidence.—1B.

▶ This study suggests that using circumferential Quickcast tape, which provides strict immobilization, may yield potentially better results than the traditional low-temperature lever-type thermoplastic orthosis (LTPP) frequently used. The authors performed a detailed and comprehensive study with focused examination of the efficacy of full-time immobilization for type I mallet finger injuries with a comparison of the 2 splint materials mentioned above. The Quickcast group initially does not remove the splint for hygiene until the first follow-up with the clinician at week 3 or 4, whereas the LTPP group is instructed to remove the orthosis on a daily basis for skin care.

Most hand therapists would concur that fabricating an effective mallet orthosis can be a challenge for even the most experienced and skilled therapist. Shortcomings of mallet splints often include difficulty with optimizing rigid, unyielding support to the distal phalanx with the distal interphalangeal (DIP) in slight hyperextension; allow for proximal interphalangeal motion, offer ventilation for adequate skin condition, and ultimately stay on! Certainly patient compliance must be given extreme consideration given that many of our patients are competitive athletes or lead very active lifestyles and participate in several intense sport and leisure activities.

This study suggests that use of the Quickcast tape might indeed offer preferable results versus the traditional thermoplastic splints that are more commonly used. The authors theorize that possibly the use of a circumferential Quickcast tape offers compression, thereby limiting edema and ultimately leading to improved DIP extension. As a clinician, it is often counterintuitive to provide a circumferential splint when edema fluctuations and skin integrity are of concern. Clearly, this article suggests that skin maceration was not a significant issue in either group and that extension lag of the DIP in the end was less in the Quickcast group. Of interest as well, the article suggests that slight DIP motion does not necessarily equate with failure.

The authors state that DIP flexion was limited in both groups after the immobilization period; however, there were no differences between the 2 groups. DIP flexion continued to improve going forward. They also state there were no differences between grip and tip to tip pinch strength between the 2 groups.

Further collection of demographic information such as age and evaluation of edema would be valuable information to facilitate optimal results for our mallet finger population. Consideration for the use of Quickcast tape is certainly foremost in my bag of tricks to consider when splinting the mallet finger.

L. Brooke, OTR/L, CHT

The Epidemiology of Reoperation After Flexor Pulley Reconstruction
Dy CJ, Lyman S, Schreiber JJ, et al (Hosp for Special Surgery, NY)
J Hand Surg 38A:1705-1711, 2013

Purpose.—We used a statewide database to determine the incidence of pulley reconstruction and to evaluate the influence of demographics on reoperation. We hypothesized that age, insurance status, and concomitant nerve or tendon procedure would influence the likelihood of reoperation.

Methods.—We used the Statewide Planning and Research Cooperative System ambulatory surgery database from New York, which represents all outpatient surgery in the state. Patients who had flexor pulley reconstruction from 1998 to 2009 were identified using Current Procedural Terminology 4 codes. Subsequent surgery records for these patients were identified through 2010, allowing at least 1 year follow-up. Concomitant nerve procedure and flexor tendon repair/reconstruction were identified. The type and timing of subsequent procedures, including tenolysis and repeat pulley reconstruction, were recorded. Univariate statistics were calculated to compare age, sex, and payer type between patients with and without reoperation. A multivariable, logistic regression model was used to evaluate the association of the demographics with the chances of having reoperation.

Results.—There were 623 patients who had flexor pulley reconstruction from 1998 to 2009. The incidence of pulley reconstruction was 0.27 per 100,000 persons, with an annual frequency of 52 procedures. There were 39 (6%) reoperations. There was no difference in age, concomitant nerve or tendon repair, or workers' compensation between patients with and without reoperation. Regression modeling showed a higher likelihood among men of having reoperation.

Conclusions.—Flexor pulley reconstructions are rare. One-quarter of surgeons performed only one flexor pulley reconstruction over a 12-year period. The 6% reoperation rate is similar to our previous findings for flexor tendon repair using similar methodology. Our report provides information that may be useful in counseling patients.

▶ Because flexor pulley reconstruction is a rarely performed procedure, data on incidence, complications, and rate of reoperation are sparse. This study was undertaken to elucidate these facts by investigating 623 patients from the Statewide Planning and Research Cooperative System ambulatory surgery database from New York.

The incidence of pulley reconstruction was 0.27 per 100 000 persons. The reoperation rate was 6%, most of which were tenolyses. One-quarter of surgeons performed the operation once during the 12-year observation period. Interestingly, the reoperation rate was not higher in those single-time surgeons compared with those who performed multiple pulley reconstructions during the same period. The mean time to pulley reconstruction (232 days) was longer than the time to flexor tendon repair (140 days). The most common cause for flexor pulley reconstruction and the predilection site was rock climbing and the A2 pulley of the middle finger, respectively. Using a multivariable logistic regression model, the authors could not find any correlation between the chance of reoperation and the demographic factors (age, sex, concomitant nerve repair, and flexor tendon repair).

Despite the inherent limitations of the use of an administrative database, this study is helpful for a better understanding of flexor pulley reconstructions.

M. Choi, MD

The Thompson Procedure for Chronic Mallet Finger Deformity

Kanaya K, Wada T, Yamashita T (Sapporo Med Univ School of Medicine, Hokkaido, Japan)
J Hand Surg 38A:1295-1300, 2013

Purpose.—To evaluate the outcomes of the Thompson procedure for chronic mallet finger deformity and review the utility of this procedure.

Methods.—Seven cases of chronic mallet finger with a swan neck deformity were treated by the Thompson procedure. Ranges of motion for the distal interphalangeal (DIP) and proximal interphalangeal (PIP) joints were measured, and complications were investigated at the final examination. Patients were evaluated using the criteria reported by Abouna and Brown.

Results.—Four patients were men, and 3 were women. The average age at the time of surgery was 44 years (range, 25 to 71 y). The middle finger was affected in 4 cases, and the index, ring, and small finger were involved in 1 case each. The average extensor lag on the DIP joint was 42° (range, 35° to 50°). All cases were treated with the Thompson procedure. The swan neck deformity was corrected in all cases. The average motion at the final examination was −4° (range, −30° to 0°) in extension and 91° (range, 85° to 110°) in flexion for the PIP joint and −5° (range, −10° to 0 °) in extension and 63° (range, 45° to 85°) in flexion for the DIP joint. A buttonhole deformity and a dimple at the proximal tied end of the graft were seen in 1 case. Assessment by the criteria of Abouna and Brown revealed that 6 of 7 patients were categorized as cured and one as improved. No patient was categorized as unchanged.

Conclusions.—The procedure provides a predictable method for correcting loss of DIP joint extension with or without PIP joint hyperextension. We believe that the Thompson procedure is an effective technique for the salvage, following failed treatment, of a closed mallet injury with an associated swan neck deformity.

▶ The authors describe their results of chronic mallet finger deformity with concomitant proximal interphalangeal (PIP) swan-neck deformity with the use of the Thompson procedure in a series of 7 patients. Originally described in 1978, the Thompson procedure consists of reconstruction of the spiral oblique retinacular ligament (SORL) with the palmaris longus tendon without repair of the terminal tendon. In effect, distal interphalangeal (DIP) and PIP joint extension are linked by virtue of SORL reconstruction, which can also simultaneously correct DIP extensor lag with associated PIP hyperextension. Another benefit of this procedure is its utility in the treatment of patients who have already failed surgical management, such as previous direct suture repair of the terminal tendon.

The authors correctly point out that there are additional treatment options for chronic mallet, which include prolonged extension splinting, tenodermodesis and Fowler central slip tenotomy. Of course, benign neglect should be mentioned because in many individuals, extensor lag at the DIP joint with a mild swan-neck deformity results in minimal functional detriment. The patients in this case series were evaluated by the criteria of Abouna and Brown, who described a 3-tiered scoring system. Six of 7 patients in this series were cured, and 1 patient was graded as improved despite experiencing a "buttonhole deformity" at the PIP joint.

Although mechanically sound, this procedure represents the need for precision graft tensioning and adjustment. With the potential morbidity of graft harvest and surgical incisions surround the middle and proximal phalanx, I consider Fowler's central slip tenotomy a preferred technique for chronic mallet finger with concomitant swan-neck deformity. The simplicity of Fowler's sectioning of the central slip at the middle phalanx base cannot rival the elegant SORL reconstruction described by Thomson and re-created by the authors of this interesting article. However, it is just that reproducible simplicity that lends itself to use in the rare circumstance of chronic mallet deformity.

S. M. Jacoby, MD

Flexor Pollicis Longus Dysfunction After Volar Plate Fixation of Distal Radius Fractures

Chilelli BJ, Patel RM, Kalainov DM, et al (Northwestern Univ Feinberg School of Medicine, Chicago, IL)
J Hand Surg 38A:1691-1697, 2013

Purpose.—To evaluate the natural history and etiology of decreased thumb interphalangeal (IP) joint flexion after volar plate fixation of distal radius fractures.

Methods.—A total of 46 patients who underwent volar plating of 48 distal radius fractures by a single surgeon were retrospectively studied. Of those patients, 24 (24 wrists) exhibited loss of thumb IP joint flexion (group 1) and 22 (24 wrists) retained thumb IP joint flexion (group 2) with attempted thumb opposition to the small finger after surgery. All patients were seen at regular intervals until IP joint flexion returned and fracture healing was confirmed radiographically. Patient demographics, fracture patterns, surgical variables, and final radiographs were compared between groups. Twenty patients in group 1 were seen after a mean of 6.5 months (range, 5—12 mo) for specific outcome measurements. Eight cadaveric specimens were used to replicate the flexor carpi radialis approach to the distal radius and evaluate flexor pollicis longus tendon excursion.

Results.—There were no significant differences in fracture pattern, patient age or sex, injured extremity dominance, time to surgery, incision length, plate composition, plate length, tourniquet time, or final wrist radiographs between groups. In group 1, active thumb IP joint flexion returned on average 52 days (range, 19–143 d) postoperatively. At final evaluation in this group, mean IP joint flexion was 11° less than the contralateral thumb IP joint; however, patient-determined outcomes were favorable in most cases. In the cadaveric specimens, excursion of the flexor pollicis longus tendon decreased with sequential soft tissue dissection and retraction.

Conclusions.—Loss of thumb IP joint flexion after volar plating of distal radius fractures was common, and motion returned to near normal in most cases within 2 months. Partial stripping of the flexor pollicis longus muscle from investing fascia and bone and retraction of soft tissues are likely etiological factors.

▶ This study is somewhat of a mixed bag. It is composed of a prospective study examining temporary decreased thumb interphalangeal (IP) flexion after distal radius open reduction and internal fixation (ORIF) as well as a cadaver study as to possible etiologies. I agree with the message that patients often have an initial decrease in active thumb metacarpophalangeal (MP) flexion (much like they have decrease in forearm supination and wrist extension relative to pronation and flexion initially). I have always simply attributed this to surgical dissection, retraction, and the proximity of the flexor pollicis longus (FPL) to the hardware.

Methodologically speaking, the article has some limitations. The largest to me is considering IP flexion as normal if the patient is able to "oppose to the small finger to the middle or proximal half of the proximal phalanx." This really speaks to carpometacarpal (CMC), MP and IP motion. Patients with excellent CMC and MP motion can often achieve opposition to this level with only 15 to 20 degrees of IP flexion. Also in many patients, "normal" can be opposition to the distal palmar crease in line with the small finger (well beyond the definition of "normal" used here). And the extent of the initial soft tissue injury (which could serve as a confounder) isn't assessed in patients.

Two patients with decreased motion were tested with electromyography and dynamic ultrasonography with normal results.

In the 8-limb cadaver portion of the study, progressive FPL release from the radius (as is required for plate application) up to 6 cm resulted in progressive decreased FPL excursion (up to a total of 4 mm additional loss). This dissection resulted in loss of roughly one-third of the bony footprint of the FPL from the radius.

In the end, this study offers an explanation for the mild temporary decrease in thumb IP flexion experienced after distal radius ORIF via a volar approach. These findings do not change my practice, however, as I will continue to carry out this surgery in the same manner and rehabilitate patients in the same manner.

G. Gaston, MD

Outcomes of Digital Zone IV and V and Thumb Zone TI to TIV Extensor Tendon Repairs Using a Running Interlocking Horizontal Mattress Technique

Altobelli GG, Conneely S, Haufler C, et al (Newton-Wellesley Hosp/Tufts Univ School of Medicine, Boston, MA; Newton-Wellesley Hosp, MA)
J Hand Surg 38A:1079-1083, 2013

Purpose.—Biomechanical evidence has demonstrated that the running interlocking horizontal mattress (RIHM) repair for extensor tendon lacerations is significantly stronger, with higher ultimate load to failure and less tendon shortening compared with other techniques. We investigated the efficacy and safety of primary extensor tendon repair using the RIHM repair technique in the fingers followed by the immediate controlled active motion protocol, and in the thumb followed by a dynamic extension protocol.

Methods.—We conducted a retrospective review of all patients undergoing extensor tendon repair from August 2009 to April 2012 by single surgeon in an academic hand surgery practice. The inclusion criteria were simple extensor tendon lacerations in digital zones IV and V and thumb zones TI to TIV and primary repair performed using the RIHM technique. We included 8 consecutive patients with 9 tendon lacerations (3 in the thumb). One patient underwent a concomitant dorsal hand rotation flap for soft tissue coverage. We used a 3−0 nonabsorbable braided suture to perform a running simple suture in 1 direction to obtain a tension-free tenorrhaphy, followed by an RIHM corset-type suture using the same continuous strand in the opposite direction. Average time to surgery was 10 days (range, 3−33 d). Mean follow-up was 15 weeks (range, 10−26 wk). We applied the immediate controlled active motion protocol to all injuries except those in the thumb, where we used a dynamic extension protocol instead.

Results.—Using the criteria of Miller, all 9 tendon repairs achieved excellent or good results. There were no tendon ruptures or extensor lags. No patients required secondary surgery for tenolysis or joint release. No wound complications occurred.

Conclusions.—The RIHM technique for primary extensor tendon repairs in zone IV and V and T1 to TIV is safe, allows for immediate controlled active motion in the fingers and an immediate dynamic extension protocol in the thumb, and achieves good to excellent functional outcomes. These clinical outcomes support prior biomechanical data.

Type of Study/Level of Evidence.—Therapeutic IV.

▶ The authors report on 9 extensor tendon laceration repairs performed by the senior author using a single technique. The running interlocking horizontal mattress suture configuration was performed with a 3-0 braided polyester suture. This method was first described by Lee et al in 2010. In this study, the included injuries were all simple, sharp, and primarily repaired. The zones of injury and postoperative therapy protocols differed between patients. The injuries were 1 each of zones T2, T3, T4, and IV with 5 zone V injuries. The zone IV and V injuries in the fingers were treated with an immediate controlled active motion protocol with digital yoke splinting to limit flexion. The thumb tendon repairs were treated with 4 weeks of extension splinting.

The results show excellent results in 7 repairs and 2 good results with 5° of flexion loss. The good results were in an index finger and middle finger, apparently zone IV and V, respectively, although the authors do not specify the zone.

These results show very good outcomes with a new technique for extensor tendon repairs performed by a surgeon other than the one who developed it. The repair is simple, strong, and effective. The strengths of this study are that it comprised 1 surgeon and 1 technique. Its weaknesses are that it is a retrospective review without a control group, and there is no blinding as to technique. The postoperative protocol differed by digit, and all of the injuries were on the flat extensor hood. Nevertheless, this study adds to the data supporting the use of this new technique and is clinically useful in that regard.

D. J. Mastella, MD

Percutaneous Release, Open Surgery, or Corticosteroid Injection, Which Is the Best Treatment Method for Trigger Digits?
Wang J, Zhao J-G, Liang C-C (Tianjin Hosp, China)
Clin Orthop Relat Res 471:1879-1886, 2013

Background.—Percutaneous A1 pulley release surgery for trigger digit (finger or thumb) has gained popularity in recent decades. Although many studies have reported the failure rate and complications of percutaneous release for trigger digit, the best treatment for trigger digit remains unclear.

Questions/Purposes.—Our aim was to identify the relative risk of treatment failure, level of satisfaction, and frequency of complications, comparing percutaneous release with open surgery or corticosteroid injections for adult patients with trigger digits.

Methods.—We searched PubMed, Embase, and the Cochrane Library for randomized controlled trials (RCTs), comparing percutaneous release with open surgery or corticosteroid injections. Seven RCTs involving 676 patients were identified. Methodologic quality was assessed by the Detsky quality scale. After data extraction, we compared results using a fixed meta-analysis model.

Results.—There were no differences in the failure rate (risk ratio [RR] = 0.93; 95% CI, 0.14–6.25) and complication frequency (RR = 0.83; 95% CI, 0.15–4.72) between patients undergoing percutaneous release and open surgery. Patients treated with percutaneous release had fewer failures (RR = 0.07; 95% CI, 0.02–0.21) and a greater level of satisfaction (RR = 2.01; 95% CI, 1.62–2.48) compared with the patients treated with corticosteroid injections. We found no difference in complication frequency between percutaneous release and corticosteroid injection (RR = 3.19; 95% CI, 0.51–19.91).

TABLE 2.—Methodologic Quality of Included Studies

Study	Adequate Randomization	Allocation Concealment	Assessor Blinding	Similar Baseline	Rate of Drop-out	Detsky Scores[†]
Gilberts et al. [14]	Yes	Yes	No	Yes	Unclear	16
Maneerit et al. [19]	Unclear	Unclear	Unclear	Yes	1.7%	14
Dierks et al. [12]	Partial*	Unclear	Unclear	Unclear	Unclear	14
Chao et al. [9]	Yes	Yes	Unclear	Yes	4.1%	18
Bamroongshawgasame [2]	Unclear	Unclear	Unclear	Yes	Unclear	13
Zyluk and Jagielski [34]	Yes	Yes	Yes	Yes	17%	15
Sato et al. [28]	Yes	Yes	Unclear	Yes	Unclear	14

Editor's Note: Please refer to original journal article for full references.

*Partial randomization (ie, patients are allocated according to known characteristics such as date of birth, day of presentation, or hospital chart number).

[†]Detsky quality score is used to assess the methodologic quality of randomized controlled trials (maximum, 21 scores).

Conclusions.—The frequencies of treatment failure and complications were no different between percutaneous release surgery and open surgery for trigger digit in adults. Patients treated with percutaneous releases were less likely to have treatment failure than patients treated with corticosteroid injections (Table 2).

▶ This is a systematic review with meta-analysis examining the potential benefits of steroid injections vs percutaneous release vs open release of trigger digits. The authors admit they are unable to make definitive conclusions about treatment preferences, as the data are predictably scant for randomized, controlled trials (RCT). The article is meaningful, however, in that it has all the qualities of a good systematic review and highlights topics that might make a better study in the future. Their findings represent a typical slice of insufficient data that can be culled from the historical literature in orthopedics and surgical sciences. From an identification pool of 123 studies, only 7 had sufficient data to address their research question. Therefore, lingering questions regarding the difference between trigger thumb vs trigger finger, type of steroid used, addition of anesthetic to the injection, type of percutaneous technique, and type of anesthesia for surgery remain unanswered.

The authors use the Detsky score to assess the quality of the reviewed articles.[1] This score provides a ranking of useful criteria when assessing RCTs, with a maximum score of 21. The average score for the 7 articles is 14.9, which indicates only fair to moderate scientific robustness. The Detsky methodology suggests a benchmark for all of us pursuing clinical research trials. At the very least, applying such rigors will likely help us design better studies for the next generation to appraise.

A. Ladd, MD

Reference

1. Detsky AS, Naylor CD, O'Rourke K, McGeer AJ, L'Abbé KA. Incorporating variations in the quality of individual randomized trials into meta-analysis. *J Clin Epidemiol*. 1992;45:255-265.

Open Versus Percutaneous Release for the Treatment of Trigger Thumb

Guler F, Kose O, Ercan EC, et al (Antalya Education and Res Hosp Orthopaedics and Traumatology Clinic, Turkey; et al)
Orthopedics 36:e1290-e1294, 2013

The purpose of this retrospective study was to compare the outcomes and complications of conventional open surgical release and percutaneous needle release in the treatment of trigger thumb. The study comprised 87 patients with trigger thumb who were treated with either open pulley (n = 52) or percutaneous (n = 32) release between 2008 and 2011. All patients were reevaluated at a mean follow-up of 22.7 ± 9.6 months (range, 9–44 months).

Main outcome measures were the rate of recurrence, pain on movement or tenderness over the pulley, infection rate, digital nerve injury, tendon bowstringing, joint stiffness or loss of thumb range of motion, and patient satisfaction. The groups were statistically similar regarding age, sex, laterality, dominant side involvement, and trigger thumb grade on initial admission. At final follow-up, no patient had recurrence, tendon bowstringing, joint stiffness, or loss of thumb range of motion. No patients in the open pulley release group and 2 (5.7%) patients in the percutaneous release group had a digital nerve injury ($P = .159$). No statistical difference was found in the infection rate between groups ($P = .354$). A total of 98.1% of patients in the open pulley release group and 97.1% of patients in the percutaneous release group were satisfied with treatment ($P = .646$). Both techniques resulted in similar therapeutic efficacy, and the rate of potential complications was also statistically similar in each group.

Although statistically insignificant, the authors believe that the 5.7% rate of iatrogenic digital nerve injury seen in the percutaneous release group is clinically significant and serious. Therefore, they advocate using open surgical release of trigger thumb.

▶ This retrospective analysis reviewed outcomes of 2 treatments for trigger thumbs: (1) percutaneous (n = 32) versus (2) open release. The authors found that both treatments were equally effective. In addition, 2 superficial infections were noted in the open group with none in the percutaneous group (statistically insignificant). There were no sequelae associated with the superficial infections. Two patients in the percutaneous group sustained a digital nerve injury compared with none in the open group. However, this difference was not statistically significant.

I think this study brings to light the realities associated with blind procedures. Although there was no significant difference, the 2 nerve injuries associated with the percutaneous technique are worrisome. Because the radial digital nerve crosses from ulnar side of the thumb base and because it runs close to the pulley, it is inherently at risk in a procedure such as percutaneous A-1 pulley release. I share the authors conclusions that despite the lack of statistical significance, the risk of nerve injury in percutaneous trigger thumb release is a real and legitimate concern.

M. Rizzo, MD

Corticosteroid Injection With or Without Thumb Spica Cast for de Quervain Tenosynovitis
Mardani-Kivi M, Karimi Mobarakeh M, Bahrami F, et al (Guilan Univ of Med Sciences, Rash; Kerman Univ of Med Sciences, Iran)
J Hand Surg 39:37-41, 2014

Purpose.—To compare the corticosteroid injection (CSI) with or without thumb spica cast (TSC) for de Quervain tendinitis.

Methods.—In this prospective trial, 67 eligible patients with de Quervain tenosynovitis were randomly assigned into CSI + TSC (33 cases) and CSI (34 cases) groups. All patients received 40 mg of methylprednisolone acetate with 1 cc lidocaine 2% in the first dorsal compartment at the area of maximal point tenderness. The primary outcome was the treatment success rate, and the secondary outcome was the scale and quality of the treatment method using Quick Disabilities of Arm, Shoulder and Hand and visual analog scale scores.

Results.—The groups had no differences in mean age, sex, and occupation. The visual analog scale and Quick Disabilities of the Arm, Shoulder and Hand scores were similar in both groups before the treatment. The treatment success rate was 93% in the CSI + TSC group and 69% in the CSI group. Although both methods improved the patients' conditions significantly in terms of relieving pain and functional ability, CSI + TSC had a significantly higher treatment success rate.

Conclusions.—The combined technique of corticosteroid injection and thumb spica casting was better than injection alone in the treatment of de Quervain tenosynovitis in terms of treatment success and functional outcomes.

Type of Study/Level of Evidence.—Therapeutic II.

▶ The authors aim to compare 2 groups of patients treated for DeQuervain's tenosynovitis prospectively: one with corticosteroid injection alone and the other with injection plus splinting. In addition to evaluating the clinical outcomes, patient subjective scores (QuickDASH and visual analog scores) were assessed. There was a significant difference in outcomes in patients treated with both splinting and injection versus those treated with injection alone.

Despite the possibility of a placebo effect from patients treated with both interventions, the study methods were excellent and the results are conclusive. In addition, even though it is more costly to consider splinting in addition to injection, it is reassuring that its use can be justified and result in superior and more predictable outcomes.

M. Rizzo, MD

Corticosteroid Injection With or Without Thumb Spica Cast for de Quervain Tenosynovitis

Mardani-Kivi M, Karimi Mobarakeh M, Bahrami F, et al (Guilan Univ of Med Sciences, Rash; Kerman Univ of Med Sciences, Iran)
J Hand Surg Am 39:37-41, 2014

Purpose.—To compare the corticosteroid injection (CSI) with or without thumb spica cast (TSC) for de Quervain tendinitis.

Methods.—In this prospective trial, 67 eligible patients with de Quervain tenosynovitis were randomly assigned into CSI + TSC (33 cases) and CSI (34 cases) groups. All patients received 40 mg of methylprednisolone acetate with 1 cc lidocaine 2% in the first dorsal compartment at the area of maximal point tenderness. The primary outcome was the treatment success rate, and the secondary outcome was the scale and quality of the treatment method using Quick Disabilities of Arm, Shoulder and Hand and visual analog scale scores.

Results.—The groups had no differences in mean age, sex, and occupation. The visual analog scale and Quick Disabilities of the Arm, Shoulder and Hand scores were similar in both groups before the treatment. The treatment success rate was 93% in the CSI + TSC group and 69% in the CSI group. Although both methods improved the patients' conditions significantly in terms of relieving pain and functional ability, CSI + TSC had a significantly higher treatment success rate.

Conclusions.—The combined technique of corticosteroid injection and thumb spica casting was better than injection alone in the treatment of de Quervain tenosynovitis in terms of treatment success and functional outcomes.

Type of Study/Level of Evidence.—Therapeutic II.

▶ This study evaluates whether the addition of a thumb spica cast to patients receiving steroid injections for de Quervains tenosynovitis improves outcomes. Although the authors identified a statistically significant difference in their primary outcome, something they call the *treatment success rate*, I am not convinced that this measure is clinically meaningful. The outcome measure is a combination of 3 things: radial-sided wrist pain, tenderness over the first dorsal compartment, and a positive Finkelstein test. It is positive when all 3 are present and negative when any one of the 3 is not. Response rate to both groups was good; 93% in the cast group and 69% in the no-cast group. In my patient population, some patients have persistent Finkelstein test results after injection but are happy and do not seek additional treatment. Using the authors' primary outcome measure, these patients would have been counted in the failure group. I suspect that the differences they identified may not be clinically relevant enough to subject patients to the additional cost and aggravation of a cast. Additionally, although the difference in QuickDASH was statistically significant, the 8-point difference is far lower than the minimal clinically important difference for this measure (MCID = 18). Lastly, the patients who were unsuccessfully treated the first time all responded to a second injection. Taken together, casting does not meaningfully improve outcomes in these patients, and I will not be adding it into my current treatment algorithm.

A. Daluiski, MD

Endoscopic *versus* open release in patients with de Quervain's tenosynovitis: a randomised trial
Kang HJ, Koh IH, Jang JW, et al (Yonsei Univ College of Medicine, Seoul, South Korea)
Bone Joint J 95-B:947-951, 2013

The purpose of this study was to compare the outcome and complications of endoscopic *versus* open release for the treatment of de Quervain's tenosynovitis. Patients with this condition were randomised to undergo either endoscopic (n = 27) or open release (n = 25). Visual Analogue Scale (VAS) pain and Disabilities of Arm, Shoulder, and Hand (DASH) scores were measured at 12 and 24 weeks after surgery. Scar satisfaction was measured using a VAS scale. The mean pain and DASH scores improved significantly at 12 weeks and 24 weeks ($p < 0.001$) in both groups. The scores were marginally lower in the endoscopic group compared to the open group at 12 weeks ($p = 0.012$ and $p = 0.002$, respectively); however, only the DASH score showed a clinically important difference. There were no differences between the groups at 24 weeks. The mean VAS scar satisfaction score was higher in the endoscopic group at 24 weeks ($p < 0.001$). Transient superficial radial nerve injury occurred in three patients in the endoscopic group compared with nine in the open release group ($p = 0.033$).

We conclude that endoscopic release for de Quervain's tenosynovitis seems to provide earlier improvement after surgery, with fewer superficial radial nerve complications and greater scar satisfaction, when compared with open release.

▶ The authors present an interesting and well-designed study comparing endoscopic and open release of first dorsal extensor compartment. They randomly assigned 30 patients to undergo either of these procedures, and assessment of Visual Analogue Scale (VAS) pain and Disabilities of Arm, Shoulder, and Hand (DASH) scores was made after 12 and 24 weeks postoperatively. The authors confirmed better outcome in the endoscopic group after 12 weeks, but there was no difference at the end of the study. They also provided additional useful information such as the number of abductor pollicis longus (APL) slips and the presence of the intracompartmental septum. Despite an elegant design of the study, there are some weaknesses. The groups seem to be well matched, but the variation of DASH scores is quite different despite similar mean values. Moreover, I think that the DASH score is also influenced by any disabilities of shoulder and elbow and it doesn't focus much on hand disabilities. I would prefer using PRWE, Mayo wrist score, or Michigan Hand Questionnaire to assess disabilities related to de Quervain's tenosynovitis. Still, the study has a great importance for surgeons who may consider endoscopic release.

I always doubt providing tourniquet time as a comparable measure of procedure time. I observe longer set-up time for endoscopic procedures when compared with open. These procedures can also be more expensive because of the use of delicate optics (easy to damage), wires, and dedicated knives. I perform an open release with a transverse 1.5-cm approach, which gives enough visualization to perform a safe approach, assess the APL slips, and complete the procedure and is very aesthetic after healing.

P. Czarnecki, MD

10 Trauma

Palmar Opening Wedge Osteotomy for Malunion of Fifth Metacarpal Neck Fractures

Zhang X, Liu Z, Shao X, et al (Second Hosp of Qinhuangdao, Changli; People's Hosp of Lulong, Qinhuangdao; Chinese Med Association in Qinhuangdao; et al)
J Hand Surg 38A:2461-2465, 2013

Malunion of fifth metacarpal neck fractures may present an aesthetic problem that needs surgical correction. This article reports palmar opening wedge osteotomy for the treatment of malunion of fifth metacarpal neck fractures in 21 hands. The length of the fifth metacarpal was increased using the technique. We also present long-term results in patients using the technique. Palmar opening wedge osteotomy is a successful surgical technique for the treatment of malunion of fifth metacarpal neck fractures.

▶ The authors describe an opening wedge osteotomy as an alternative technique to treat malunions of the fifth metacarpal (MCP) neck. The advantage of this technique over previously described techniques is that, in addition to correcting angulation, it also corrects length of the shortened MCP. Although statistical analysis was not performed, the authors found that this technique did improve patients' MCP arc of motion, thumb to little finger pinch strength, and length and angulation of the MCP neck. All patients' bones healed at an average of 8 weeks.

Strengths of this study include the novel technique, use of standardized patient-reported questionnaire, and little finger MCP-specific clinical outcomes. Additionally, patients were followed up for a minimum of 1 year, enabling ample time to assess bone healing and MCP-associated outcomes and complications. Weaknesses of this study include the small number of patients, lack of statistical analysis, relatively short-term follow-up preventing assessment of the longevity of this technique, and lack of a control group or technique.

The technique described in this study has multiple advantages when treating these malunions. The ability to correct length, in addition to angulation, is an important consideration and advantage of previously described closing wedge osteotomies. The opening wedge osteotomy is designed to correct the volar comminution and collapse from the original injury, restoring close to anatomic alignment of the fifth MCP. Furthermore, the authors describe a relatively simple and reproducible technique with an ulno-dorsal approach to the fifth MCP.

There is debate as to the acceptable angulation and shortening for malunions or nonunions of the fifth MCP neck. With biomechanical studies suggesting

MCP shortening has an important impact on function, this opening wedge technique should be a consideration. However, long-term studies are needed to assess the longevity, refracture rates, and maintenance of motion and angulation for both opening and previously described closing wedge osteotomies to truly determine the optimal technique.

E. R. Wagner, MD

Stability of Acute Dorsal Fracture Dislocations of the Proximal Interphalangeal Joint: A Biomechanical Study
Tyser AR, Tsai MA, Parks BG, et al (MedStar Union Memorial Hosp, Baltimore, MD)
J Hand Surg Am 39:13-18, 2014

Purpose.—We performed a cadaveric biomechanical study to characterize proximal interphalangeal joint stability after an injury to different amounts of the volar articular base of the middle phalanx (intact, 20%, 40%, 60%, and 80% volar defects).

Methods.—Eighteen digits on 6 hands were tested through full proximal interphalangeal joint range of motion using computer-controlled flexion and extension via the digital tendons. We collected proximal interphalangeal joint kinematic cine data in a true lateral projection with minifluoroscopy. We measured the amount of dorsal middle phalanx translation in full proximal interphalangeal joint extension. As we cycled the joint from full flexion into extension, we recorded the angle at which subluxation occurred.

Results.—No specimens with 20% volar bony defect subluxated. All specimens in the 60% and 80% groups subluxated at an average flexion angle of 67° (range, 10° to 90°) in the 60% group and at all degrees of flexion in the 80% group. In the 40% group, 28% of specimens demonstrated subluxation at an average flexion angle of 14° (range, 4° to 40°). Mean dorsal translation of the middle phalanx in relation to the proximal phalanx at full digital extension was 0.2 mm in the 20% group, 0.8 mm in the 40% group, 3.2 mm in the 60% group, and 3.1 mm in the 80% group.

Conclusions.—Simulated volar articular bony defects of 20% were stable, whereas those with 60% and 80% defects were unstable during digital motion. Stability in the 40% group was variable and appeared to be the threshold for stability.

Clinical Relevance.—Knowledge of the typical amount of middle phalanx defect and degree of proximal interphalangeal joint extension that can lead to joint instability may improve management of mechanically important proximal interphalangeal joint fracture dislocations.

▶ This is an interesting cadaveric study that defines the degree of middle phalangeal volar bony defect responsible for proximal interphalangeal joint instability. Similar to what has been written in clinical reports, 20% of the volar lip or less was stable, 40% was stable in some positions, and anything over 60% was unstable. As with many cadaveric studies, the methodology does not recapitulate the clinical reality of these injuries. The soft tissue component of the injury is not adequately accounted for in this model, a weakness the authors address. Despite this, the study reminds us of the inherent instability of larger injuries and the capacity for displacement if treated nonoperatively. Often, the presenting postreduction lateral radiograph will dictate treatment. If the joint is held in a flexed position and there is persistent dorsal translation, I typically stabilize the joint with a distraction fixator made from k-wires. I have found that the difficulty in treating these injuries comes not from predicting stability at the time of presentation but from patients presenting weeks or months after their injury. Unlike treating these joint injuries acutely, chronic fracture subluxations require much more extensive dissection and lead to less optimal results, which is often surprising to patients who believed they had a simple jammed finger.

A. Daluiski, MD

Ultrasound of displaced ulnar collateral ligament tears of the thumb: the Stener lesion revisited
Melville D, Jacobson JA, Haase S, et al (Univ of Michigan, Ann Arbor)
Skeletal Radiol 42:667-673, 2013

Purpose.—To retrospectively characterize the ultrasound appearance of displaced ulnar collateral ligament (UCL) tears that are proven at surgery, and then determine the accuracy of the resulting ultrasound criteria in differentiating displaced from non-displaced UCL tears.

Materials and Methods.—After institutional review board approval, 26 patients were identified from the radiology information system over a 10-year period that had ultrasound evaluation of the thumb and surgically proven UCL tear. Retrospective review of the displaced full-thickness tears was carried out to characterize displaced tears and to establish ultrasound criteria for such tears. A repeat retrospective review 4 months later of all UCL tears applied the criteria to determine accuracy of ultrasound in the diagnosis of displaced full-thickness UCL tear.

Results.—The 26 subjects consisted of 17 displaced full-thickness UCL tears, seven non-displaced full-thickness tears, and two partial-thickness tears at surgery. Retrospective ultrasound review of displaced full-thickness tears identified two criteria present in all cases: non-visualization of the UCL ligament and presence of a heterogeneous mass-like area proximal to the first metacarpophalangeal joint. Applying these criteria at the second retrospective review resulted in 100 % sensitivity, specificity, positive predictive value, negative predictive value, and accuracy.

Conclusions.—The ultrasound findings of absent UCL fibers and presence of a heterogeneous mass-like abnormality proximal to the first metacarpophalangeal joint achieved 100 % accuracy in differentiating displaced from non-displaced full-thickness UCL tear of the thumb.

Displaced full-thickness UCL tears most commonly were located proximal to the adductor aponeurosis.

▶ This retrospective study demonstrates that ultrasound can diagnose a Stener lesion of the ulnar collateral ligament at the metacarpophalangeal joint with 100% accuracy. It does not demonstrate that the ultrasound should replace a good examination with or without local anesthesia. The study adds to the information as to when one should consider surgical care because a Stener lesion will not allow for healing ligament to bone. Ultrasound remains an adjunct with specific indications when considering the surgical care of these ligament tears. A good history and examination can be supplemented by the judicious use of ultrasound. It is not necessary for all patients. As health care resources diminish in the future, judicious use of this modality should be considered.

C. Carroll, MD

Acute Compartment Syndrome After Intramedullary Nailing of Isolated Radius and Ulna Fractures in Children
Blackman AJ, Wall LB, Keeler KA, et al (Washington Univ School of Medicine, St Louis, MO)
J Pediatr Orthop 34:50-54, 2014

Background.—There exist varying reports in the literature regarding the incidence of compartment syndrome (CS) after intramedullary (IM) fixation of pediatric forearm fractures. A retrospective review of the experience with this treatment modality at our institution was performed to elucidate the rate of postoperative CS and identify risk factors for developing this complication.

Methods.—In this retrospective case series, we reviewed the charts of all patients treated operatively for isolated radius and ulnar shaft fractures from 2000 to 2009 at our institution and identified 113 patients who underwent IM fixation of both-bone forearm fractures. There were 74 closed fractures and 39 open fractures including 31 grade I fractures, 7 grade II fractures, and 1 grade IIIA fracture. If the IM nail could not be passed easily across the fracture site, a small open approach was used to aid reduction.

Results.—CS occurred in 3 of 113 patients (2.7%). CS occurred in 3 of 39 (7.7%) of the open fractures compared with none of 74 closed fractures ($P = 0.039$), including 45 closed fractures that were treated within 24 hours of injury. An open reduction was performed in all of the open fractures and 38 (51.4%) of the closed fractures. Increased operative time was associated with developing CS postoperatively (168 vs. 77 min, $P < 0.001$). CS occurred within the first 24 postoperative hours in all 3 cases.

Conclusion.—CS was an uncommon complication after IM fixation of pediatric diaphyseal forearm fractures in this retrospective case series. Open fractures and longer operative times were associated with developing CS after surgery. None of 45 patients who underwent IM nailing of closed fractures within 24 hours of injury developed CS; however, 51.4% of these patients required a small open approach to aid reduction and nail passage. We believe that utilizing a small open approach for reduction of one or both bones, thereby avoiding the soft-tissue trauma of multiple attempts to reduce the fracture and pass the nail, leads to decreased soft-tissue trauma and a lower rate of CS. We recommend a low threshold for converting to open reduction in cases where closed reduction is difficult.

▶ Compartment syndrome in children merits special attention because children are often unable to voice their concerns or their symptoms effectively. Unlike adults who develop the "5 Ps," children will manifest a compartment syndrome with the "3 As": anxiety, agitation, and increased analgesic requirements. One important finding of this study was that the compartment syndrome in 2 of 3 cases occurred the day after the initial fixation. In all 3 cases, forearm compartment syndrome was heralded by increasing pain.

In this study, nearly 10% of patients with open fractures developed a compartment syndrome after intramedullary fixation of both radial and ulnar shaft fractures. These patients were more likely to present with a nerve palsy compared with those who did not develop a compartment syndrome. Surgical times were also more than double on average than for patients who did not develop a compartment syndrome.

In summary, this study should serve as a warning to all orthopedic surgeons who care for children. Compartment syndrome can occur with any pediatric forearm fracture, but those with increasing pain, open fractures, and prolonged surgical times are at highest risk. The authors' recommendations of limiting the number of attempts at passing the intramedullary rod to 3 and to observing all children for at least 24 hours after fixation are probably prudent. Ignore the child with increasing pain at your own (and the patient's) peril.

D. A. Zlotolow, MD

Fingertip Reconstruction With Simultaneous Flaps and Nail Bed Grafts Following Amputation
Hwang E, Park BH, Song SY, et al (CHA Univ, Seongnam, Korea; Konkuk Univ School of Medicine, Chungju, Korea)
J Hand Surg 38A:1307-1314, 2013

Purpose.—To report our technique and results with treating fingertip amputations with flaps and simultaneous nailbed grafts.

Methods.—We reconstructed 20 fingertip amputations with loss of bone and nail with flaps combined with nailbed grafts. We reconstructed the volar side of the fingertip with a flap, and the dorsal side of the fingertip with a nailbed grafted to the raw inner surface of the flap. We employed volar V-Y advancement flaps for transverse or dorsal oblique fingertip injuries and generally used abdominal flaps for volar oblique fingertip injuries. We harvested nailbeds from the amputated finger or from the patient's first toe.

Results.—The length of the amputated fingertips was restored with the flaps, and the lost nailbeds were restored to their natural appearance with the nailbed grafts. We classified the results according to the length of the reconstructed fingertip and the appearance of the nail. Excellent or good results were achieved in 16 cases. Three cases had fair results and 1 had a poor result. We observed favorable results for distal fingertip amputations (Allen type II or III). In particular, most cases that were reconstructed with volar V-Y advancement flaps combined with nailbed grafts demonstrated favorable results.

Conclusions.—This method is useful for the restoration of dorsal oblique or transverse type fingertip amputations and is a good alternative when replantation is not an option.

▶ This report introduces a novel approach to fingertip injuries with a focus on nail reconstruction. The authors report excellent results after use of nail bed grafts and flaps for palmar soft tissue replacement.

Despite the fact that bony reconstruction was not done in any of the cases, the authors claim that no hook nail deformity was seen. This is surprising, because most of the reported cases (15 of 20) had bone loss. In some them, the loss of bone was substantial. It is known that hook nail deformity occurs if the nail bed is not supported by bone. The authors explain the nonoccurrence of hook nails by the sufficient support of soft tissue and the use of tightening sutures between the remnant lateral nail fold and the flap. They actually had a case of severe hook nail deformity in a case in which they had used a thenar flap as soft tissue cover, but that case was excluded from the series. The authors believe that the thin soft tissue padding was the cause for hook nail formation.

This problem remains unsolved, especially because in one of the figures (Fig 1 in the original article) a case with bone loss is presented; however, the drawing illustrates the reconstruction with the amputated bone portion under the nail bed. This is in contradiction to the authors' writing.

It may be possible that the authors have found a new method of fingertip reconstruction without hook nail deformity even in cases of substantial bone loss. To prove that this is possible without any additional bony support, however, further reports from other centers will be necessary to support this paradigm shift.

Another question that remains unsolved is how patients pinched with a fingertip that is composed of supple soft tissue but lacks bony support.

M. Choi, MD

A Nationwide Review of the Treatment Patterns of Traumatic Thumb Amputations
Shale CM, Tidwell JE III, Mulligan RP, et al (Scott and White Healthcare, Temple, TX; Texas A&M Health Sciences Ctr, Temple)
Ann Plast Surg 70:647-651, 2013

Traumatic thumb amputations are a common problem with significant associated cost to patients, hospitals, and society.

The purpose of this study was to review practice patterns for traumatic thumb amputations using the National Trauma Data Bank. By using a large nationwide database, we hoped to better understand the epidemiology and predictors of attempts and successful replantation.

The design was a retrospective review of the National Trauma Data Bank between the years 2007 and 2010, investigating patients with traumatic thumb amputations. Analyses of these patients based on replantation attempt, mechanism of injury, and demographics were performed. Comparisons were made between hospitals based on teaching status and on patient volume for replant attempt and success rates.

There were 3341 traumatic thumb amputations with 550 (16.5%) attempts at replantation and an overall success rate of 84.9%. Nonteaching hospitals treated 1238 (37.1%) patients, and attempted 123 (9.9%) replantations with a success rate of 80.5%. Teaching hospitals treated 2103 (63.0%) patients, and attempted 427 (20.3%) replantations with a success rate of 86.2%. Being in a teaching hospital increased the odds of attempted replantation by a factor of 3.1 ($P < 0.001$) when compared to a nonteaching hospital. Treatment at a high-volume center increased the rate of attempted replantation by a factor of 3.4 ($P < 0.001$), as compared to low-volume hospitals.

Practice patterns show that teaching and high-volume hospitals attempt to replant a higher percentage of amputated thumbs. Success rates are similar across practice settings.

▶ The authors have reported on the incidence of traumatic thumb amputations and the rates of attempted and successful replantations at both teaching and nonteaching hospitals. There are several limitations to this study as is expected. Their outcome data are only as good as the data input. There may be local hospitals that are regional hand centers that are not classified as trauma centers but care for isolated traumatic hand injuries. In addition, there may be nonteaching (community) hospitals that have hand fellowships and residency programs, and there are likely trauma centers included in the database that do not have hand surgery fellowship programs, making the comparison between the 2 institution types difficult to interpret.

In addition, the ICD 9 codes for thumb amputation can include everything from a soft tissue amputation or amputation of the bony tip to complete amputation at the carpometacarpal joint region. Finally, they include successful replantations as those that are discharged from the hospital without the code for amputation during the same admission. It is possible that some of these patients had attempted replantation of multiple digits, with subsequent amputation of a finger, but not the thumb, as well as revision of the thumb amputation after hospital discharge.

These shortcomings are inherent to any database query. Fortunately, insurance status did not seem to be a factor in whether replantation was attempted.

Although this report does not do anything to change current practice, it is a potential beginning in reviewing patients with traumatic amputations and hopefully modifying the current system or creating a new system to ensure all patients who are candidates for replantation of digital amputations receive the best possible treatment.

W. C. Hammert, MD

Opinions Regarding the Management of Hand and Wrist Injuries in Elite Athletes

Dy CJ, Khmelnitskaya E, Hearns KA, et al (Hosp for Special Surgery, NY)
Orthopedics 36:815-819, 2013

Injuries to the hand and wrist are commonly encountered in athletes. Decisions regarding the most appropriate treatment, the timing of treatment, and return to play are made while balancing desires to resume athletic activities and sound orthopedic principles. Little recognition in the literature exists regarding the need for a different approach when treating these injuries in elite athletes and the timing to return to play.

This study explored the complexities of treating hand and wrist injuries in the elite athlete. Thirty-seven consultant hand surgeons for teams in the National Football League, National Basketball Association, and Major League Baseball completed a brief electronic survey about the management of 10 common hand injuries. Notable variability existed in responses for initial management, return to protected play, and return to unprotected play for all injuries, aside from near consensus agreement (94%) that elite athletes with stable proximal interphalangeal dislocations could immediately return to protected play. Basketball surgeons were less likely to recommend early return to protected play than non-basketball surgeons. Baseball surgeons were more likely to recommend early unprotected play after scaphoid fixation. Football surgeons were more likely to recommend earlier return to protected play after thumb ulnar collateral ligament injuries, whereas basketball surgeons were less likely to recommend earlier return to protected play.

This study demonstrated wide variability in how consultant hand surgeons approach the treatment of hand and wrist injuries. The findings emphasize the need to individually tailor treatment decisions to the patient's desires and demands, particularly in high-performance athletes.

▶ The most significant aspect of this article is the conclusion that for most hand and wrist injuries, there is no clear consensus on the type of treatment and timing regarding return to play, even among consultant hand surgeons of professional teams.

One of this study's strengths was the ability to get 37 consultant hand surgeons of professional teams to complete a survey on the management of hand and wrist injuries in elite athletes. A weakness of this study is seen in some of the clinical scenarios and choices presented. For example, the consultant hand surgeon was asked his or her opinion on timing of return to protected play versus unprotected play in a player with a nondisplaced scaphoid fracture; however, there was no mention of the location of the fracture, such as distal pole versus waist versus proximal pole, which may determine the chosen treatment. Another example is the presented choices of timing of return to play after a nondisplaced scaphoid fracture. Less than 4 to 6 weeks with or without protected play was not presented as an option. Rather, immediately and when healed, 4 to 6 weeks were the only 2 options of return to play after the nondisplaced scaphoid fracture.

Although this was a very simple study performed to get some baseline information from consultant hand surgeons regarding their preferences in the management of hand and wrist injuries in elite athletes, the study's conclusion that there was such variability and no clear consensus on the treatment and timing of return to play for many of these injuries is important for all those who have a stake in the athlete's well being, such as the treating hand surgeon, team physician, trainer, coach, agent, and team owner.

In my experience treating many professional athletes from a variety of sports and as a consultant hand surgeon to several different professional teams, I am not at all surprised by the findings of this study. The treatment of a specific athlete's injury depends on different factors, such as type of injury, type of sport, position, and timing of injury during the season and during the career. As the study states, the treatment of an athlete's injury must be tailored to the individual athlete; in other words, there is no "cookie-cutter" approach to the treatment of these injuries in elite athletes.

S. S. Shin, MD, MMSc

Hand and Wrist Injuries in Golf
Ek ETH, Suh N, Weiland AJ (Hosp for Special Surgery, NY; Monash Univ, Melbourne, Australia)
J Hand Surg 38A:2029-2033, 2013

Background.—Golf is now played by persons of every socioeconomic class and age and both genders, and golf-related injuries are prevalent. The coordinated, synchronized movements of the entire body in golf swings most often cause injuries to the hand and wrist, as well as the lumbar spine. Professional and high-level golfers usually sustain overuse injuries and amateur golfers injuries caused by poor swing mechanics, overzealous play, or sudden trauma such as hitting a tree. After a detailed history, a careful examination is needed to reach an accurate diagnosis. Golfers should report the characteristics of the injury, level of play (often revealed by the golfer's handicap), onset of symptoms, whether he or she is right- or left-handed, and when during the golf swing the symptoms are most notable. Most golf injuries affect the lower hand. The phase of the golf swing can indicate the nature of the injury. The most common golf-related injuries to the hand and wrist were discussed, along with their evaluation and treatment.

Injuries.—A sudden forceful impact can produce instability of the extensor carpi ulnaris (ECU) tendon. In the golf swing, when the wrist supinates, ulnar deviates, and flexes during impact, a painful snapping or clicking can occur over the wrist's dorso-ulnar side. Voluntary subluxation is often seen. The diagnosis is confirmed on dynamic ultrasound and magnetic resonance imaging (MRI). Treatment includes rest and strict long-arm splinting for 4 to 6 weeks with the wrist in extension, radial deviation, and supination. A removal splint is used for 4 weeks thereafter. Recurrent instability may require repair or reconstruction of the tendon sheath.

Tears of the triangular fibrocartilage complex (TFCC) result from excessive repetitive rotational motions in the wrist joint. Symptoms include ulnar-sided wrist pain, tenderness in the fovea area, and a palpable click with forearm rotation. The distal radioulnar joint may be unstable in larger tears. MRI is highly accurate diagnostically. Treatment consists of immobilization of the wrist and forearm, nonsteroidal anti-inflammatory drugs, and corticosteroid injection. In patients whose nonsurgical methods fail and for high-level athletes, wrist arthroscopy may be performed. Treatment depends on the type of TFCC tear and its location. Debridement is used for central tears, with arthroscopic or open repair for peripheral tears, followed by immobilization.

Hook of hamate fractures are the most common bony injuries in golfers and usually affect the lead hand, often when the golfer abruptly strikes the ground. Patients usually complain of focal tenderness over the hook when gripping the club and pain with ball strike. Paresthesia into the ulnar two digits occurs with irritation of the adjacent ulnar nerve. Clicking and the risk for rupture caused by abrasion of the tendons on the raw bone surface of the fracture are also seen. The use of plain radiographs with a carpal tunnel view can be improved by adding computed tomography (CT) to detect the fracture's size and location. Union can be challenging. Excision of the hook of the hamate may be needed if pain persists, neurological symptoms develop, or the flexor tendons are at risk. Recovery from surgery with no significant complications is expected.

Golfers rarely develop triquetro-hamate impingement, but this can create ulnar-sided wrist pain of the lead hand. Point tenderness is apparent over the hamate, but specific diagnosis is difficult. Arthroscopy through the mid-carpal portal may help diagnostically and clinically, permitting debridement of any chondromalacia present. Treatment includes modifying the swing mechanics, use of anti-inflammatory drugs, and arthroscopy and debridement should these nonsurgical methods fail.

Ulnar-sided wrist pain can also result from pisotriquetral arthritis. Direct palpation of the pisiform elicits tenderness that is exacerbated by the pisotriquetral shear test. The clinician should obtain a 30-degree oblique wrist radiograph centered through the pisotriquetral joint and confirmatory MRI or CT. Diagnosis and therapy are aided by a differential lidocaine injection (with or without corticosteroids) into the joint. Persistent pain may prompt surgical excision of the pisiform.

With maximal ulnar deviation of the wrist, ulnar styloid impingement may occur, usually at the point of impact. Confirmatory symptoms are elicited with forced ulnar deviation of the wrist, causing tenderness over the ulnar styloid. Neutral posteroanterior radiographs can reveal ulnar

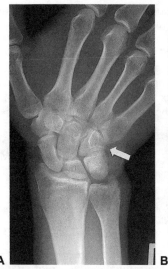 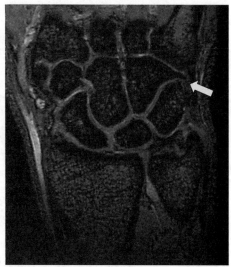

A **B**

FIGURE 3.—A Plain radiograph showing impaction of the triquetrum against the hamate in extreme ulnar deviation (arrow). B The T1-weighted, 3-dimensional, fat-suppressed MRI images demonstrating degenerative changes at the ulnar aspect of the triquetro-hamate articulation (arrow) with overhanging osteophyte formation due to chronic impaction. (Reprinted from Ek ETH, Suh N, Weiland AJ. Hand and wrist injuries in golf. *J Hand Surg.* 2013;38A:2029-2033, with permission from the American Society for Surgery of the Hand)

variance. The ulnar styloid's morphology should be evaluated, and MRI can detect edema in the ulnar carpals, which confirms impaction. Correction of the swing mechanics, anti-inflammatory drugs, and rest may resolve the problem; if not, arthroscopic or open ulnar styloidectomy may work.

Conclusions.—Most golfing injuries can be prevented through proper swing mechanics, avoidance of repetitive and/or excessive practice or play, and placing the hands properly on the club (Fig 3).

▶ The authors review common golf hand and wrist injuries and highlight poor mechanics of the golf swing and overuse as primary culprits. Personally and professionally, I can add a few comments, having grown up in a golf family and being married to a golf pro, studying the biomechanics of the golf swing,[1] and seeing enthusiastic golfer-patients of all backgrounds over the years. The poor mechanics typically, in my experience, occur with 4 common occurrences: (1) overgripping the club; (2) hands not working together as an end unit from a solid core; (3) pre-impact maneuvers such as jumping, casting, or chunking the club; and (4) hitting off mats, invariably thin pieces of artificial turf over a slab of concrete. The authors highlight 5 common entities: (1) extensor carpi ulnaris instability, (2) triangular fibrocartilage complex tear, (3) hook of hamate fracture, (4) triquetrohamate impingement, and (5) pisotriquetral arthritis. I agree to the frequency of these with the exception of triquetrohamate impingement (Fig 3), which I will now look for in the future. I would add to these (1) trigger finger; (2) flexor carpi ulnaris tendinitis, which may be an extension of the pisotriquetral inflammation;

and (3) extensor carpi radialis and brevis tendinitis, perhaps an extension of lateral epicondylitis (as common if not more in my practice than medial epicondylitis, so-called golfer's elbow). Overly tight grip in conjunction with an errant shot or club-vs-ground event explains most of golfers' ills about the wrist. Core stabilization, stretching, and repetition of good mechanics go a long way to injury prevention. Lowering golf scores, however, is another thing altogether. Unfortunately, the more swing thoughts invading your mind as you address the ball, the more the swing deteriorates. To paraphrase the great Bobby Jones, the longest distance in golf is the 6 inches between your ears. Here's to the KISS principle—in golf and in surgery!

A. Ladd, MD

Reference

1. Meister DW, Ladd AL, Butler EE, et al. Rotational biomechanics of the elite golf swing: benchmarks for amateurs. *J Appl Biomech*. 2011;27:242-251.

Reconstruction of Chronic Thumb Metacarpophalangeal Joint Radial Collateral Ligament Injuries With a Half-Slip of the Abductor Pollicis Brevis Tendon

Iba K, Wada T, Hiraiwa T, et al (Sapporo Med Univ School of Medicine, Japan)
J Hand Surg 38A:1945-1950, 2013

Purpose.—To evaluate a reconstructive method for chronic radial collateral ligament (RCL) injuries of the thumb metacarpophalangeal (MCP) joint using a combination of RCL advancement and the transfer of a half-slip of the abductor pollicis brevis tendon.

Methods.—Eight patients (4 male and 4 female; mean age, 25 y) with chronic RCL injury of the thumb MCP joint were enrolled. All patients were referred to our institution because of continuing pain and instability on the radial side of the MCP joint when grasping or pinching objects. The mechanism of the injury was adduction stress to the thumb during sporting activities in 5 patients, a heavy object falling on the thumb in 1, and a fall in 2. The mean duration from RCL injury to surgery was 20 weeks. The average postoperative follow-up was 51 months. We evaluated postoperative outcomes including pain, range of motion of the thumb MCP joint, grip strength, key pinch strength, Disabilities of the Arm, Shoulder, and Hand score, and ability to return to preinjury work or sporting activities.

Results.—No patients demonstrated continuing symptoms, and the MCP joint was stable after surgery. Postoperative grip and pinch strength (37 and 6.3 kg, respectively) were increased compared with preoperative values (34 and 3.9 kg, respectively). All patients returned fully to their preinjury work or sporting activities within 6 months after surgery. Although postoperative flexion was decreased by an average of 6°, no patients noted functional deficiency.

Conclusions.—We recommend the reconstructive method of RCL advancement and transfer of a half-slip of the abductor pollicis brevis tendon to alleviate pain and improve grip and pinch strength in chronic RCL injuries of the thumb MCP joint.

▶ The authors present an interesting technique for the treatment of chronic injuries of the radial collateral ligament of the metacarpophalangeal (MCP) joint of the thumb. They report a series of 8 patients with chronic radial collateral ligament injury who underwent a reconstructive procedure using a combination of radial collateral ligament (RCL) advancement and the transfer of a half-slip of the abductor pollicis brevis tendon. Regardless of its small sample size and retrospective design, this study adds another interesting technique to the armamentarium of the hand surgeon. The authors report encouraging results despite a significant loss of flexion at the MCP joint. Unstable injuries to the RCL are relatively rare but may be as debilitating as tears of the ulnar collateral ligament. The treatment of chronic complete ruptures is similar to that for the ulnar collateral ligament (UCL). However, in contrast to the UCL, a torn RCL almost always lies beneath the abductor aponeurosis. Therefore, it is possible that the ends of the RCL can be mobilized and repaired in the chronic situation. In case the RCL is fibrotic or cannot be mobilized, a free tendon graft or an augmentation/reinforcement technique such as the one described by the authors can be used. Currently, I use a free tendon graft for the reconstruction of chronic RCL injuries of the MCP joint of the thumb. The authors' technique might be an interesting alternative in patients with an absent palmaris longus and will prevent any donor site scar or morbidity. Despite the limitations of the study, this technique is an interesting addition to the current techniques of treatment of this uncommon injury.

A. L. Wahegaonkar, MD, FACS, MCh (Orth)

Reconstruction of Chronic Thumb Metacarpophalangeal Joint Radial Collateral Ligament Injuries With a Half-Slip of the Abductor Pollicis Brevis Tendon
Iba K, Wada T, Hiraiwa T, et al (Sapporo Med Univ School of Medicine, Japan)
J Hand Surg 38A:1945-1950, 2013

Purpose.—To evaluate a reconstructive method for chronic radial collateral ligament (RCL) injuries of the thumb metacarpophalangeal (MCP) joint using a combination of RCL advancement and the transfer of a half-slip of the abductor pollicis brevis tendon.

Methods.—Eight patients (4 male and 4 female; mean age, 25 y) with chronic RCL injury of the thumb MCP joint were enrolled. All patients were referred to our institution because of continuing pain and instability on the radial side of the MCP joint when grasping or pinching objects. The mechanism of the injury was adduction stress to the thumb during sporting activities in 5 patients, a heavy object falling on the thumb in 1, and a fall in 2. The mean duration from RCL injury to surgery was 20 weeks. The average postoperative follow-up was 51 months. We evaluated postoperative outcomes including pain, range of motion of the thumb MCP joint, grip strength, key pinch strength, Disabilities of the Arm, Shoulder, and Hand score, and ability to return to preinjury work or sporting activities.

Results.—No patients demonstrated continuing symptoms, and the MCP joint was stable after surgery. Postoperative grip and pinch strength (37 and 6.3 kg, respectively) were increased compared with preoperative values (34 and 3.9 kg, respectively). All patients returned fully to their preinjury work or sporting activities within 6 months after surgery. Although postoperative flexion was decreased by an average of 6°, no patients noted functional deficiency.

Conclusions.—We recommend the reconstructive method of RCL advancement and transfer of a half-slip of the abductor pollicis brevis tendon to alleviate pain and improve grip and pinch strength in chronic RCL injuries of the thumb MCP join.

▶ Treatment of chronic collateral ligament injuries at the thumb metacarpophalangeal (MP) joint can be difficult and often require the use of a tendon graft or off-the-shelf allograft.

The authors report on a series of 8 patients who underwent treatment of chronic radial collateral ligament injuries of the thumb by locally rotating a slip of the abductor pollicis brevis in addition to advancement of the radial collateral ligament. This method involves leaving the abductor at its insertion in the proximal phalanx and creating a slip (the dorsal 50% of the tendon). The slip is released proximally and secured into the metacarpal head and radial collateral ligament.

The technique has afforded a stable construct in all patients with no pain and return to full unrestricted activities and employment.

The advantages of this method are that it is convenient and avoids donor site morbidity. It is worth considering in these often-challenging cases.

M. Rizzo, MD

Comparison of *In Vitro* Motion and Stability Between Techniques for Index Metacarpophalangeal Joint Radial Collateral Ligament Reconstruction
Dy CJ, Tucker SM, Hearns KA, et al (Hosp for Special Surgery, NY)
J Hand Surg 38A:1324-1330, 2013

Purpose.—To evaluate a technique using interference screws to secure a tendon graft for reconstruction of the radial collateral ligament (RCL) of the index finger metacarpophalangeal (MCP) joint. We hypothesized that this technique would provide equivalent stability and flexion as a 4-tunnel reconstruction.

Methods.—We isolated the RCL in 17 cadaveric index fingers. A cyclic load was applied to the intact RCL across the MCP joint to assess flexion, ulnar deviation at neutral (UD 0), and ulnar deviation at 90° of MCP joint flexion (UD 90). The RCL was excised from its bony origin and insertion. We performed each reconstruction (4-tunnel and interference screw) sequentially on each specimen in a randomized order using a palmaris longus tendon graft. We repeated testing after each reconstruction and compared differences from the intact state between techniques using paired *t*-tests for all joint positions (flexion/UD 0/UD 90).

Results.—There was no statistically significant difference in UD 0 or UD 90 between the intact state and after interference screw reconstruction. Compared with the intact state, there was significantly less UD 0 and significantly more UD 90 after 4-tunnel reconstruction. There was no statistically significant difference between techniques when we compared changes in −UD 0 or UD 90. Change in flexion was statistically significantly different, which indicates that the interference screw technique better replicated intact MCP joint flexion compared with the 4-tunnel technique.

Conclusions.—Interference screw reconstruction of the index RCL provides stability comparable to 4-tunnel reconstruction and is less technically challenging. These results substantiate our clinical experience that the interference screw technique provides an optimal combination of stability and flexion at the index MCP joint.

Clinical Relevance.—Using an interference screw to reconstruct the index RCL is less challenging than 4-tunnel reconstruction and provides stability and range of motion that closely resemble the native MCP joint.

▶ The authors present an *in vitro* study of 2 techniques for radial collateral ligament reconstruction for the instability of index metacarpophalangeal (MP) joint. The study was well designed and clearly described, and the thesis was to prove that a simpler technique with 2 interference screws is reliable and effective compared with 4-tunnel reconstruction. The described technique was more stable but provides less motion, which can be a disadvantage. Second, using interference screws is much more expensive and should be used with caution in patients with poor bone stock. Interference screws certainly simplify the technique and approach, which can be an advantage in clinical conditions. The data presented are clear and well described and the techniques nicely illustrated and commented, which makes this study much more relevant for clinical practice.

I rarely see injuries and instability of index MP joint, and the low frequency of those injuries was also pointed out by the authors. These few patients I have encountered did not require operative treatment. I also agree that there is a group of underdiagnosed patients. When considering operative technique in this particular situation, I would go for the tunneled reconstruction because, in my opinion, slightly better stability and a simple approach don't justify the higher cost and possible implant-related problems of interference screws.

P. Czarnecki, MD

11 Distal Radius Fractures

Current Concepts in the Treatment of Distal Radial Fractures
Ipaktchi K, Livermore M, Lyons C, et al (Denver Health Med Ctr, CO; Univ of Colorado School of Medicine, Aurora)
Orthopedics 36:778-784, 2013

Distal radial fractures are among the most commonly encountered traumatic fractures of the upper extremity. Initial trauma mechanism, fracture pattern, associated injuries, and patient age influence treatment and outcome. Although stable fractures are commonly treated conservatively, the past decade has seen changes in surgical practice and techniques. Indications for surgery have been extended and refined based on new insight into the pathophysiology of the distal end of the forearm and technological advances in implant design. Despite the frequency of this fracture, only limited higher-level evidence exists to guide practitioners in decision making for this injury. This article highlights key concepts in the treatment of distal radial fractures and summarizes current evidence.

▶ This article provides an excellent review of a common but often difficult problem. The article highlights the issues and solutions. It is well written and informative. It is a useful article when considering care of a distal radius fracture. Outcome studies will come in the future that will lead the surgeon to advise optimal care. This review adds to the data on treatment and surgical indications for open reduction and fixation. Multiple approaches are highlighted, as a volar locked plate cannot be the solution for all distal radius fractures. The article reviews pertinent anatomy and parameters of a satisfactory reduction in the young and considers issues in the elderly.

Fixation techniques covered range from pins to external fixators and beyond to minimally invasive techniques and hardware. The role of open reduction and internal fixation is discussed as well. The article presents a good review of the topic and can be helpful in considering an approach for any fracture of the distal radius.

C. Carroll, MD

An investigation of the effect of AlloMatrix bone graft in distal radial fracture: a prospective randomised controlled clinical trial

D'Agostino P, Barbier O (Cliniques Universitaires St-Luc, Brussels, Belgium)
Bone Joint J 95-B:1514-1520, 2013

The osteoinductive properties of demineralised bone matrix have been demonstrated in animal studies. However, its therapeutic efficacy has yet to be proven in humans. The clinical properties of AlloMatrix, an injectable calcium-based demineralised bone matrix allograft, were studied in a prospective randomised study of 50 patients with an isolated unstable distal radial fracture treated by reduction and Kirschner (K-) wire fixation. A total of 24 patients were randomised to the graft group (13 men and 11 women, mean age 42.3 years (20 to 62)) and 26 to the no graft group (8 men and 18 women, mean age 45.0 years (17 to 69)).

At one, three, six and nine weeks, and six and 12 months postoperatively, patients underwent radiological evaluation, assessments for range of movement, grip and pinch strength, and also completed the Disabilities of Arm, Shoulder and Hand questionnaire. At one and six weeks and one year post-operatively, bone mineral density evaluations of both wrists were performed.

No significant difference in wrist function and speed of recovery, rate of union, complications or bone mineral density was found between the two groups. The operating time was significantly higher in the graft group (p = 0.004). Radiologically, the reduction parameters remained similar in the two groups and all AlloMatrix extraosseous leakages disappeared after nine weeks.

This prospective randomised controlled trial did not demonstrate a beneficial effect of AlloMatrix demineralised bone matrix in the treatment of this category of distal radial fractures treated by K-wire fixation.

▶ The authors fashioned a level-1 study to evaluate the efficacy of the use of allograft bone (AlloMatrix) as an adjunct in the management of distal radius fractures. They found no difference in clinical outcomes and patient subjective outcomes and radiographic healing between groups. In fact, the operating time was greater in the bone graft group.

I applaud the authors in helping to sort out this area of longstanding controversy. The findings mirror those of my own clinical experience. Although it can be tempting to fill defects in cases of severe comminution, most cases of distal radius appear to do fine without bone grafting. In most distal radius fractures, today's plates and screws afford rigid fixation and support the fracture sufficiently to allow enough time for the bone to knit together.

M. Rizzo, MD

Predictors of Distal Radioulnar Joint Instability in Distal Radius Fractures
Fujitani R, Omokawa S, Akahane M, et al (Affiliated Hosp of Nara Med Univ, Osaka, Japan; Nara Med Univ, Kashihara, Japan)
J Hand Surg 36A:1919-1925, 2011

Purpose.—A tear of the triangular fibrocartilage complex (TFCC) is the most frequent soft tissue injury associated with fractures of the distal radius, and repair of the deep ligamentous portion of the TFCC is considered when the tear contributes to instability of the distal radioulnar joint (DRUJ). The purpose of this prospective cohort study was to identify predictors of DRUJ instability accompanying unstable distal radius fractures.

Methods.—Between 2002 and 2007, we prospectively treated 163 consecutive patients with unstable distal radius fractures with the volar locking plating system. Complete radioulnar ligament tears representing DRUJ instability were present in 11 of 163 distal radius fractures. We tested univariate associations between DRUJ instability and potential predictors and conducted multivariate analysis to establish independent predictors of instability. We applied receiver operating characteristics curves within the significant risk factors to determine threshold values.

Results.—In univariate analyses, only the radial and sagittal translation ratios of the fracture site were significant predictors of DRUJ instability. Multivariate logistic regression analysis confirmed that the radial translation ratio, which corresponds to a normalized DRUJ gap, was a significant risk factor. According to the receiver operating characteristics curve for the radial translation ratio, the area under the curve was 0.89. A cutoff value of 15% for the radial translation ratio showed the highest diagnostic accuracy rate.

Conclusions.—A radiographic finding of a normalized DRUJ gap on posteroanterior views was the most important predictor to identify DRUJ instability accompanying unstable distal radius fractures. The relative risk of instability increases by 50% when the ratio of DRUJ widening increases by 1%.

▶ Injury to the triangular fibrocartilage complex is the most frequent injury associated with fractures of the distal radius. Previous studies have indicated that patients who had distal radioulnar joint (DRUJ) instability after distal radius fractures went on to a worse functional outcome.

In this prospective study, 163 patients with displaced fractures of the distal radius underwent open reduction and internal fixation and clinical examination for DRUJ instability under anesthesia. DRUJ instability with complete radioulnar ligament tears, confirmed with open surgery, was identified in 11 of the 163 patients.

The authors concluded that an increase of the radioulnar gap on the posterior-anterior (PA) radiographic projection was an important predictor for DRUJ instability. They also found that radial (PA projection) and sagittal plain (lateral projection) translation were also predictors of DRUJ instability. In contrast, ulnar styloid fractures were not a predictor of DRUJ instability.

The primary limitation of this study is that a highly subjective manual clinical test was performed to screen patients for DRUJ instability. This study should not, therefore, be regarded as an incidence study for DRUJ instability after distal radius fractures. This study serves to remind us that the incidence of functionally relevant DRUJ instability after displaced distal radius fractures has likely been overstated in the past.

A future study using an automated clinical evaluation tool that reliably and accurately measures the amount of DRUJ displacement, with dorsally and volarly applied forces, coupled with dynamic imaging of the DRUJ during forearm rotation may help increase our understanding of DRUJ instability after displaced distal radius fractures. The authors have reinforced the prevailing current thinking that not all styloid base fractures, in the setting of displaced distal radius fractures, need surgical repair.

P. Murray, MD

A new radiological method to detect dorsally penetrating screws when using volar locking plates in distal radial fractures: The dorsal horizon view
Haug LC, Glodny B, Deml C, et al (Med Univ of Innsbruck, Austria)
Bone Joint J 95-B:1101-1105, 2013

Penetration of the dorsal screw when treating distal radius fractures with volar locking plates is an avoidable complication that causes lesions of the extensor tendon in between 2% and 6% of patients. We examined axial fluoroscopic views of the distal end of the radius to observe small amounts of dorsal screw penetration, and determined the ideal angle of inclination of the x-ray beam to the forearm when making this radiological view.

Six volar locking plates were inserted at the wrists of cadavers. The actual screw length was measured under direct vision through a dorsal approach to the distal radius. Axial radiographs were performed for different angles of inclination of the forearm at the elbow.

Comparing axial radiological measurements and real screw length, a statistically significant correlation could be demonstrated at an angle of inclination between 5° and 20°. The ideal angle of inclination required to minimise the risk of implanting over-long screws in a dorsal horizon radiological view is 15°.

▶ The authors investigate a previously published method[1] to correctly determine screw lengths in distal radius fractures. Their study shows that a longitudinal angle of 15° is ideal to identify screw protrusion.

Although the study is solid, I don't agree with the authors that the method is simple; I find it actually quite difficult or even impossible to perform with smaller fluoroscopes. My preferred method is to put in screws that are 2 to 4 mm shorter than the actual measurement. I think that this is possible for 2 reasons. First, there is solid biomechanic evidence that screws that are only 75% of the ideal length provide the same strength as bicortical fixation. Second, in many fractures there is no true bicortical fixation anyway. For me, choosing shorter screws seems much less cumbersome than the dorsal horizon view.

K. Megerle, MD, PhD

Reference

1. Wall LB, Brodt MD, Silva MJ, Boyer MI, Calfee RP. The effects of screw length on stability of simulated osteoporotic distal radius fractures fixed with volar locking plates. *J Hand Surg Am.* 2012;37:446-453.

A Simple Method for Choosing Treatment of Distal Radius Fractures
Kodama N, Imai S, Matsusue Y (Shiga Univ of Med Science, Japan)
J Hand Surg 38A:1896-1905, 2013

Purpose.—To design an easy-to-use guide for decision making in distal radius fractures in patients older than 50 years and to retrospectively analyze its ability to predict treatment in 164 patients.

Methods.—The present study consisted of 4 parts. The first part was a review of the literature to identify possible important factors that predict treatment outcome of distal radius fractures in patients 50 years old and older. The second part identified which of these first-tier factors that orthopedic surgeons consider to be important by a questionnaire that was sent to 83 orthopedic surgeons qualified by the Japanese Orthopedic Association with response rate of 61%. The third part further identified which of the subsets of factors best predict outcome in a retrospective study of 41 patients 50 years old or older, yielding a final subset of factors to create a scoring system. The fourth part of the study then evaluated the ability of this scoring system to predict the outcome as evaluated by the modified Mayo wrist score and the Disabilities of the Arm, Shoulder and Hand score in a retrospective study of 164 distal radius fractures in patients 50 years old or older.

Results.—The 164 patients were divided into 4 groups by the present scoring system: conservative group, relative conservative group, relative surgical group, and surgical group according to the recommended therapeutic modalities. Clinical outcomes of those that followed the recommendation of the present scoring system resulted in favorable consequences. In contrast, the outcomes of those not following the recommendation were inferior.

Conclusions.—The present scoring system may be used as an easy-to-use decision-making tool when choosing conservative or surgical treatment for distal radius fractures.

▶ The authors present a guide to aid decision making in older patients with fractures of the distal radius. Personally, I think that the scientific value of this study is limited. The authors performed a survey in the Japanese community regarding which factors the members thought were pertinent to the treatment of distal radius fractures and then weighted some of the factors subjectively to construct the scoring system. The scoring system, therefore, might be broken down to this: all fractures that are unstable or show intra-articular displacement should be treated operatively. The (well-known) main problem with distal fractures remains that there is no recognized relationship between suboptimal reduction and clinical outcome. Personally, I aim to restore the original anatomy as well possible with the idea that the original anatomy will have the highest probability of a good clinical outcome. Interestingly, this seems to be consistent with the authors' findings, because patients treated operatively (assuming that the anatomy could be improved) showed equal or better outcomes in all subgroups.

K. Megerle, MD, PhD

Volar Plate Position and Flexor Tendon Rupture Following Distal Radius Fracture Fixation

Kitay A, Swanstrom M, Schreiber JJ, et al (Hosp for Special Surgery, NY)
J Hand Surg 38A:1091-1096, 2013

Purpose.—To determine whether there were differences between plate position in patients who had postoperative flexor tendon ruptures following volar plate fixation of distal radius fractures and those who did not.

Methods.—Three blinded reviewers measured the volar plate prominence and position on the lateral radiographs of 8 patients treated for flexor tendon ruptures and 17 matched control patients without ruptures following distal radius fracture fixation. We graded plate prominence using the Soong grading system, and we measured the distances between the plate and both the volar critical line and the volar rim of the distal radius.

Results.—A higher Soong grade was associated with flexor tendon rupture. Patients with ruptures had plates that were more prominent volarly and more distal than matched controls without ruptures. Plate prominence projecting greater than 2.0 mm volar to the critical line had a sensitivity of 0.88, a specificity of 0.82, and positive and negative predictive values of 0.70 and 0.93, respectively, for tendon ruptures. Plate position distal to 3.0 mm from the volar rim had a sensitivity of 0.88, a specificity of 0.94, and positive and negative predictive values of 0.88 and 0.94, respectively, for tendon ruptures.

Conclusions.—We identified plate positions associated with attritional flexor tendon rupture following distal radius fracture fixation with volar plates. To decrease rupture risk, we recommend considering elective hardware removal after union in symptomatic patients with plate prominence greater than 2.0 mm volar to the critical line or plate position within 3.0 mm of the volar rim.

Type of Study/Level of Evidence.—Therapeutic III.

▶ This article is significant in that it essentially deconstructs the Soong grade into 2 important parameters (plate to volar critical line [PCL] distance and plate to volar rim [PVR] distance) the high values of which may predict the incidence of flexor tendon rupture after volar plate fixation of distal radius fractures.

Strengths of this study include the relatively larger number of cases with flexor tendon ruptures compared with those of previous studies and the methodical calculation of the discussed parameters. A weakness is its retrospective design.

Like the Soong grade, these parameters are important to keep in mind during the repair of distal radius fractures to prevent the devastating complication of flexor tendon rupture. To decrease the chance of flexor tendon rupture, the authors recommend elective hardware removal after a minimum of 6 months after fracture repair in those cases in which the plate prominence is greater than 2.0 mm volar to the critical line or the plate position is within 3.0 mm of the volar rim.

Like most other surgeons who fix distal radius fractures, I am extremely aware of where I position the volar plate relative to the volar rim to minimize the risk of flexor tendon rupture. I always err on making the plate more proximal than distal when possible, although there are sometimes cases in which you have no choice but to position the plate as distally as possible to capture distal fragments, such as the lunate facet. In these cases, I routinely remove the plate 6 months after repair.

S. S. Shin, MD, MMSc

Volar Plate Fixation for the Treatment of Distal Radius Fractures: Analysis of Adverse Events

Tarallo L, Mugnai R, Zambianchi F, et al (Univ of Modena and Reggio Emilia, Italy; et al)
J Orthop Trauma 27:740-745, 2013

Objectives.—Determining the rate of specific adverse events after volar plating performed for distal radius fractures.

Design.—Retrospective.

Setting.—University level I trauma center.

Patients.—We searched the electronic database of all surgical procedures performed in our department using the following keywords: distal radius fracture, wrist fracture, and plate fixation. We identified 315 patients, 12 of whom were lost at follow-up.

Intervention.—Volar plate fixation for the treatment of distal radius fractures.

Main Outcome Measurements.—At an average follow-up of 5 years, 303 patients were evaluated through medical records and clinical and radiographic assessment for specific adverse events after volar plate fixation.

Results.—Adverse events were observed in 18 patients (5.9%). Implant-related adverse events, including tendon impairments, intra-articular screws, and screw loosening, were observed in 15 patients (5.0%). Extensor tendon impairments were represented by 5 cases of extensor tenosynovitis and 3 cases of rupture of the extensor pollicis longus due to screws protruding dorsally. Flexor impairments were represented by 2 cases of tenosynovitis and 2 cases of flexor pollicis longus rupture. Screw penetration into the radioulnar joint was observed in 1 case. Loss of reduction was identified in 3 cases. One patient had a deep postoperative infection treated with operative debridement. One patient experienced injury to the median nerve during routine implant removal unrelated to tendon issues.

Conclusions.—The majority of adverse events after volar plate fixation were due to technical errors in implant placement. In our cohort, tendon impairments were the most frequently observed; among these, extensor tendon impairments were the most represented (50% of all adverse events). All 12 tendon-related adverse events were due to technical shortcomings with implant placement.

Level of Evidence.—Therapeutic Level IV. See Instructions for Authors for a complete description of levels of evidence.

▶ The authors report a retrospective review of patients treated at their institution and find (like other recent reviews) that the bulk of a relatively low complication rate of 5.9% may be attributed to primarily technical errors. Most are problems and ruptures of the dorsal tendons. Whereas this might be counterintuitive, as volar positioning has likely issues related to volar tendon problems, it speaks to the need for vigilance with plate and screw fixation. Special views such as an angled lateral and an axial view that provide more information about the dorsal anatomy are worth heeding. The median nerve damage at incidental hardware removal requiring nerve grafting is vexing. The authors deserve a nod for telling the story.

A. Ladd, MD

Comparison of a New Intramedullary Scaffold to Volar Plating for Treatment of Distal Radius Fractures

van Kampen RJ, Thoreson AR, Knutson NJ, et al (Mayo Clinic, Rochester, MN; Conventus Orthopaedics, Inc, Maple Grove, MN)
J Orthop Trauma 27:535-541, 2013

Objectives.—To compare the biomechanical properties of a new nitinol intramedullary (IM) scaffold implant with those of volar plates for the treatment of dorsally comminuted extra-articular distal radius fractures using an established model.

Methods.—A dorsal wedge osteotomy was performed on a bone model to simulate a dorsally comminuted extra-articular distal radius fracture. This model was used to compare stiffness of 3 different distal radius fixation devices—an IM scaffold implant, a commercially available titanium volar locking plate, and a stainless steel non-locking T-plate. Six constructs were tested per group. Tolerance for physiological loading was assessed by applying 10,000 cycles of axial loading up to 100 N applied at 2 Hz. Axial and eccentric load stiffness were assessed before cyclic loading and axial stiffness again after cyclic loading. Groups were compared using analysis of variance.

Results.—Initial axial stiffness (in Newton per millimeter) was significantly $(P = 0.011)$ different only between the volar locking plate (427 ± 43) and non-locking T-plate (235 ± 69). After cyclic loading, axial stiffness was not significantly different between the volar locking plate (392 ± 67) and IM scaffold implant (405 ± 108), but both were significantly $(P < 0.001)$ stiffer than the non-locking T-plate (187 ± 53). Eccentric loading stiffness was not significantly different between the IM scaffold implant (67 ± 140) and volar locking plate (63 ± 5), but both were significantly $(P < 0.001)$ stiffer than the non-locking T-plate (25 ± 4).

Conclusions.—Stiffness of the IM scaffold implant and volar locking plate fracture model constructs was equivalent. Biomechanical testing suggests that this novel IM scaffold provides sufficient stability for clinical use, and further testing is warranted.

▶ This is a report examining the biomechanical properties of a relatively novel implant designed for distal radius fracture fixation in an artificial bone fracture model. Conceptually, the novel implant, DRS System by Conventus, supports fractured distal radii via an intramedullary nitinol scaffold and cannulated screws placed after the implant is expanded to fill the metaphyseal defect. The hypothetical advantage of this implant is avoiding a high percentage of the metal external to the distal radius, as is required in all forms of distal radius plating, hypothetically minimizing the resultant soft tissue complications. Minimizing tendon complications is one of the reasons behind the trend in the last decade or more of increasing use of volar locking plates. However, complications have been reported with all forms of distal radius plating. With this one biomechanical model, the DRS implant appeared to have similar biomechanical characteristics to a commonly used titanium volar locking plate and to be superior to a conventional stainless steel volar plate. It is unclear why the authors chose a volar nonlocking plate, as there is very little or no role for that type of implant for fractures that are simulated by this model. Nevertheless, the biomechanical results are similar enough to the volar locking plate that a clinical series of fractures comparing the 2 types of fixation is expected. This article does not address in any way some of the clinical concerns with this implant including its performance in very osteoporotic bone and in fractures with non-displaced or displaced intra-articular fractures.

P. Blazar, MD

Prospective Evaluation of Pronator Quadratus Repair Following Volar Plate Fixation of Distal Radius Fractures
Tosti R, Ilyas AM (Temple Univ School of Medicine, Philadelphia, PA; Thomas Jefferson Univ, Philadelphia, PA)
J Hand Surg 38A:1678-1684, 2013

Purpose.—To evaluate the efficacy of pronator quadratus (PQ) repair after volar plating of distal radius fractures.

Methods.—All consecutive distal radius fractures treated operatively with a volar plate during a 1-year period were assigned to receive a repair of the PQ versus no repair. Surgical exposure, reduction, and postoperative rehabilitation were equivalent in both groups. Clinical outcomes with a minimum follow-up of 12 months were assessed via range of motion; grip strength; Disabilities of the Arm, Shoulder, and Hand (DASH) scores; and visual analog scale (VAS) scores.

Results.—A total of 60 consecutive distal radius fractures were treated operatively with a locking volar plate. Full follow-up data were available for 33 patients in the PQ repair group and 24 patients in the control group. At 12 months, the mean DASH score was 8 for the repair group and 5 for the control group. Range of motion at the wrist, grip strength, and VAS scores were also not significantly different between groups. In addition, we found no significant differences in any of the parameters at the 2-, 6-, or 12-week intervals, although we observed greater grip strength and wrist flexion in the repair group at 6 weeks. Reoperation was required for 4 patients in the repair group and 1 in the control group.

Conclusions.—Pronator quadratus repair after volar plating of a distal radius fractures did not significantly improve postoperative range of motion, grip strength, or DASH and VAS scores at 1 year. The rates of reoperation between groups were not significantly different.

▶ This article prospectively evaluated 60 consecutive operatively treated distal radius fractures using 2 different variable angle volar plating systems, with or without pronator quadratus (PQ) repair. The authors followed up with 57 of 60 patients for 1 year, with outcomes measures including range of motion, grip strength, Disabilities of the Arm, Shoulder, and Hand scores, and visual analog scale (VAS) scores. They report no statistically significant differences except for greater grip strength and wrist flexion in the PQ repair group at 6 weeks. At 1 year, however, no differences were noted. They also report no statistically significant differences in reoperation rates, although 4 patients in the repair group required reoperation compared with one in the control group. None of the patients suffered any flexor tendon-related issues. The authors conclude that there is no scientific evidence to support PQ repair. The authors appropriately point out that 1-year follow-up may not be long enough to show late flexor tendon rupture or tenosynovitis.

This reasonably well-done study calls into question the routine PQ repair after volar plate fixation of the distal radius fracture. It is clear that plates should be positioned proximal to the watershed line, and volar tilt must be restored to avoid plate prominence and likely subsequent flexor tendon-related complications. These 2 principles are far more important than PQ repair, but, as surgeons, I believe we should strive to restore anatomy as best as possible, and thus I continue to routinely repair the PQ where possible.

D. Zelouf, MD

Outcomes After Volar Plate Fixation of Low-grade Open and Closed Distal Radius Fractures Are Similar

Kim JK, Park SD (Ewha Womans Univ School of Medicine, Seoul, Korea)
Clin Orthop Relat Res 471:2030-2035, 2013

Background.—Low-grade (Gustilo and Anderson Type I or II) open distal radius fractures (DRFs) have been treated by volar locking plate fixation. However, it is unclear whether the outcomes after volar locking plate fixation for low-grade open DRFs are comparable to those for closed DRFs.

Questions/Purposes.—We asked whether low-grade open DRFs had worse DASH scores and higher infection rates than closed DRFs when the DRFs were treated by volar plate fixation.

Methods.—Twenty consecutive patients treated by volar locking plate fixation for low-grade open DRFs constituted the open fracture group, and 40 patients were selected from among the total number of patients treated by volar, locking plate fixation for closed DRFs as the closed fracture group. Complications including infection were recorded. Clinical outcomes and radiographic assessments were performed postoperatively at 3 months and 1 year.

Results.—At 3 postoperative months, wrist flexion and extension, grip strengths, and DASH scores were better in the closed fracture group; however, no difference was observed postoperatively between the two groups in terms of any functional outcome measure at 1 year. Any of the radiographic parameters were not different between the groups. There were no differences in infection rate and in any other complication rate between the groups.

Conclusions.—Although functional outcomes of open DRFs were inferior to those of closed DRFs at 3 months, at 1 year, outcomes of low-grade open DRFs were found to be comparable to those of closed DRFs when volar plate fixation was used.

▶ This article assessed the effect of a low-grade open injury on outcomes with distal radius fractures treated with volar plate fixation. This study has several strengths. The matched design helps eliminate bias from other factors that may affect outcome, a reliable outcome measure (Disabilities of the Arm, Shoulder and Hand [DASH]) was used, and a blinded assessor was used to evaluate outcomes. Unfortunately, this study was only powered for the primary outcome (DASH scores) and not adequately powered to assess infection rates (66% power). The authors state that all open fractures were treated within 48 hours; however, the mean time to open reduction and internal fixation was not given, and it would be interesting to know how urgently these injuries were taken to the operating room. Overall, this study helps surgeons inform patients with low-grade open injuries that they may have a slower recovery of pain and function. However, in the long term (1 year), they can expect good outcomes. Unfortunately, we cannot definitively say that the infection risk is not increased, as the study was underpowered for this finding. Further evidence is needed to determine how urgently these injuries need to be taken to the operating room, as the risk of infection still worries most surgeons.

R. Grewal, MD, MSc

Effect of early administration of alendronate after surgery for distal radial fragility fracture on radiological fracture healing time
Uchiyama S, Itsubo T, Nakamura K, et al (Shinshu Univ School of Medicine, Matsumoto, Japan)
Bone Joint J 95-B:1544-1550, 2013

This multicentre prospective clinical trial aimed to determine whether early administration of alendronate (ALN) delays fracture healing after surgical treatment of fractures of the distal radius. The study population comprised 80 patients (four men and 76 women) with a mean age of 70 years (52 to 86) with acute fragility fractures of the distal radius requiring open reduction and internal fixation with a volar locking plate and screws. Two groups of 40 patients each were randomly allocated either to receive once weekly oral ALN administration (35 mg) within a few days after surgery and continued for six months, or oral ALN administration delayed until four months after surgery. Postero-anterior and lateral radiographs of the affected wrist were taken monthly for six months after surgery. No differences between groups was observed with regard to gender ($p = 1.0$), age ($p = 0.916$), fracture classification ($p = 0.274$) or bone mineral density measured at the spine ($p = 0.714$). The radiographs were assessed by three independent assessors. There were no significant differences in the mean time to complete cortical bridging observed between the ALN group (3.5 months (SE 0.16)) and the no-ALN group (3.1 months (SE 0.15)) ($p = 0.068$). All the fractures healed in the both groups by the last follow-up. Improvement of the Quick-Disabilities of the Arm, Shoulder and Hand (QuickDASH) score, grip strength, wrist range of movement, and tenderness over the fracture site did not differ between the groups over the six-month period. Based on our results, early administration of ALN after surgery for distal radius fracture did not appear to delay fracture healing times either radiologically or clinically.

▶ This randomized trial by Uchiyama et al concludes that early initiation of bisphosphonate treatment has no effect on the clinical or radiographic outcomes of distal radius fractures treated with volar plate fixation. Because bisphosphonates suppress both bone resorption and formation, controversy surrounds their use in the immediate postfracture period. Most patients with distal radius fractures have osteopenia or osteoporosis at the time of injury and benefit from treatment for their low bone mineral density.

This study adds to a growing body of literature supporting the use of bisphosphonates after fracture without any detrimental effects on fracture healing. This report is unique in that it includes patients with normal bone density and osteopenia in addition to those with an established diagnosis of osteoporosis.

Because most patients with distal radius fractures are osteopenic, the study provides important evidence that treatment with alendronate is safe in this specific patient population. Demonstrating that immediate postoperative treatment with alendronate does not impair fracture healing will hopefully ensure that orthopedic surgeons do not miss a valuable opportunity to initiate treatment for underlying abnormalities in bone metabolism immediately after a fracture occurs. Additional strengths include a comprehensive definition of fracture healing, including both clinical and radiographic criteria.

Weaknesses include short follow-up, which does not allow an assessment of long-term complications associated with bisphosphonate use (eg, atypical fractures). Also, the authors treated patients with 35 mg of alendronate weekly rather than the typical dose of 70 mg recommended to treat osteoporosis. Their rationale for this and the rationale for continuing treatment for only 6 months are not clear. Furthermore, the authors included both men and women in their analysis despite the fact that 95% of patients were women. Despite these limitations, this study supports the early initiation of bisphosphonate treatment after operative fixation for distal radius fractures in patients older than 50.

T. D. Rozental, MD

The Mechanical Stability of Extra-Articular Distal Radius Fractures With Respect to the Number of Screws Securing the Distal Fragment
Crosby SN, Fletcher ND, Yap ER, et al (Vanderbilt Univ Med Ctr, Nashville, TN)
J Hand Surg 38A:1097-1105, 2013

Purpose.—The treatment of distal radius fractures with volar locked plating (VLP) has gained popularity. Many different designs and sizes of plates afford a wide variety of configurations of locking screws that can be placed into the distal fracture fragment. The purpose of this study was to determine whether using half of the distal locking screws decreased stability when compared with using all possible distal locking screws with 4 different VLP systems.

Methods.—Twenty-four identical synthetic distal radius sawbone models were instrumented with 1 of 4 designs of VLP devices over a standardized dorsal wedge osteotomy to simulate a dorsally comminuted, extra-articular distal radius fracture. Distal locking screws were placed in varying configurations. Six radii per plate model with different screw configurations then underwent axial loading, volar bending, and dorsal bending using a servohydraulic machine. Distal fragment displacement was recorded using a differential variable reluctance transducer.

Results.—There was no significant difference in fracture fragment displacement when using half of the distal locking screw set compared with using the full screw set. Mean differences in displacement between half and full screws were less than 0.1 mm. All configurations had the greatest magnitude of displacement during axial loading. Mean displacement was less in plates containing 2 rows of distal locking screws (−0.4 mm) compared with plates containing 1 row (−0.6 mm).

Conclusions.—Using half of the distal locking screws in VLP in an extra-articular, nonosteoporotic distal radial fracture model with noncyclical, nondestructive loading does not decrease construct stability compared with using all of the screws. Not filling all holes in VLP is more cost effective and does not sacrifice plate stiffness or construct stability. Plates with 2 rows of distal locking screws create more stable fixation than plates with 1 row of distal locking screws.

▶ This study compares construct stability in saw bones with simulated extra-articular distal radius fractures treated with volar locking plates with the use of either all or half of the distal bicortical locking screws. The authors tested 4 different volar locking plates and report no clinically significant differences in fracture displacement in constructs in which all distal screws were placed vs those that had only half of the distal locking screws placed.

In the current health care climate in which cost is of paramount importance, this study reinforces prior work[1] showing that it is not necessary to fill every plate hole with a screw in order to achieve stability. Furthermore, there are few differences between plates, leaving the choice of implant to the individual surgeon's choice.

The study limitations include the fact that the model simulated extra-articular fractures, yet prior work has found similar results in cadaveric models with intra-articular injuries. As the authors correctly point out, it is difficult to determine whether their findings can be extrapolated to osteoporotic bone or more comminuted fracture patterns. In addition, the authors did not study the influence of screw length on construct stability. For simple fractures in healthy bone, however, the results indicate that limited use of distal screws may provide adequate fixation at a lower cost and with fewer potential complications.

T. Rozental, MD

Reference

1. Moss DP, Means KR Jr, Parks BG, Forthman CL. A biomechanical comparison of volar locked plating of intra-articular distal radius fractures: use of 4 versus 7 screws for distal fixation. *J Hand Surg Am.* 2011;36:1907-1911. Epub 2011 Oct 22. Source: Curtis National Hand Center, Union Memorial Hospital, Baltimore, MD 21218, USA.

Volar Locking Plates Versus External Fixation and Adjuvant Pin Fixation in Unstable Distal Radius Fractures: A Randomized, Controlled Study

Williksen JH, Frihagen F, Hellund JC, et al (Oslo Univ Hosp, Norway)
J Hand Surg 38A:1469-1476, 2013

Purpose.—To determine whether volar locking plates are superior to external fixation with adjuvant pins in the treatment of unstable distal radius fractures.

Methods.—A total of 111 unstable distal radius fractures were randomized to treatment with external fixation (EF) using adjuvant pins or with a volar locking plate (VLP). The mean age of the patients was 54 years (range, 20—84 y). Seven patients were lost to follow-up. At 1 year, 104 patients were assessed with a visual analog scale pain score, Mayo wrist score, Quick-Disabilities of the Arm, Shoulder, and Hand (*Quick*DASH), range of motion, and radiological evaluation. The *Quick*DASH score at 52 weeks was the primary outcome measure.

Results.—The operative time in the EF group was 77 minutes, compared with 88 minutes in the VLP group. At 52 weeks, patients with VLPs had a higher Mayo wrist score (90 vs 85), better supination (89° vs 85°), and less radial shortening (+1.4 mm vs +2.2 mm). There were more patients with pain over the ulnar styloid in the EF group (16 vs 6 patients). For AO type C2/C3, the patients with VLPs had better supination (90° vs 76°) and less ulnar shortening (+1.1 mm vs +2.8 mm). The complication rate was 30% in the EF group, compared with 29% in the VLP group. Eight (15%) plates were removed due to complications. The *Quick*DASH score was not significantly different between the groups.

Conclusions.—Although we did not find a significant difference between the groups for the *Quick*DASH score, we believe that our results support the use of VLPs for the treatment of unstable distal radius fractures. A serious concern is that some patients will have to have their plates removed; therefore, improving the surgical technique is important.

Type of Study/Level of Evidence.—Therapeutic I.

▶ The study present results from a randomized trial comparing volar plate fixation with external fixation and pinning for AO type A and C fractures of the distal radius. The trial demonstrated no difference in the primary outcome (*Quick*DASH score) between groups at one year. The volar plate group did, however, have higher Mayo wrist scores and better radiographic reductions than the external fixation group, particularly for more complex fracture patterns. Complications were similar among groups.

The authors are to be commended for designing and executing a successful clinical trial. They were able to enroll a large number of patients and achieved excellent follow-up. The study adds to an expanding body of literature showing that outcomes one year after operative treatment for distal radius fractures are similar irrespective of the type of fixation used.

Study limitations include the lack of a comparison between groups to ensure that the demographic and fracture characteristics were similar as well as the lack of an intermediate time point to determine whether early outcomes are different between groups. This would support the current belief that volar plate fixation allows a faster return to function and that most of the benefit with plate fixation is seen in the first few months after injury. Furthermore, the authors provide little detail surrounding complications. In particular, the reasons for which plates necessitated removal are not clearly described. Details would be helpful in substantiating the authors' comment that the surgical technique requires improvement.

T. D. Rozental, MD

The Effect of Acute Distal Radioulnar Joint Laxity on Outcome After Volar Plate Fixation of Distal Radius Fractures

Kim JK, Yi JW, Jeon SH (Ewha Womans Univ, Seoul, Korea)
J Orthop Trauma 27:735-739, 2013

Objectives.—The objective of this study was to determine whether intraoperative laxity of the distal radioulnar joint (DRUJ) is associated with adverse postoperative outcomes after volar plate fixation of a distal radius fracture (DRF) and 4 weeks of immobilization.

Designs.—Prospective study with clinical and radiographic assessment.

Setting.—Level 1 trauma center.

Patients.—One hundred consecutive patients were treated by volar locking plate fixation at our institution for an unstable DRF from April 2007 to November 2009. Of these patients, 84 patients with a minimum follow-up of 12 months were enrolled in this study.

Intervention.—Intraoperative DRUJ laxity was evaluated using a radio-ulnar stress test after fixation of DRF using volar locking plate and splint immobilization of the forearm for 1 month in patients with intraoperative DRUJ laxity. Patients were allocated to an unstable group or stable group according to the presence of intraoperative DRUJ laxity.

Main Outcome Measurements.—Our primary outcome measure was disabilities of arm, shoulder, and hand score and the secondary outcome measures were wrist motion, grip strength, modified Mayo wrist score, visual analogue scale for wrist pain, and ongoing pain in the DRUJ.

Results.—Nineteen of the 84 study subjects were allocated to the unstable group and 65 to the stable group. No significant differences were observed between 2 groups in wrist range of motion, grip strength, modified Mayo wrist score, disabilities of arm, shoulder, and hand score, visual analogue scale score, and ongoing pain in the DRUJ at 1 year postoperatively.

Conclusions.—In our series of patients treated with volar locking plate and immobilization of the forearm for 1 month in patients with intraoperative laxity of the DRUJ, laxity did not affect impairment, pain, or disability 1 year after fracture. However, the role of postoperative immobilization of the forearm is debatable and merits additional study.

Level of Evidence.—Prognostic Level I.

▶ This prospective study looking at the nonoperative management of distal radioulnar joint (DRUJ) laxity after volar plate fixation of distal radius fractures is a very good study in my opinion. Strengths of this study include its prospective nature, the consistent management strategy, validated outcome measurements, the use of arthroscopy to identify triangular fibrocartilage complex (TFCC) tears, and the correlation of DRUJ laxity with TFCC tears (including type of tear), ulnar styloid fractures (including base vs distal), and 1-year follow-up data. This study corroborates the growing body of literature in a well-designed study supporting nonoperative management of DRUJ laxity as well as associated ulnar styloid and TFCC tears.

Perhaps the biggest concern I have with this study is the widespread application of this message and not discussing the difference between laxity and instability. We have all stressed the DRUJ after surgery and find it increased in laxity compared with the opposite side, but I would argue this is very different from true DRUJ instability. When the DRUJ can be dislocated and reduced with stress, I feel it is a different scenario that warrants a different treatment strategy (open reduction and internal fixation of the styloid base fracture or TFCC repair). The authors do not attempt to grade the laxity (admittedly very subjective) but also do not report any cases of instability.

This report also shows some interesting associations. I was surprised to see that they found no association between ulnar styloid base fractures and DRUJ laxity. Furthermore, the presence of an ulnar styloid fracture wasn't statistically associated with the presence of a TFCC tear.

My practice has been evolving in this area over the last few years. I used to routinely fix all ulnar styloid base fractures, then only those with laxity or instability. Recently I have begun only treating those with an unstable DRUJ and simply splinting DRUJ laxity for 4 to 6 weeks similar to the authors' strategy. This report makes me feel more comfortable with this approach, although I still feel true instability should be approached in a different manner.

G. Gaston, MD

A descriptive study on wrist and hand sensori-motor impairment and function following distal radius fracture intervention
Karagiannopoulos C, Sitler M, Michlovitz S, et al (OrthopediCare Clinic, Chalfont, PA; Temple Univ, Philadelphia, PA; Cayuga Hand Therapy PT, Ithaca, NY)
J Hand Ther 26:204-215, 2013

Study Design.—Descriptive cross-sectional design.

Introduction.—Wrist and hand sensori-motor impairment have been observed after distal radius fracture (DRF) treatment. This impairment and its relationship to function lack research.

Purpose of the Study.—The primary aim of this exploratory study was to determine the magnitude of wrist and hand sensori-motor impairment following surgical and non-surgical treatment among older patients following DRF. Secondary aims were to determine the relationship between wrist and hand sensori-motor impairment with function and pain as well as the relationships among wrist and hand sensori-motor impairment and function and age following DRF.

Methods.—Ten Test (TT), active joint position sense (JPS), electromyography (EMG), computerized hand-grip dynamometer (CHD), and the Patient-Rated Wrist Evaluation (PRWE) were used to assess twenty-four female participants 8 weeks following DRF treatment and their 24 matched-control healthy counterparts on wrist and hand sensibility, proprioception, muscle recruitment, grip force, muscle fatigue, and functional status.

Results.—Participants following DRF demonstrated significantly (p <.05) greater sensory (i.e., JPS, TT), and motor (i.e., EMG, CHD) deficits than their control counterparts. A significantly higher functional deficit (i.e., PRWE) also existed among participants following DRF than the control group. Participants following surgical and non-surgical DRF treatment were found to be statistically different only on total grip force. Group differences on JPS and total grip force revealed the strongest effect size with the highest correlations to PRWE. EMG and muscle fatigue ratio group differences revealed a weaker effect size with a fair degree of correlation to PRWE. Pain significantly correlated with sensori-motor function. Age did not correlate with any measured variable.

Conclusions.—Significant wrist and hand sensori-motor impairment and functional deficits among older females 8 weeks following DRF surgical and non-surgical interventions were revealed. JPS and total grip force were the most clinically meaningful tests for assessing the sensori-motor status as well as explaining functional disability and pain levels for these patients.

Level of Evidence.—2c.

▶ In this descriptive cross-sectional study, the authors were primarily trying to determine the magnitude of wrist and hand sensorimotor impairment after surgical and nonsurgical treatment among older patients after distal radius fractures (DRFs). The sample was comprised of 48 female participants ranging in age from 50 to 83 years. All participants were tested 8 weeks after their respective DRF treatment. They were equally divided into surgical, nonsurgical, and control groups. Sensory function was assessed using the Ten Test and joint position sense (JPS), and motor function was tested via muscle electromyography, muscle coactivations, and computerized hand grip dynamometer (total grip force, muscle fatigue). The Patient-Rated Wrist Evaluation questionnaire was used to determine function. The authors concluded that both the surgical and nonsurgical groups showed significant wrist and hand sensorimotor impairment and functional deficits compared with their control group counterpart. They found that the JPS and total grip force were the most clinically useful tools in assessing the sensorimotor status and explaining the functional disability levels for these patients.

The surgical group in this study had therapy initiated starting 7 days postoperatively, and the nonsurgical group did not have any therapy until 6 weeks after casting intervention of the DRF. This left a noted difference in time in which the surgical group had 50% longer period before study testing to participate in physical therapy compared with the nonsurgical group that had only 2 weeks of therapy before testing (specific therapeutic treatment was not revealed). Participants in the nonsurgical group would most likely present with greater deficits in stiffness, swelling, and muscular atrophy compared with the surgical group. This, in turn, could contribute to sensorimotor deficits and would account for the greater deficit found in grip force compared with the surgical group (35% and 65%, respectively).

The study did not state this, but I wonder how patients with underlying carpometacarpal osteoarthritis (CMC OA) fared in this study. In assessing total grip force area and muscle fatigue ratio, participants were asked to sustain their grip force as hard as possible for 30 seconds on the computerized handgrip dynamometer (CHD). This can be very challenging and painful for the patient with CMC OA, and, as we know, the propensity of women over the age of 50 who have CMC OA is quite high.

I found it interesting that the JPS test was one of the most clinically meaningful indicators of impairment assessed in the study. This is not something we typically perform in our clinic when treating DRF, but given the simplicity of the test, it may be worthwhile to add to our regime as an additional useful assessment tool in our clinic.

C. Gordon, OTR/L, CHT

A retrospective cohort investigation of active range of motion within one week of open reduction and internal fixation of distal radius fractures
Driessens S, Diserens-Chew T, Burton C, et al (Logan Hosp, Queensland, Australia; et al)
J Hand Ther 26:225-231, 2013

Distal radius fractures stabilized by open reduction internal fixation (ORIF) have become increasingly common. There is currently no consensus on the optimal time to commence range of motion (ROM) exercises post-ORIF.

A retrospective cohort review was conducted over a five-year period to compare wrist and forearm range of motion outcomes and number of therapy sessions between patients who commenced active ROM exercises within the first seven days and from day eight onward following ORIF of distal radius fractures.

One hundred and twenty-one patient cases were identified. Clinical data, active ROM at initial and discharge therapy assessments, fracture type, surgical approaches, and number of therapy sessions attended were recorded.

One hundred and seven (88.4%) cases had complete datasets. The early active ROM group ($n = 37$) commenced ROM a mean (SD) of 4.27 (1.8) days post-ORIF. The comparator group ($n = 70$) commenced ROM exercises 24.3 (13.6) days post-ORIF. No significant differences were identified between groups in ROM at initial or discharge assessments, or therapy sessions attended. The results from this study indicate that patients who commenced active ROM exercises an average of 24 days after surgery achieved comparable ROM outcomes with similar number of therapy sessions to those who commenced ROM exercises within the first week.

Level of Evidence.—2B, retrospective cohort.

▶ This retrospective study out of Australia focuses on the timeframes of initiating active range of motion (AROM) after open reduction internal fixation (ORIF) for distal radius fractures. The authors chose to compare 2 groups:

the early AROM group, which began ROM exercises within 7 days postoperative, at a mean of 4.27 days, and the group that began AROM after the first 7 days postoperative, at a mean of 24.3 days. They hypothesized that early intervention with controlled AROM exercises may lead to improved function and that prolonged rest may slow recovery of function. The study was limited to measures of ROM only. The authors found that the early AROM group had similar ROM at discharge to those who started therapy later and that the groups required the same number of therapy sessions to achieve results. However, because no outcome studies were used, they were unable to determine functional levels during therapy and after discharge.

This study allows the hand therapist to appreciate early referrals for therapy post-ORIF for distal radius fracture and not become overly concerned if therapy is unable to be initiated until later in the healing phase. The authors note that their study results do not justify early AROM when there may be a risk because of concurrent injuries or when there are scheduling or transportation issues. However, early referrals may have benefits not addressed in this study, such as earlier return to function including work and overall patient satisfaction. Pain issues often reported postsurgically are not addressed in this study.

I was impressed that in this study the "late" group was determined to be those who started therapy from day 8 post-ORIF compared with an entire early group that started therapy within the first 7 days. More often it seems that referrals to therapy are received after suture removal at 10 to 14 days postoperative. It is good to know that many surgeons are now referring their postsurgical patients within the first 2 weeks, allowing for therapy to begin during the initial phase of tissue healing. Timely referral is certainly appreciated by hand therapists, as it allows us to encourage early mobility, often preventing long-term stiffness and delayed functional return. I look forward to more research from this group of authors.

S. J. Clark, OTR/L, CHT

Improved Fracture Risk Assessment Based on Nonlinear Micro-Finite Element Simulations From HRpQCT Images at the Distal Radius
Christen D, Melton LJ III, Zwahlen A, et al (Inst for Biomechanics, Zurich, Switzerland; Mayo Clinic, Rochester, MN)
J Bone Miner Res 28:2601-2608, 2013

More accurate techniques to estimate fracture risk could help reduce the burden of fractures in postmenopausal women. Although micro-finite element (µFE) simulations allow a direct assessment of bone mechanical performance, in this first clinical study we investigated whether the additional information obtained using geometrically and materially nonlinear µFE simulations allows a better discrimination between fracture cases and controls. We used patient data and high-resolution peripheral quantitative computed tomography (HRpQCT) measurements from our previous clinical study on fracture risk, which compared 100 postmenopausal women with a distal forearm fracture to 105 controls. Analyzing these data with

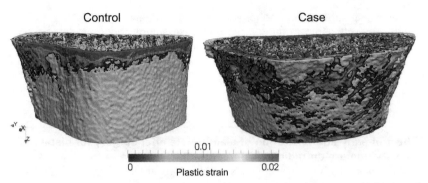

FIGURE 2.—Large plastic regions in the cortical bone. (Reproduced from Journal of Bone and Mineral Research. Christen D, Melton III LJ, Zwahlen A, et al. Improved fracture risk assessment based on nonlinear micro-finite element simulations from HRpQCT images at the distal radius. *J Bone Miner Res.* 2013;28:2601-2608, with permission from the American Society for Bone and Mineral Research.)

the nonlinear μFE simulations, the odds ratio (OR) for the factor-of-risk (yield load divided by the expected fall load) was marginally higher (1.99; 95% confidence interval [CI], 1.41−2.77) than for the factor-of-risk computed from linear μFE (1.89; 95% CI, 1.37−2.69). The yield load and the energy absorbed up to the yield point as computed from non-linear μFE were highly correlated with the initial stiffness ($R^2 = 0.97$ and 0.94, respectively) and could therefore be derived from linear simulations with little loss in precision. However, yield deformation was not related to any other measurement performed and was itself a good predictor of fracture risk (OR, 1.89; 95% CI, 1.39−2.63). Moreover, a combined risk score integrating information on relative bone strength (yield load-based factor-of-risk), bone ductility (yield deformation), and the structural integrity of the bone under critical loads (cortical plastic volume) improved the separation of cases and controls by one-third (OR, 2.66; 95% CI, 1.84−4.02). We therefore conclude that nonlinear μFE simulations provide important additional information on the risk of distal forearm fractures not accessible from linear μFE nor from other techniques assessing bone microstructure, density, or mass (Fig 2).

▶ This highly technical article is notable for 2 reasons: It highlights the importance of distal radius fractures as important predictors of osteoporosis (and future fractures) and suggests improved fragility fracture prediction based on the distal radius. Briefly, high-resolution peripheral quantitative computed tomography (HRpQCT) is more precise than dual-energy x-ray absorptiometry (DXA) in assessing bone mineral density. It is more expensive and largely relegated to research studies and has yet to attain clinically relevant status. HRpQCT provides more quantitative information, including regional differences such as cortical vs medullary bone and subchondral characteristics, whereas DXA measures an average of these features. As such, a DXA is largely useless for the distal radius; typically the shaft, not the critical metaphyseal subchondral bone, is measured if ordered on a DXA scan. This study suggests clinical utility based on reassessment of current data of distal radii (Fig 2) that will improve prediction and, ideally, treatment. As usual, the sticky wicket in changing the paradigm will likely be cost to institution and insurer alike.

A. Ladd, MD

Effect of early administration of alendronate after surgery for distal radial fragility fracture on radiological fracture healing time

Uchiyama S, Itsubo T, Nakamura K, et al (Shinshu Univ School of Medicine, Matsumoto, Japan)

Bone Joint J 95-B:1544-1550, 2013

This multicentre prospective clinical trial aimed to determine whether early administration of alendronate (ALN) delays fracture healing after surgical treatment of fractures of the distal radius. The study population comprised 80 patients (four men and 76 women) with a mean age of 70 years (52 to 86) with acute fragility fractures of the distal radius requiring open reduction and internal fixation with a volar locking plate and screws. Two groups of 40 patients each were randomly allocated either to receive once weekly oral ALN administration (35 mg) within a few days after surgery and continued for six months, or oral ALN administration delayed until four months after surgery. Postero-anterior and lateral radiographs of the affected wrist were taken monthly for six months after surgery. No differences between groups was observed with regard to gender ($p = 1.0$), age ($p = 0.916$), fracture classification ($p = 0.274$) or bone mineral density measured at the spine ($p = 0.714$). The radiographs were assessed by three independent assessors. There were no significant differences in the mean time to complete cortical bridging observed between the ALN group (3.5 months (SE 0.16)) and the no-ALN group (3.1 months (SE 0.15)) ($p = 0.068$). All the fractures healed in the both groups by the last follow-up. Improvement of the Quick-Disabilities of the Arm, Shoulder and Hand (QuickDASH) score, grip strength, wrist range of movement, and tenderness over the fracture site did not differ between the groups over the six-month period. Based on our results, early administration of ALN after surgery for distal radius fracture did not appear to delay fracture healing times either radiologically or clinically.

▶ This is a well-structured multicenter study evaluating the effects of early administration of alendronate (ALN) following distal radius fracture fixation. It is well established that many patients who sustain distal radius fractures are osteoporotic and will likely be candidates for pharmacologic treatment with bisphosphonates (eg, ALN). However, starting soon (while fracture is still healing) may delay union.

The authors were pleased to note that delayed union did not occur in patients treated with ALN within a few days of surgery versus placebo.

This study helps answer an important question and helps us feel more comfortable with treating patients with osteoporosis sooner rather than later, minimizing concerns of delayed union at the distal radius fracture site.

M. Rizzo, MD

Complications after volar locking plate fixation of distal radius fractures
Johnson NA, Cutler L, Dias JJ, et al (Leicester Royal Infirmary, UK)
Injury 45:528-533, 2014

Volar locking plates are an increasingly popular treatment for distal radius fractures. We reviewed complications observed after volar locking plate fixation in a busy teaching hospital. The purpose of the study was to assess whether complication rates after volar locking plate use in general, routine trauma practice were higher than published literature from expert users.

A retrospective review was carried out of patients treated with a volar locking plate between January 2009 and December 2010. The series included 206 procedures in 204 patients (77 males and 127 females) with mean age of 55 years (range 16—94). Surgery was performed by 18 different consultant surgeons and 11 registrars.

A total of 22 complications were observed in 20 patients with an overall complication rate of 9.7%. Seven (3.4%) patients developed tendon problems including four (1.9%) tendon ruptures. Four (1.9%) patients required re-operation for metalwork problems; four patients developed complex regional pain syndrome (CRPS). Three fracture reduction problems were noted. A total of 16 further operations were carried out for complications.

The overall complication rate was low even when surgery was done by many surgeons, suggesting that this is a safe and reproducible technique. This study provides information which can be used to counsel patients about risks, including those of tendon and metalwork problems. This allows patients to make an informed decision. Surgeons must have specific strategies to avoid these complications and remain vigilant so that these can be identified and managed early.

▶ Locked volar plating in the treatment of distal radius fractures has become the most common surgical method of fixation over the past 10 years. Like all surgeries, however, these procedures and method of fixation are not without risk. The aim of this retrospective study was to evaluate the complications associated with volar locking plate fixation among a cohort of multiple surgeons who were not expert users.

The study included 204 patients who underwent 206 surgeries. Twenty-two complications were noted, as follows: tendon injury in 7 cases (3.4%), hardware complications in 4 wrists (1.9%), complex regional pain syndrome in 4 wrists (1.9%), fractures with loss of reduction in 3 patients (1.4%), wound healing problems in 1 patient (.5%), 1 vascular injury (.5%), and irritation from the hardware after fixation of the ulnar styloid in 2 patients (1%).

The authors felt the complication rates were low enough to conclude that volar plate fixation method, even in the hands of surgeons who are not considered "experts" in the field, is a safe and reproducible technique.

M. Rizzo, MD

Intense Pain Soon After Wrist Fracture Strongly Predicts Who Will Develop Complex Regional Pain Syndrome: Prospective Cohort Study

Moseley GL, Herbert RD, Parsons T, et al (The Univ of South Australia, Adelaide; Neuroscience Res Australia, Randwick, New South Wales; Univ of Oxford, UK; et al)
J Pain 15:16-23, 2014

Complex regional pain syndrome (CRPS) is a distressing and difficult-to-treat complication of wrist fracture. Estimates of the incidence of CRPS after wrist fracture vary greatly. It is not currently possible to identify who will go on to develop CRPS after wrist fracture. In this prospective cohort study, a nearly consecutive sample of 1,549 patients presenting with wrist fracture to 1 of 3 hospital-based fracture clinics and managed nonsurgically was assessed within 1 week of fracture and followed up 4 months later. Established criteria were used to diagnose CRPS. The incidence of CRPS in the 4 months after wrist fracture was 3.8% (95% confidence interval = 2.9–4.8%). A prediction model based on 4 clinical assessments (pain, reaction time, dysynchiria, and swelling) discriminated well between patients who would and would not subsequently develop CRPS (c index .99). A simple assessment of pain intensity (0–10 numerical rating scale) provided nearly the same level of discrimination (c index .98). One in 26 patients develops CRPS within 4 months of nonsurgically managed wrist fracture. A pain score of ≥ 5 in the first week after fracture should be considered a "red flag" for CRPS.

Perspective.—This study shows that excessive baseline pain in the week after wrist fracture greatly elevates the risk of developing CRPS. Clinicians can consider a rating of greater than 5/10 to the question "What is your average pain over the last 2 days?" to be a "red flag" for CRPS.

▶ A prospective analysis was undertaken in 3 clinics to determine factors associated with the development of complex regional pain syndrome (CRPS) after distal radius fracture. The authors examined 4 clinical assessments: pain, reaction time, dysynchiria, and swelling. All fractures were treated conservatively, and all patients were assessed within 1 week of injury and at 4 months postinjury via phone conversation.

The authors concluded that higher pain levels (> 5 on 1–10 scale) were associated with increased risk of development of CRPS.

I applaud the prospective nature and volume of patients accumulated for this study. In addition, the statistical analysis seems valid. However, given that pain is subjective, one could conclude that the findings are intuitive and not surprising.

M. Rizzo, MD

A Simple Method for Choosing Treatment of Distal Radius Fractures
Kodama N, Imai S, Matsusue Y (Shiga Univ of Med Science, Japan)
J Hand Surg 38A:1896-1905, 2013

Purpose.—To design an easy-to-use guide for decision making in distal radius fractures in patients older than 50 years and to retrospectively analyze its ability to predict treatment in 164 patients.

Methods.—The present study consisted of 4 parts. The first part was a review of the literature to identify possible important factors that predict treatment outcome of distal radius fractures in patients 50 years old and older. The second part identified which of these first-tier factors that orthopedic surgeons consider to be important by a questionnaire that was sent to 83 orthopedic surgeons qualified by the Japanese Orthopedic Association with response rate of 61%. The third part further identified which of the subsets of factors best predict outcome in a retrospective study of 41 patients 50 years old or older, yielding a final subset of factors to create a scoring system. The fourth part of the study then evaluated the ability of this scoring system to predict the outcome as evaluated by the modified Mayo wrist score and the Disabilities of the Arm, Shoulder and Hand score in a retrospective study of 164 distal radius fractures in patients 50 years old or older.

Results.—The 164 patients were divided into 4 groups by the present scoring system: conservative group, relative conservative group, relative surgical group, and surgical group according to the recommended therapeutic modalities. Clinical outcomes of those that followed the recommendation of the present scoring system resulted in favorable consequences. In contrast, the outcomes of those not following the recommendation were inferior.

Conclusions.—The present scoring system may be used as an easy-to-use decision-making tool when choosing conservative or surgical treatment for distal radius fractures.

▶ The decision of when to choose surgery in the treatment of distal radius fractures continues to evolve and remains (at times) challenging, especially for surgeons early in practice or those who rarely see these injuries. The authors attempt to define a scoring system as a guide to help clarify the role for surgical treatment. Their methods included an extensive review of the literature as well as a questionnaire for candidate factors. Point scoring was based on 19 factors such as hand dominance, presence of dorsal cortical comminution, articular step-off, and ulnar variance before attempted closed reduction. They prioritized the numbers based on surgeon questionnaires and they statistically validated an algorithm. Finally, the authors retrospectively trialed the scoring system for more than 150 patients (76 treated vs 88 open reduction, internal fixation), and outcomes were similar, supporting the validity of the system.

I applaud the effort of the authors and appreciate that a better validation will come with prospectively utilizing the scoring system. Many of these scoring markers are fairly intuitive for seasoned surgeons, but I feel that a scoring system such as this helps younger surgeons or surgeons in training.

M. Rizzo, MD

12 Tumor

Limited Arthrodesis of the Wrist for Treatment of Giant Cell Tumor of the Distal Radius
Flouzat-Lachaniette C-H, Babinet A, Kahwaji A, et al (AP-HP/Université Paris Descartes, France)
J Hand Surg 38A:1505-1512, 2013

Purpose.—To present the functional results of a technique of radiocarpal arthrodesis and reconstruction with a structural nonvascularized autologous bone graft after *en bloc* resection of giant cell tumors of the distal radius.

Methods.—A total of 13 patients with a mean age of 37 years with aggressive giant cell tumor (Campanacci grade III) of distal radius were managed with *en bloc* resection and reconstruction with a structural nonvascularized bone graft. The primary outcome measure was the disability evaluated by the Musculoskeletal Tumor Society rating score of limb salvage. Secondary outcomes included survival of the reconstruction measured from the date of the operation to revision procedure for any reason (mechanical, infectious, or oncologic). Other outcomes included active wrist motion and ability to resume work.

Results.—Mean follow-up period was 6 years (range, 2-14 y). The median arc of motion at the midcarpal joint was 40°, median wrist flexion was 20°, and median extension was 10°. The median Musculoskeletal Tumor Society score based on the analysis of factors pertinent to the patient as a whole (pain, functional activities, and emotional acceptance) and specific to the upper limb (positioning of the hand, manual dexterity, and lifting ability) was 86%. Five patients underwent a second surgical procedure. The cumulative probability of reoperation for mechanical reason was 31% at similar follow-up times at 2, 5, and 10 years.

Conclusions.—This technique provided a stable wrist and partially restored wrist motion with limited pain. However, further surgical procedures may be necessary to reach this goal.

Type of Study/Level of Evidence.—Therapeutic IV.

▶ Treatment of aggressive giant cell tumors of bone at the distal radius are frequently challenging to achieve oncologically successful treatment without significant loss of wrist motion and function. The literature reports moderate rates of nonunion and reoperation and the frequent need for wrist arthrodesis. This study provides intermediate-length follow-up for en bloc resection of giant cell tumors of the distal radius reconstructed with autograft corticocancellous bone grafts from the tibia. The included tumors either presented with significant soft tissue mass or had failed prior surgical treatment with recurrence of the tumor including soft tissue mass or with insufficient bone to permit curettage and grafting. Their technique involved 2 corticocancellous strips taken from the anteromedial tibia and fixed proximally and distally in a sandwich fashion with screws to the radial shaft and the scaphoid and lunate. Additional cancellous bone graft was applied to both sites, and an external fixator was used to span the construct for an average of 16 weeks.

The primary distinction of this series/technique is that the nonunion rate (2 of 13) was significantly lower than with other techniques using nonvascularized bone graft (40%–60%) and that all patients did come to union eventually. Functional recovery was reasonable as measured using the Musculoskeletal Tumor Society score. It is unfortunate from the hand surgeon's perspective that a Disabilities of the Arm, Shoulder, and Hand score or other functional scoring system more familiar to the hand surgery audience was not used to better understand comparable functional deficits. However, the preservation of an average of 40° of wrist motion in other clinical situations has led to superior function to total wrist fusion, which is the relevant standard for these complex reconstructions. Further, one wonders if a spanning wrist plate as is sometimes used for complex distal radial fractures might have led to more rapid recovery of function for patients. However, this technique appears to be a helpful addition to caring for a complicated problem allowing for oncologic success and what appears to be reasonable functional preservation.

P. Blazar, MD

The Association Between Glomus Tumors and Neurofibromatosis

Harrison B, Moore AM, Calfee R, et al (Univ of Texas Southwestern Med School, Dallas; Mayo Clinic, Rochester, MN; Washington Univ School of Medicine, St Louis, MO)
J Hand Surg 38A:1571-1574, 2013

Purpose.—To determine whether an epidemiologic association exists between glomus tumors and neurofibromatosis.

Methods.—Using a pathology database, we established a study cohort consisting of all patients who had undergone excision of a glomus tumor of the hand between 1995 and 2010. We created a control cohort by randomly selecting 200 patients who had undergone excision of a ganglion cyst over the same period. We reviewed medical records for each cohort to identify patients with a diagnosis of neurofibromatosis. We calculated the odds ratio was calculated and performed Fisher's exact test to determine the significance of the association.

Results.—We identified 21 patients with glomus tumors of the hand. Six of these patients carried the diagnosis of neurofibromatosis (29%). In contrast, no patients in the control group carried the diagnosis of neurofibromatosis. The odds ratio for a diagnosis of neurofibromatosis in association with a glomus tumor compared with controls was 168:1.

Conclusions.—This study provides evidence of a strong epidemiologic association between glomus tumors and neurofibromatosis. Glomus tumor should be included in the differential diagnosis in neurofibromatosis patients who present with a painful lesion of the hand or finger.
Type of Study/Level of Evidence.—Diagnostic III.

▶ Glomus tumors were previously thought to occur in isolation without any known associations. However, case reports and molecular genetics studies have found a relationship between neurofibromatosis I and glomus tumors.

This is an interesting case-control study comparing a group of patients with glomus tumors of the hand with a group of patients with ganglion cysts. The age and sex distributions of the 2 groups are similar. The authors found that there was an epidemiologic association between glomus tumors in the hand and neurofibromatosis (odds ratio, 168:1; 95% confidence interval of 9 to 3128). This provides additional evidence that there is a relationship between the 2 conditions.

This article provides an estimate of the relative risk (based on the odds ratio) of a diagnosis of neurofibromatosis in association with a glomus tumor. The authors feel that this association is clinically relevant. It can help suggest the diagnosis of a glomus tumor in a patient with neurofibromatosis who presents with a painful lesion in the finger or hand. However, because most patients with neurofibromatosis are diagnosed young, the chance of the glomus tumor being the first presentation of neurofibromatosis is low. The limitations of the study are well discussed in the article.

The article provides additional evidence of this association, which has not been well described in hand surgery textbooks.

A. Chong, MD

Chondrosarcoma of the head of the fifth metacarpal treated with an iliac crest bone graft and concurrent Swanson's arthroplasty
Hills AJ, Tay S, Gateley D (St George's Hosp, London, UK)
J Plast Reconstr Aesthet Surg 67:e84-e87, 2014

Chondrosarcomas are rare malignant tumours of the bone with hyaline cartilage differentiation — only 1.5% affect the hands. Currently there is a limited range of techniques available to reconstruct the metacarpophalengeal joints affected by such neoplasias.

We report a 30-year-old lady who presented with a grade 2 chondrosarcoma in the epiphseal region of her fifth metacarpal who underwent enbloc resection of the affected metacarpal and immediate reconstruction, using a Swansons arthroplasty and non-vascularised iliac crest bone graft. Our findings are presented after follow-up of 9 years and we review the current reconstructive options available.

▶ The authors share a case, with nearly 10-year follow-up, of chondrosarcoma of bone reconstructed with iliac crest corticocancellous graft and Swanson silicone metacarpophalangeal joint arthroplasty. This method of reconstruction has been able to preserve function and motion. This is an interesting and creative solution for a situation that would normally be treated with either fusion or ray deletion.

M. Rizzo, MD

13 Vascular

The Impact of Antiplatelet Medication on Hand and Wrist Surgery
Bogunovic L, Gelberman RH, Goldfarb CA, et al (Washington Univ, School of Medicine, St Louis, MO)
J Hand Surg 38A:1063-1070, 2013

Purpose.—To quantify the impact of maintaining antiplatelet medication during hand and wrist surgery on bleeding and functional outcomes.

Methods.—This prospective cohort trial compared operative outcomes and complications of hand and wrist surgery in patients without interruption of daily antiplatelet medications (n = 107 procedures) with control patients (n = 107 procedures). We determined rates of complications requiring reoperation for each group. We compared measures of surgical site bleeding (extent of ecchymosis or hematoma formation), patient-rated outcome assessment (Quick Disabilities of the Arm, Shoulder, and Hand score and visual analog scales of pain and swelling), and 2-point discrimination between groups. Data were collected preoperatively and postoperatively at 2 and 4 weeks. We confirmed control and antiplatelet populations to be similar for data analysis according to health status (Short Form-12) and percentage of bony procedures.

Results.—One patient receiving antiplatelet medication required reoperation for surgical site bleeding after wrist arthrodesis (0.9%). There were no complications in the control group. The extent of postoperative ecchymosis was similar in the antiplatelet and control patients at 2 weeks (16 vs 19 mm) and 4 weeks (1 vs 1 mm). Hematoma rates were not increased for patients receiving antiplatelet medication (17% vs 14% at 2 wk). Patient-rated function scores were equivalent at baseline and at follow-up between groups. A total of 22 control patients and 20 patients receiving antiplatelet medication had transiently increased 2-point discrimination (≥ 2-mm change) postoperatively.

Conclusions.—Bleeding-related perioperative complications were rare when continuing antiplatelet medications without interruption for hand and wrist surgery. Maintenance of antiplatelet medication does not appear to negatively affect patient-rated or objective measures of function, although surgical-site bleeding may be greatest in patients taking higher-dose antiplatelet medication and undergoing bony procedures.

Type of Study/Level of Evidence.—Therapeutic II.

▶ In their article, The Impact of Antiplatelet Medication on Hand and Wrist Surgery, Bogunovic et al present a comparison of 2 cohorts of patients to shed some light on the importance of considering a patient's antiplatelet status before

181

performing hand surgery. They test 2 hypotheses: first that hand surgery can be performed while maintaining antiplatelet medication with minimal risk of complication and, second, that noncatastrophic bleeding at the surgical site would be affected by the medications but without a difference in the QuickDASH. The inclusion and exclusion criteria are well defined. They conclude that postoperative complications were rare in patients on antiplatelet therapy and that antiplatelet therapy does not have a negative effect on functional measures.

The study has significant weaknesses. The antiplatelet group includes patients who were taking 81 mg of aspirin as their antiplatelet therapy. There is no reason to think that 81 mg of aspirin treatment is similar to clopidogrel; 81 mg aspirin has been used for prevention of heart attack for years and is not sufficient to prevent clotting of coronary stents. Clearly, treatment with clopidogrel changes primary coagulation much more effectively and is the main concern with antiplatelet therapy. And indeed, the subgroup analysis of high-dose aspirin and clopidogrel versus low-dose aspirin supports a true difference in hematoma formation when none was reported, giving some credence to the notion that the group stratification may lead to confounding.

Additionally, nonsteroidal anti-inflammatory drug (NSAID) use was not considered, and the antiplatelet effects of these drugs may significantly confound the results. No consideration of their use or dosage was taken. Could these drugs have a greater effect in this study than the 60 of 92 patients in the cohort taking only 81 mg aspirin? Given the potential large size of the effect of NSAID use and the potential small size of the effect of 81 mg aspirin in the cohort, this issue would need greater investigation to support the authors' findings.

The timing of release of tourniquet was not controlled. In patients on antiplatelet treatment, the tourniquet was more often deflated to control bleeding, further confounding the results.

In practice, we do not discontinue antiplatelet medications for hand and wrist surgery. When a significant dissection is planned proximal to the wrist, we will work with the physician prescribing the antiplatelet regimen to decide whether to discontinue the medication and, if so, whether coverage with heparin and the use of a heparin window is warranted. In no cases have we had complications from bleeding in the face of aspirin use, although clopidogrel has caused what we consider to be more bruising than expected.

Overall, this worthy study has significant flaws in its design. The number of confounding factors is significant and questions the validity of the conclusions.

D. J. Mastella, MD

Lymphedema After Upper Limb Transplantation: Scintigraphic Study in 3 Patients

Cavadas PC, Thione A, Carballeira A, et al (Hosp de Manises, Valencia, Spain; et al)
Ann Plast Surg 71:114-117, 2013

Lymphatic vasculature is known to spontaneously reconnect after hand replantation. Nonetheless, lymphatic outflow has not been specifically studied in hand transplantation.

Lymphedema was studied clinically and scintigraphically in 3 bilateral upper limb transplants performed in Valencia, Spain, since 2006. Case 1 was a radiocarpal level, case 2 midforearm and proximal forearm, and case 3 was a transhumeral transplantation. Follow-up was 5, 4, and 3 years, respectively. Clinically, in case 1, there was a left-sided moderate lymphedema, case 2 was normal, and a right-sided moderate lymphedema was present in case 3. Lymphoscintigraphy results were consistent with the clinical findings. It was normal in the 4 nonedematous limbs. In the 2 affected limbs, there were scintigraphic findings of lymphatic block and lymphangiectasia.

The study demonstrates objectively that lymphatic circulation can reconnect spontaneously in hand transplantations, although not in a homogeneously efficient way.

▶ The authors raise an interesting point that the intact dermis can take over the lymphatic drainage in replant/transplant but not in lymphadenectomy. This has been shown clinically, but the mechanism remains unclear. Further study in this area, on a histologic or molecular level, may help prevent disabling lymphedema in patients who undergo axillary dissections or irradiation.

J. Toto, MD

Brachial Artery Catheterization: An Assessment of Use Patterns and Associated Complications
Handlogten KS, Wilson GA, Clifford L, et al (Mayo Clinic College of Medicine, Rochester, MN; Mayo Clinic, Rochester, MN)
Anesth Analg 118:288-295, 2014

Background.—Although studies have compared safety and outcomes of radial artery cannulation with other arterial catheterization locations, there is insufficient information describing brachial artery catheterization. In this study, we characterized the perioperative use patterns and the complication rates associated with brachial arterial catheterization and compared these outcomes with radial artery catheterization.

Methods.—We performed a retrospective analysis of adult patients (age ≥18 years) undergoing surgical procedures at an academic medical center from January 1, 2008, to December 31, 2011. An institutional database containing information on anesthetic care was queried to identify all brachial artery catheterizations. Baseline characteristics, details relating to the surgical and catheterization procedures, and catheter-related complications were collected and compared with a random sample of patients receiving radial artery catheterization.

Results.—We identified 858 patients receiving brachial catheterization perioperatively. An additional 3432 patients receiving radial catheterization were identified. Patients receiving brachial catheterization were more often women, had a lower body mass index, had more comorbidities, and had longer anesthetic and catheterization durations. Three vascular complications were identified in the cohort receiving brachial artery catheterization compared with 1 patient with a peripheral neuropathy in the radial artery catheterization cohort (unadjusted complication incidence [95% confidence intervals] brachial artery catheterization, 0.35% [0.12%−1.02%] vs radial artery catheterization, 0.03% [0.005%−0.16%], respectively; $P = 0.030$; relative risk [95% confidence interval] = 12.0 [1.7−83.4]). There were no catheter-related bloodstream infections.

Conclusions.—We found that brachial artery catheterization is used in more medically complex patients and for longer duration than radial artery catheterizations. Although the limited number of adverse outcomes precluded statistical adjustments in this investigation, the observed differences in complication rates between cannulation methods suggest that brachial artery catheterization may be a suitable alternative to radial artery catheterization in patients with complex medical comorbidities.

▶ Although retrospective in nature and lacking the numbers for statistical conclusions, this study provides, in my opinion, valuable information regarding outcomes and complications associated with brachial artery catheterization. Whereas radial artery cauterization complications are well documented and better understood, surprisingly little is known about complications associated with cannulization of the brachial artery. In addition to exploring this question, a second aim of the study was to examine patterns of use for brachial artery catheterization. The authors also compared their results with those of patients who underwent radial artery catheterization.

The authors reviewed 4 years of database entries from anesthesia records at the Mayo Clinic and were able to identify 858 patient who received brachial catheters perioperatively.

Compared with the radial artery group, the patients who underwent brachial artery catheterization had more comorbidities (such as coronary artery disease, kidney dysfunction, chronic obstructive pulmonary disease, congestive heart failure), were female and had lower body mass indices. No infections were noted in the brachial group versus 2 in the radial artery cohort. However, 3 brachial artery patients had vascular ischemia, of which 2 required thrombectomy and the other thrombolysis; no cases of vascular ischemia were noted in the radial artery group. One patient in the radial artery cohort did have the neurologic complication of transient paresthesias in the thumb that resolved with time.

Overall, the rates of complication are low in both groups with higher risk of vascular complications with brachial artery catheterizations. Nonetheless, it appears that brachial artery cannulization is a reasonable alternative to radial artery catheterization.

M. Rizzo, MD

Upper Extremity Thromboembolism in a Patient With Subclavian Steal Syndrome

Yamaguchi DJ, Matthews TC (Univ of Alabama at Birmingham)

Ann Vasc Surg 27:673.e9-673.e11, 2013

Subclavian steal is the physiologic process whereby blood flow through a vertebral artery is reversed at the level of the basilar artery as a means of supplying arterial inflow to the ipsilateral subclavian artery. This occurs in the setting of ipsilateral subclavian artery origin occlusion. We describe a case in which a patient with subclavian steal syndrome developed acute upper extremity ischemia secondary to thromboemboli from a chronically occluded ipsilateral subclavian stent (at the origin of the left subclavian artery). He subsequently underwent staged left upper extremity arterial thromboembolectomy followed by definitive revascularization via carotid—subclavian bypass. In addition, subclavian artery ligation proximal to the ipsilateral vertebral artery was performed. The patient's sensory and motor neurologic hand function returned to baseline with restoration of symmetric upper extremity arterial occlusion pressures and pulse volume recordings. A search of the literature revealed that this was the first case report of acute thromboembolic hand ischemia in the setting of subclavian steal.

▶ This article presents a case report of acute limb ischemia in the setting of a chronically thrombosed subclavian stent and subclavian steal. The patient had > 12 hours of ischemia time with reported paresthesias. A thrombectomy was performed with resulting improved flow to the hand, although postoperative assessment showed brachial pressure of 89 on the surgical side vs 146 on the nonsurgical side, which normalized after carotid-subclavian bypass. Fasciotomies were discussed as an option but not performed.

The authors report a subjective decrease sensation and paresis but do not elaborate. In addition, they subjectively report a full return of function at 3 days but do not provide any objective data except for the vascular assessment postoperatively.

This is an interesting case report, although it is difficult to draw any conclusions from the article except the addition of subclavian steal and stent thrombosis to the differential diagnosis of an acutely ischemic hand.

C. Heinrich, MD

Arm lymphoedema after axillary surgery in women with invasive breast cancer

Sackey H, Magnuson A, Sandelin K, et al (Karolinska Inst and Karolinska Univ Hosp, Stockholm, Sweden; Örebro Univ Hosp, Sweden; et al)

Br J Surg 101:390-397, 2014

Background.—The primary aim was to compare arm lymphoedema after sentinel lymph node biopsy (SLNB) alone *versus* axillary lymph node dissection (ALND) in women with node-negative and node-positive breast cancer. The secondary aim was to examine the potential association between self-reported and objectively measured arm lymphoedema.

Methods.—Women who had surgery during 1999—2004 for invasive breast cancer in four centres in Sweden were included. The study groups were defined by the axillary procedure performed and the presence of axillary metastases: SLNB alone, ALND without axillary metastases, and ALND with axillary metastases. Before surgery, and 1, 2 and 3 years after operation, arm volume was measured and a questionnaire regarding symptoms of arm lymphoedema was completed. A mixed model was used to determine the adjusted mean difference in arm volume between the study groups, and generalized estimating equations were employed to determine differences in self-reported arm lymphoedema.

Results.—One hundred and forty women had SLNB alone, 125 had node-negative ALND and 155 node-positive ALND. Women who underwent SLNB had no increase in postoperative arm volume over time, whereas both ALND groups showed a significant increase. The risk of self-reported arm lymphoedema 1, 2 and 3 years after surgery was significantly lower in the SLNB group compared with that in both ALND groups. Three years after surgery there was a significant association between increased arm volume and self-reported symptoms of arm lymphoedema.

Conclusion.—SLNB is associated with a minimal risk of increased arm volume and few symptoms of arm lymphoedema, significantly less than after ALND, regardless of lymph node status.

▶ Hand surgeons have expressed concern regarding procedures performed on the ipsilateral arm after treatment of breast cancer, particularly after lymph node dissections. The literature suggests a low rate of precipitating lymphedema after modern breast cancer treatment; this study investigates the incidence of self-reported symptoms of lymphedema and arm volume after either axillary node dissection or sentinel lymph node biopsy (SLNB). The study reports a significant increase in self-reported symptoms of lymphedema and arm volume after axillary dissection relative to SLNB.

However, a year after surgery (in distinction to findings at 2 and 3 years), women who reported symptoms of lymphedema and those who did not had no difference in arm volume. One of the major confounding issues is a reliable and appropriate way to measure arm volume. In addition, patient-reported (subjective) symptoms alone are notoriously subject to many confounding factors. Women have been more or less told for decades to expect lymphedema after breast cancer treatment, and this has become a part of their expectations, which may lead to altered perceptions of their arm symptoms. Likewise, the questions listed on the patient survey are vague and could apply to many symptoms that arise outside the realm of lymphedema. Thus, I think it is difficult to arrive at any conclusions after review of this study given the flaws.

J. E. Adams, MD

14 Diagnostic Imaging

The Role of Magnetic Resonance Imaging in Scaphoid Fractures
Murthy NS (Mayo Clinic, Rochester, MN)
J Hand Surg 38A:2047-2054, 2013

Fractures of the scaphoid are the most common surgically treated carpal fracture, and early diagnosis is critical to minimize complications including osteonecrosis. If the initial radiographs after the injury are inconclusive, early magnetic resonance imaging (MRI) provides an immediate diagnosis to allow for proper management. This has been shown to be cost effective both in direct measureable costs and likely in difficult-to-measure indirect costs related to lost productivity. In the cases in which no scaphoid fracture is present, MRI provides alternate diagnoses such as identification of other fractures (eg, other carpals and distal radius), osseous contusions, and soft tissue injuries (preferably $\geq 1.5T$). When MRI is contraindicated, computed tomography (CT) is a reasonable alternative after the initial and repeat negative radiographs. MRI is the best imaging modality for assessing osteonecrosis of the proximal pole in a scaphoid nonunion. Unfortunately, the most useful imaging sequences remain controversial. My institution relies on the noncontrast T1-weighted images for the primary diagnosis of osteonecrosis with dynamic contrast enhancement used in a supplemental fashion.

▶ The author presents us with a current concept review on the use of magnetic resonance imaging (MRI) in scaphoid fractures. The author, a radiologist, gives the hand surgeon a concise well-written summary of the relevant literature. He outlines the role of MRI in establishing the diagnosis of a scaphoid fracture in cases in which radiographs are inconclusive. The cost effectiveness of this approach is also discussed. The author also discusses the role of MRI in identifying areas of avascularity, a relevant question for those treating scaphoid nonunions. Many illustrative cases are included and the current controversies in the literature presented and explained in an easy-to-read manner. The authors also touch on the cost effectiveness of MRI, which is important in today's health care climate. A review of what is done at the author's center proves useful and provides a practical guideline for the hand surgeon who deals with scaphoid fractures and nonunions.

R. Grewal, MD

Accuracy of Ultrasonography and Magnetic Resonance Imaging in Diagnosing Carpal Tunnel Syndrome Using Rest and Grasp Positions of the Hands

Horng Y-S, Chang H-C, Lin K-E, et al (Buddhist Tzu Chi General Hosp, Taipei Branch, Taiwan; Tzu Chi Univ, Hualien, Taiwan; Natl Taiwan Univ, Taipei; et al)
J Hand Surg 37A:1591-1598, 2012

Purpose.—To compare the accuracy of ultrasonography and magnetic resonance imaging (MRI) in diagnosing carpal tunnel syndrome (CTS) in both the rest and grasp positions. We postulated that the diagnostic accuracy could be improved by imaging hands in the grasp position rather than in the rest position.

Methods.—Fifty patients with CTS and 45 healthy volunteers received a package of questionnaires and had a physical examination and a nerve conduction study. Ultrasonography and MRI images were recorded in both the rest and grasp positions for each participant.

Results.—There were significant differences between the patients and the healthy volunteers regarding patient-reported outcomes, the results of physical examinations, the nerve conduction studies, and the ultrasonography and MRI imaging. The area under the receiver operating characteristic curve of ultrasonography was significantly improved by measuring the bowing of the flexor retinaculum in the grasp position than by measuring that in the rest position. The diagnostic accuracy of ultrasonography was similar to that of MRI when we used a combination of the measurements of the cross-sectional area of the median nerve in the rest position and the bowing of the flexor retinaculum in the grasp position.

Conclusions.—The accuracies of MRI and ultrasonography for diagnosing CTS were improved by measuring the bowing of the flexor retinaculum in the grasp position. Ultrasonography can be an adequate screening method for CTS if clinicians combine the cross-sectional area of the median nerve in the rest position and the bowing of the flexor retinaculum in the grasp position.

Type of Study/Level of Evidence.—Diagnostic I (Table 2).

▶ This is a well-written, retrospective study of characteristic ultrasound findings associated with an ulnar collateral ligament (UCL) tear of the thumb

TABLE 2.—Comparison of the Results of Physical Examinations Between Hands With Carpal Tunnel Syndrome and Healthy Hands

Variables	CTS Hands (n = 91) (mean ± SD)	Healthy Hands (n = 91) (mean ± SD)
Wrist circumference (cm)*	15.7 ± 1.2	14.8 ± 1.1
Grasp strength (kg)*	17.1 ± 7.5	22.9 ± 7.8
Palmar pinch strength (kg)*	2.7 ± 1.6	3.8 ± 1.4
Lateral pinch strength (kg)*	4.1 ± 2.3	5.3 ± 1.7
Monofilament sensory test*	29.7 ± 3.5	32.3 ± 3.1

*Indicates statistical significance between the groups; $P < .05$; t-test of mixed effects model.

consistent with the Stener lesion. This group retrospectively reviewed the ultrasound imaging of 26 patients who had undergone surgical repair of UCL tears. By manipulating the criteria and reanalyzing their images, they were able to accurately identify if a UCL tear existed. Their ultrasound diagnosis of displaced UCL tears consisted of (1) absence of normal UCL fibers spanning the first metacarpophalangeal joint and (2) heterogeneous well-defined mass-like abnormality at least in part proximal to the apex of the metacarpal lateral tubercle. When these criteria were used, the authors were able to achieve 100% sensitivity and specificity with ultrasound imaging of surgically identified UCL tears (Table 2).

This study is very interesting in the fact that ultrasound scan can easily be performed in the office setting after an acute thumb injury. Utilizing the well-established ultrasound criteria presented, it would be possible to accurately identify these UCL tears for possible surgical intervention. Research in this area needs to continue, as the numbers used for establishment of these criteria were fairly low. It does, however, show an interesting and useful method of utilizing ultrasound scan as an office-based diagnostic tool.

J. Brault, MD

Is dynamic contrast-enhanced MRI useful for assessing proximal fragment vascularity in scaphoid fracture delayed and non-union?

Ng AWH, Griffith JF, Taljanovic MS, et al (The Chinese Univ of Hong Kong, People's Republic of China; The Univ of Arizona Health Network, Tucson)
Skeletal Radiol 42:983-992, 2013

Objective.—To assess dynamic contrast-enhanced magnetic resonance imaging (DCE MRI) as a measure of vascularity in scaphoid delayed-union or non-union.

Materials and Methods.—Thirty-five patients (34 male, one female; mean age, 27.4 ± 9.4 years; range, 16–51 years) with scaphoid delayed-union and non-union who underwent DCE MRI of the scaphoid between September 2002 and October 2012 were retrospectively reviewed. Proximal fragment vascularity was classified as good, fair, or poor on unenhanced MRI, contrast-enhanced MRI, and DCE MRI. For DCE MRI, enhancement slope, E_{slope} comparison of proximal and distal fragments was used to classify the proximal fragment as good, fair, or poor vascularity. Proximal fragment vascularity was similarly graded at surgery in all patients. Paired t test and McNemar test were used for data comparison. Kappa value was used to assess level of agreement between MRI findings and surgical findings.

Results.—Twenty-five (71 %) of 35 patients had good vascularity, four (11 %) had fair vascularity, and six (17 %) had poor vascularity of the proximal scaphoid fragment at surgery. DCE MRI parameters had the highest correlation with surgical findings (kappa = 0.57). Proximal scaphoid fragments with surgical poor vascularity had a significantly lower E_{max} and E_{slope} than those with good vascularity ($p = 0.0043$ and 0.027).

The sensitivity, specificity, positive and negative predictive value and accuracy of DCE MRI in predicting impaired vascularity was 67, 86, 67, 86, and 80 %, respectively, which was better than that seen with unenhanced and post-contrast MRI. Flattened time intensity curves in both proximal and distal fragments were a feature of protracted non-union with a mean time interval of 101.6 ± 95.5 months between injury and MRI.

Conclusions.—DCE MRI has a higher diagnostic accuracy than either non-enhanced MRI or contrast enhanced MRI for assessing proximal fragment vascularity in scaphoid delayed-union and non-union. For proper interpretation of contrast-enhanced studies in scaphoid vascularity, one needs to incorporate the time frame between injury and MRI.

▶ For me, this article out of China in skeletal radiology is neither good nor bad, but rather it is irrelevant. The authors explore the use of dynamic contrast-enhanced magnetic resonance imaging (MRI) to look into the vascular status of the proximal pole in scaphoid nonunions. I agree with the authors that perfect imaging is not currently available to assess this, and the gold standard is intraoperative punctuate bleeding. I applaud the authors for looking at this imaging option but do not envision this changing my practice for many reasons.

From a methodologic perspective, the study has many flaws. First, of the 35 patients, only 10 had surgical evidence of fair or poor vascularity (vs 25 patients with well-perfused proximal poles). I don't think a 10-patient imaging study is close to adequate to answer this question. Second, some scans were done on a 3-telsa (T) magnet (which in the United States is only typically available in some academic centers and not widespread) and others on a 1.5-T magnet. The data were not subanalyzed to see if this made any difference. Lastly, plain films were not analyzed and compared first. In cases of plain film evidence of avascular necrosis, all MRI techniques would be expected to report poor flow, and really only cases of questionable flow are of interest. This could alter the sensitivity and specificity for the real desired cases.

Furthermore, from a practical standpoint, adoption of this technique would require some additional technical training and is unlikely to be popular in the United States, as there would be no additional reimbursement compared with a standard contrast-enhanced MRI because there is no modifier for this technique. Also unlike a computed tomography (CT) scan, which can be converted to a 3-dimensional (CT) at a later time point, this technique must be decided on in advance to capture the necessary data points.

In short, the technique is early even in a research arena with only now 2 published studies on the technique (incidentally both with conflicting results). Although it could improve diagnostic accuracy, ultimately it is intraoperative findings that should influence surgeons as to the appropriate graft for a particular case.

G. Gaston, MD

Intrinsic ligament and triangular fibrocartilage complex tears of the wrist: comparison of MDCT arthrography, conventional 3-T MRI, and MR arthrography

Lee RKL, Ng AWH, Tong CSL, et al (The Chinese Univ of Hong Kong, Shatin)
Skeletal Radiol 42:1277-1285, 2013

Purpose.—This study compares the diagnostic performance of multidetector CT arthrography (CTA), conventional 3-T MR and MR arthrography (MRA) in detecting intrinsic ligament and triangular fibrocartilage complex (TFCC) tears of the wrist.

Materials and Methods.—Ten cadaveric wrists of five male subjects with an average age 49.6 years (range 26—59 years) were evaluated using CTA, conventional 3-T MR and MRA. We assessed the presence of scapholunate ligament (SLL), lunotriquetral ligament (LTL), and TFCC tears using a combination of conventional arthrography and arthroscopy as a gold standard. All images were evaluated in consensus by two musculoskeletal radiologists with sensitivity, specificity, and accuracy being calculated.

Results.—Sensitivities/specificity/accuracy of CTA, conventional MRI, and MRA were 100%/100%/100%, 66%/86%/80%, 100%/86%/90% for the detection of SLL tear, 100%/80%/90%, 60%/80%/70%, 100%/80%/90% for the detection of LTL tear, and 100%/100%/100%, 100%/86%/90%, 100%/100%/100% for the detection of TFCC tear. Overall CTA had the highest sensitivity, specificity, and accuracy among the three investigations while MRA performed better than conventional MR. CTA also had the highest sensitivity, specificity, and accuracy for identifying which component of the SLL and LTL was torn. Membranous tears of both SLL and LTL were better visualized than dorsal or volar tears on all three imaging modalities.

Conclusion.—Both CT and MR arthrography have a very high degree of accuracy for diagnosing tears of the SLL, LTL, and TFCC with both being more accurate than conventional MR imaging.

▶ This is a thought-provoking study examining the issue of diagnostic imaging for soft lesions of the carpus (specifically scapholunate ligament, lunotriquetral ligament, and triangular fibrocartilage complex). Imaging modalities reported in the literature and still in use include arthrography, magnetic resonance imaging (MRI), MR arthrography, and computed tomographic (CT) arthrography. All the MRIs were obtained using a 3-T magnet and a dedicated wrist coil. To compare these modalities, the authors examined 10 cadaver wrists for the presence of these lesions and used a combination of arthrography and arthroscopy as the gold standard; if a lesion was seen at either arthrography or arthroscopy, this was regarded as pathologic. Overall, this study found CT arthrography to be superior with 100% sensitivity, specificity, and accuracy rates for scapholunate ligament and triangular fibrocartilage complex lesions, and 100%, 80%, and 90%, respectively, for lunotriquetral ligament lesions. The authors report superior sensitivity, specificity, and accuracy than most reports in the literature for conventional MRI, and they attribute this to the use of a 3-T imaging system.

One of the major concerns for hand surgeons with this report is that a moderate percentage of the lesions described as pathologic (4 of 11) were not seen at arthroscopy. This is a concern, as most clinicians have regarded arthroscopy as the true gold standard, and a surgeon faced with the scenario of a positive test and a normal arthroscopy would almost certainly treat the patient as if the test result was a false-positive. Further problems include the limited number of wrists examined (10) and the limited total number of pathologic lesions as well as some differences in imaging cadaver wrists from patients (eg, lack of motion artifacts and no limitations in positioning).

This study adds to the literature on this topic but does little to clarify the conundrum clinicians face when ordering diagnostic imaging for soft tissue lesions of the wrist. There is additional morbidity from arthrography and the use of ionizing radiation, and although this study shows superior numbers for the use of both, with the limitations above, it has not convinced me that overall it is superior to MRI for imaging in my patients.

P. Blazar, MD

15 Elbow: Trauma

Clinical Outcomes After Chronic Distal Biceps Reconstruction With Allografts

Snir N, Hamula M, Wolfson T, et al (New York Univ Hosp for Joint Diseases)
Am J Sports Med 41:2288-2295, 2013

Background.—Chronic ruptures of the distal biceps are often complicated by tendon retraction and fibrosis, precluding primary repair. Reconstruction with allograft augmentation has been proposed as an alternative for cases not amenable to primary repair.

Purpose.—To investigate the clinical outcomes of late distal biceps reconstruction using allograft tissue.

Study Design.—Case series; Level of evidence, 4.

Methods.—A total of 20 patients who underwent distal biceps reconstruction with allograft tissue between May 2007 and May 2012 were identified. Charts were retrospectively reviewed for postoperative complications, gross flexion and supination strength, and range of motion. Subjective functional outcomes were assessed prospectively with the Mayo Elbow Performance Score (MEPS) and Disabilities of the Arm, Shoulder and Hand (DASH) questionnaire.

Results.—Eighteen patients with adequate follow-up were included in the study. All had undergone late distal biceps reconstruction with allografts (Achilles [n = 15], semitendinosus [n = 1], gracilis [n = 1], or anterior tibialis [n = 1]) for symptomatic chronic ruptures of the distal biceps. At a mean office follow-up of 9.3 months (range, 4-14 months), all patients had full range of motion and mean gross strength of 4.7 of 5 (range, 4-5) in flexion and supination. After a mean out-of-office follow-up at 21 months (range, 7-68.8 months), the mean DASH score was 7.5 ± 17.9, and the mean MEPS increased from 43.1 preoperatively to 94.2 postoperatively (P < .001). The only complication observed was transient posterior interosseous nerve palsy in 2 patients. Additionally, all but 1 patient reported a cosmetic deformity. However, all patients found it acceptable.

Conclusion.—Late reconstruction for chronic ruptures of the distal biceps using allograft tissue is a safe and effective solution for symptomatic patients with functional demands in forearm supination and elbow flexion. While there are several graft options, the literature supports good results with Achilles tendon allografts. Further studies are needed to evaluate the clinical outcomes of other allograft options.

▶ The purpose of the study was to retrospectively review the outcomes of patients undergoing allograft reconstruction of chronic rupture of the distal biceps tendon at the authors' institution. A total of 20 patients underwent distal biceps tendon reconstruction and, of the 18 available for follow-up, all but 3 had Achilles tendon allografts used. Patients were evaluated with the Mayo Elbow Performance Score and the Disabilities of the Arm, Shoulder, and Hand (DASH) score.

Interestingly, reconstructions of the distal biceps tendon amounted to 14% of all distal biceps repair surgeries at their institution. Of the selected cases, retraction of the chronic rupture was universally noted and documented on magnetic resonance imaging. Most cases were performed through a single-incision technique, and the average time for surgery was 20.1 weeks, with a standard deviation of 14.8 weeks. Only 2 patients underwent surgery through a 2-incision technique, and those patients both had transient posterior interosseous nerve (PIN) palsies.

This study represents the largest series of late distal biceps tendon reconstructions in the literature. It is significant because all patients receiving allograft reconstructions had recovery of their range of motion and, although subjectively evaluated, recovery of their strength as well. The measurement of strength is not compared with the opposite side, but on a 5-point strength scale, patients achieved an impressive 4.7. Preoperative Mayo Elbow Performance Score improved significantly, preoperative pain resolved in all but 4 patients, and, perhaps most impressively, postoperative DASH scores had a mean of 7.5. All 18 patients reported that they would undergo the procedure again if necessary.

The issue of distal biceps tendon ruptures presenting after the acute rupture is an open one. Nonoperative management of distal biceps tendon ruptures has been shown to be reasonable, although the authors of this article do not agree with that opinion. However, patients universally want their biceps tendon rupture fixed independent of when they present to the orthopedist. This article is significant because it presents a large cohort of patients from an institution that is clearly seeing a large proportion of patients with chronic biceps tendon ruptures, all of whom do reasonably well despite 2 postoperative PIN palsies. The study has the ability to change current practice in 2 important ways: first, it may embolden orthopedists to attempt repair with allograft augmentation as part of the preoperative plan in patients who present with chronic biceps tendon ruptures with the knowledge that a reasonably good result is possible afterward. Second, it may allow the delay of a distal biceps tendon rupture surgery from the acute to the chronic phase in the presence of mitigating circumstances with the knowledge that surgery is possible later. This latter point may be most relevant in the treatment of elite athletes in whom in-season biceps tendon reconstruction or repair may be impossible.

The data from this article and its contribution to the literature cannot be underestimated because, when allograft reconstruction is attempted in the case of chronic distal biceps tendon rupture, this study provides the most reliable data on outcomes currently available for this relatively common presentation. Perhaps we can look forward to a sister surgical technique article to accompany this contribution to the literature with pictures to describe the authors' technique in more detail, because it will likely become one that many of us use in the treatment of these patients.

J. Elfar, MD

Effect of Elbow Flexion on the Proximity of the PIN During 2-incision Distal Biceps Repair
Jones JA, Jones CM, Grossman MG (Lenox Hill Hosp, NY; SUNY at Stony Brook Univ Med Ctr, NY)
Orthopedics 36:e931-e935, 2013

The posterior interosseous nerve (PIN) is at risk for injury during surgical dissection for distal biceps repair, yet the optimal position of elbow flexion to avoid a PIN injury has never been established for the 2-incision approach. The purpose of this study was to determine the proximity of the PIN to the radial tuberosity during surgical dissection in different degrees of elbow flexion.

Ten cadaveric specimens with an intact elbow and forearm were dissected in full pronation using a modified Boyd-Anderson approach. Half of the dissections were completed in 90° of flexion and the other half were completed in maximal flexion. To simulate the location of the PIN during a single-incision biceps repair, the distance of the PIN to the radial tuberosity was recorded in full extension and supination. Results from these measurements were assessed for differences using paired t tests, with differences deemed significant for P values less than .05. The PIN was not identified in any of the 2-incision surgical dissections.

Based on these findings, the proximity of the PIN to the radial tuberosity is not significantly affected by the degree of elbow flexion in the muscle-splitting 2-incision approach. In addition, a safe zone exists for avoiding PIN injury in a single-incision technique for distal biceps repair because a drill bit exiting the radial tuberosity greater than 1 cm in a distal-radial direction would place the PIN at risk.

▶ This study attempts to measure the distance between the posterior interosseous nerve (PIN) exit point from the supinator and the radial tuberosity in 3 conditions. The first condition is 90° of flexion with pronation, the second is hyperflexion with pronation, and the third is full supination in extension. The reason this is relevant is because both of the most utilized techniques for reinserting a distal biceps tendon onto the tuberosity involve these positions. The first 2 positions are commonly used in the 2-incision approach, and the last position is commonly utilized in the 1-incision approach. The goal of this study is to note whether there is any advantage in distance between the PIN and the radial tuberosity with any of these positions. If there were, it would favor one or another approach during reimplantation of the distal biceps tendon onto its target radial tuberosity. The results show that there is no statistically significant advantage for any of the positions or approaches with regard to the PIN. The authors note that no study has previously investigated the relationship of the PIN to the radial tuberosity in varying degrees of elbow flexion. They never encountered the nerve during their routine dissections, perhaps because the average distance between the nerve and the dissection is more than 1.5 cm. The position of the PIN did not increase or decrease to an extent greater than 2.0 mm independent of elbow flexion position.

Although this report does not serve as a tie breaker in the never-ending struggle between those who prefer 1-incision or 2-incision techniques for the repair of the biceps tendon, it does serve a significant purpose of outlining that elbow flexion really does not affect the position of the PIN with respect to the radial tuberosity to any significant degree. However, the report fails to mention the likely significant role that retraction plays in the development of postoperative PIN palsies. Even in the authors' citation of the relevant literature, the paucity of actual direct PIN injuries encountered after distal biceps tendon rupture does argue for a traction mechanism for postoperative PIN palsies, which are not uncommon after distal biceps tendon reattachments with any technique. If the placement of the retractors and their use in an aggressive manner is the likely cause of most PIN injuries during distal biceps tendon reattachment, then one would expect the results of a report like this to show that the PIN is not at high risk for direct injury using either approach. It stands to reason that the study of traction forces on the PIN in a cadaveric model would be a logical next step in the debate between those who favor 1- or 2-incision techniques.

J. Elfar, MD

Can Ulnar Variance Be Used to Detect Overstuffing After Radial Head Arthroplasty?
Moon J-G, Hong J-H, Bither N, et al (Korea Univ Guro Hosp, Seoul)
Clin Orthop Relat Res 472:727-731, 2014

Background.—Overstuffing of the radiocapitellar joint during metallic radial head arthroplasty has been reported to cause loss of elbow flexion, capitellar erosion, and early-onset osteoarthritis. Although this is known, there is no agreed-on measurement approach to determine whether overstuffing has occurred.

Questions/Purposes.—We therefore hypothesized that overlengthening the radial head during radial head arthroplasty changes the ulnar variance in the wrist.

Methods.—Seven cadaveric radii were implanted with radial head prostheses of increasing thickness. Each specimen was implanted successively with increasingly thick radial head prostheses measuring 2, 4, and 6 mm thicker than the native radial head, and radiographs were taken after implantation of each prosthesis. The ulnar variance with each prosthesis was measured using the method of perpendiculars.

Results.—The ulnar variance of the native and 2-mm ($p = 0.04$), 4-mm ($p = 0.008$), and 6-mm ($p = 0.008$) overly thick radial head prosthesis-implanted states decreased significantly with each incremental increase in prosthetic head thickness.

Conclusions.—Implantation of thicker radial head prostheses decreased the ulnar variance. Our results indicate ulnar variance could be used to detect overstuffing of radial head prostheses.

Clinical Relevance.—The simplicity and reliability of ulnar variance make it a potentially useful indicator of overlengthening after radial head arthroplasty.

▶ Overstuffing of the radial head is a common problem in radial head replacement. It can be difficult to determine the appropriate-sized implant, particularly in the setting of ligament injury. If the implant is too large, instability, pain, and accelerated joint degenerative changes can occur. Prior studies have documented that x-rays of the elbow fail to diagnose radial head overstuffing until grossly oversized implants are placed. This study assessed ulnar variance as a method to determine radial head proper sizing. It found that even with a +2 mm of overstuffing, ulnar variance significantly decreased. Issues with this study are that the native ulnar variance may already be altered by the injury, particularly in the setting of injury to the Triangular fibrocartilage complex and/or the interosseous ligament (ie, Essex-Lopresti injuries). Although ulnar variance is commonly symmetric between sides, it is not always. In addition, ulnar variance was measured in forearm films that included both the wrist and the elbow. Because of variance in positioning, this can substantially alter the perceived ulnar variance depending on where exactly the beam is placed. Overall, this report provides another option to help the surgeon place the appropriately sized radial head; in my own practice, I will continue to rely on replication of the excised portion of the proximal radius and assessment intraoperatively of the relationship between the radial head and the proximal ulna and coronoid.

J. E. Adams, MD

Effect of Elbow Flexion on the Proximity of the Pin During 2-Incision Distal Biceps Repair

Jones JA, Jones CM, Grossman MG (Lenox Hill Hosp, NY; SUNY at Stony Brook Univ Med Ctr, NY)
Orthopedics 36:e931-e935, 2013

The posterior interosseous nerve (PIN) is at risk for injury during surgical dissection for distal biceps repair, yet the optimal position of elbow flexion to avoid a PIN injury has never been established for the 2-incision approach. The purpose of this study was to determine the proximity of the PIN to the radial tuberosity during surgical dissection in different degrees of elbow flexion.

Ten cadaveric specimens with an intact elbow and forearm were dissected in full pronation using a modified Boyd-Anderson approach. Half of the dissections were completed in 90° of flexion and the other half were completed in maximal flexion. To simulate the location of the PIN during a single-incision biceps repair, the distance of the PIN to the radial tuberosity was recorded in full extension and supination. Results from these measurements were assessed for differences using paired t tests, with differences deemed significant for P values less than .05. The PIN was not identified in any of the 2-incision surgical dissections.

Based on these findings, the proximity of the PIN to the radial tuberosity is not significantly affected by the degree of elbow flexion in the muscle-splitting 2-incision approach. In addition, a safe zone exists for avoiding PIN injury in a single-incision technique for distal biceps repair because a drill bit exiting the radial tuberosity greater than 1 cm in a distal-radial direction would place the PIN at risk.

▶ This cadaveric anatomic dissection evaluated the effect of elbow flexion on the relationship between the radial tuberosity and the posterior interosseous nerve (PIN) during biceps tendon repair utilizing a modified Boyd-Anderson 2-incision approach. No significant difference was shown in the radial tuberosity to PIN distance at 90° of elbow flexion and hyperflexion. These measurements were done in full forearm pronation. An additional measurement for consideration would have been the radial tuberosity to PIN distance in varying degrees of forearm rotation and 90° elbow flexion and hyperflexion. However, as the authors state, there has been a trend toward 1-incision distal biceps repair. They measured the radial tuberosity to PIN distance with the elbow extended and forearm supinated after the previous 2 incisions had been created. Their findings support previously published data regarding the relationship.[1] The article addresses the importance of knowing the anatomy of the PIN and its relationship to surrounding structures during biceps tendon repair. They have concluded that the degree of elbow flexion does not affect the proximity of the PIN to the radial tuberosity. However, the study was underpowered and subject to cadaveric constraints. Therefore, I am cautious with interpreting these results. I will continue to be cognizant of the PIN during biceps tendon repair, which I perform through a single-incision approach. This article has not provided new information that will change my current practice routine.

A. Moeller, MD

Reference

1. Lo EY, Li CS, Van den Bogaerde JM. The effect of drill trajectory on proximity to the posterior interosseous nerve during cortical button distal biceps repair. *Arthroscopy*. 2011;27:1048-1054.

Radial Head Replacement for Radial Head Fractures
El Sallakh S (Tanta Univ, Egypt)
J Orthop Trauma 27:e137-e140, 2013

Objective.—This study aimed to analyze the clinical results after treatment of complex elbow injuries with modular anatomic radial head prosthesis (MARHP), along with ligament repair and fracture fixation.

Design.—Retrospective.

Setting.—District teaching hospital.

Patients/Participants.—The inclusion criteria were all patients with traumatic elbow instability after acute fracture or fracture dislocation, where the radial head was comminuted and irreparable at the time of surgery (Mason type III) and there was associated valgus laxity of the elbow. Of 14 patients, 12 with radial head prosthesis were available for the study.

Intervention.—MARHP (Acumed, Hillsboro, OR) was used to replace irreparable and comminuted radial head fractures when it was associated with valgus instability.

Main Outcome Measurements.—All patients were evaluated clinically and radiographically for a mean follow-up of 42 months (range, 22–58 months).

Results.—Patients recovered a similar range of motion between affected and unaffected elbows. Stability was restored to all 12 elbows, and all patients had a good or excellent result according to Mayo Elbow Performance Index and a disability of the arm, shoulder, and hand survey. Radiographic measurement revealed a congruent elbow joint.

Conclusion.—The MARHP is effectively restoring stability and congruency to the elbow joint. There was no evidence of arthritic radiocapitellar joint, capitellar osteopenia, significant proximal radial migration of the implant, or any major complications. Outcomes were optimized by recognition and addressing the associated injuries.

Level of Evidence.—Therapeutic Level IV. See Instructions for Authors for a complete description of levels of evidence.

▶ The literature has shown that radial head excision is contraindicated for patients with an incompetent medial collateral ligament, disrupted forearm interosseous ligament, or elbow dislocation. Radial head excision has fallen out of favor as a result of complications, such as valgus elbow instability, elbow stiffness, and proximal migration of the radius. The radial head has been recognized as an important stabilizer of the elbow and forearm in both clinical and biomechanical studies. This is a small retrospective cohort study of 12 elbows, which showed short-term to mid-term results of the clinical and radiologic outcome of a modular grit-blasted radial head prosthesis in the setting of comminuted radial head fractures with valgus laxity. There was no evidence of capitellar osteopenia or significant proximal radial migration of the implant, or loosening, despite prior separate reports suggestive of such. Other than having a significant difference between the affected and unaffected sides in range of motion, the patients recovered the functional range of motion of the elbow.

E. Cheung, MD

The effect of excision of the radial head and metallic radial head replacement on the tension in the interosseous membrane

Lanting BA, Ferreira LM, Johnson JA, et al (St. Joseph's Health Care, London, Ontario, Canada)
Bone Joint J 95-B:1383-1387, 2013

We measured the tension in the interosseous membrane in six cadaveric forearms using an *in vitro* forearm testing system with the native radial head, after excision of the radial head and after metallic radial head replacement. The tension almost doubled after excision of the radial head during simulated rotation of the forearm ($p = 0.007$). There was no significant difference in tension in the interosseous membrane between the native and radial head replacement states ($p = 0.09$). Maximal tension occurred in neutral rotation with both the native and the replaced radial head, but in pronation if the radial head was excised. Under an increasing axial load and with the forearm in a fixed position, the rate of increase in tension in the interosseous membrane was greater when the radial head was excised than for the native radial head or replacement states ($p = 0.02$). As there was no difference in tension between the native and radial head replacement states, a radial head replacement should provide a normal healing environment for the interosseous membrane after injury or following its reconstruction. Load sharing between the radius and ulna becomes normal after radial head Replacement. As excision of the radial head significantly increased the tension in the interosseous membrane it may potentially lead to its attritional failure over time.

▶ Excision of the radial head markedly increases loading on the interosseous membrane and alters load sharing across the radius and ulna. In this study, mean changes in the tension at the interosseous membrane were more than double the values when the radial head was excised compared with when the radial head was intact or replaced. Insertion of a correctly sized metallic radial head replacement recreates near-normal biomechanics of the forearm, with no change in the loading characteristics of the interosseous membrane. This is clinically important, indicating that radial head replacement may allow the forearm to maintain normal biomechanics and load transfer between the radius and ulna. If the interosseous membrane was damaged at the time of injury that causes a radial head fracture, it may be able to heal normally if the radial head is replaced. Given the challenges when treating chronic longitudinal radio-ulnar dissociation, this might eliminate a significant clinical complication. This was an in vitro cadaveric study with elderly specimens, which has inherent limitations. Whether these results can be directly applied to younger patients in vivo remains to be confirmed.

E. Cheung, MD

Clinical results after different operative treatment methods of radial head and neck fractures: A systematic review and meta-analysis of clinical outcome
Zwingmann J, Welzel M, Dovi-Akue D, et al (Univ of Freiburg, Med Ctr, Germany)
Injury 44:1540-1550, 2013

Introduction.—There is no consensus on optimal treatment strategy for Mason type II-IV fractures. Most recommendations are based upon experts' opinion.

Methods.—An OVID-based literature search were performed to identify studies on surgical treatment of radial head and neck fracture. Specific focus was placed on extracting data describing clinical efficacy and outcome by using the Mason classification and including elbow function scores. A total of 841 clinical studies were identified describing in total the clinical follow-up of 1264 patients.

Results.—For type II radial head and neck fractures the significant best treatment option seems to be ORIF with an overall success rate of 98% by using screws or biodegradable (polylactide) pins. ORIF with a success rate of 92% shows the best results in the treatment of type III fractures and seem to be better than resection and implantation of a prosthesis. For this fracture type the ORIF with screws (96%), biodegradable (polylactide) pins (88%) and plates (83%) showed the best results. In the treatment of type IV fractures similar results could be found with a tendency of the best results after ORIF followed by resection and implantation of a prosthesis. If a prosthesis was implanted, the primary implantation seems to be associated with a better outcome after type III (87%) and IV (82%) fractures compared to the results after a secondary implantation.

Discussion.—Recommendations for surgical treatment of radial head and neck fractures according to the Mason classification can now be given with the best available evidence.

Level of evidence.—IV.

▶ The optimal treatment strategy for radial head fractures is controversial. The authors have conducted a systematic review and meta-analysis of the literature in an attempt to develop evidence-based treatment guidelines. A thorough review of the literature was conducted and articles included from 1948 to 2011. In recent years, we have learned that radial head excision and SILASTIC implants have poor results and are not recommended, despite published reports that may have shown good short-term results. The effect inclusion of studies conducted in the distant past has on the overall results of this study is unknown. The included studies were generally of low levels of evidence, and this limits the strength of the study conclusions. As a result, the recommendations must be taken very cautiously. It is my personal experience that many Mason II fractures can be treated nonoperatively, and a randomized controlled trial is needed before we can definitively say that open reduction, internal fixation (ORIF) offers superior results. Mason type III fractures are often best treated with metallic prosthesis, especially when the head is fractured into greater than 3 fragments. Again, until a randomized, controlled trial comparing ORIF with primary prosthetic replacement is conducted, we cannot say that one treatment modality is superior to another.

R. Grewal, MD

Repairing the annular ligament is not necessary in the operation of Mason type 2, 3 isolated radial head fractures if the lateral collateral ligament is intact: Minimum 5 years follow-up
Han SH, Lee SC, Ryu KJ, et al (CHA Univ School of Medicine, Seongnam-si, Gyeonggi-do, Republic of Korea)
Injury 44:1851-1854, 2013

Introduction.—The repair of annular ligament after open reduction and internal fixation of radial head fracture could produce the irritation or crepitation during range of motion exercise. The purpose of this study is to evaluate the significance of unrepaired annular ligament during fixation of isolated radial head fractures.

Materials and Methods.—Retrospectively we reviewed the twenty-five patients who underwent surgical fixation with a plate for Mason type 2, 3 isolated radial head fracture without annular ligament repair. All the radial head fracture did not have the associated injuries which could cause the elbow instabilities. The average length of follow-up was 6.9 years. The outcomes were evaluated clinically (range of motions, instabilities, pain VAS, Broberg & Murrey functional rating score, DASH score) and radiographically (bony union, arthritic change, lateral translation of the radial head, humero-ulnar angle with maximum varus stress of elbow, ulnar variance).

Results.—The range of motions between affected and contralateral side were not significantly different at last follow-up. No one showed the instabilities of elbow. The mean pain VAS, Broberg & Murrey functional rating score, and DASH score were 2.7 ± 0.5, 95.3 ± 2.5, and 14.8 ± 5.3 points respectively. Bony union was observed for all cases. There was no significant difference in the lateral translation of the radial head, humero-ulnar angle with maximum varus stress of elbow, and ulnar variance between the affected and the contralateral arm.

Conclusion.—The isolated role of the annular ligament seems overestimated. We scrutinize that the annular ligament repair is not essential in the operative treatment of isolated radial head fractures if the lateral collateral ligament is intact.

▶ This study aims to address the role of the unrepaired annular ligament in elbow stability in the setting of an isolated radial head fracture. A range of outcome measures are used, including the DASH score, a valid and reliable measure. The follow-up is excellent at a mean of nearly 7 years and a minimum of 5 years. The authors state that the role of the annular ligament is overestimated, and they feel that repair is not essential in the setting of an isolated radial head fracture with an intact lateral ulnar collateral ligament. It should be noted however, that these conclusions are based on a retrospective study. Limitations also include the lack of a comparison or control group and small sample size (n = 25). In this series, it seems that the annular ligament was not repaired in each case or stability tested intraoperatively, and unstable elbows were excluded from this series. This may have led to the risk of selection bias. My personal practice is to repair the annular ligament and aim to restore normal anatomy. However, care must be taken not to overtighten and shorten this ligament during repair, as that may be more detrimental than leaving it unprepared.

R. Grewal, MD

16 Elbow: Miscellaneous

Nonsurgical Treatment of Elbow Stiffness
Paul R, Chan R (Univ of Alberta, Edmonton, Canada)
J Hand Surg 38A:2002-2004, 2013

Background.—It is common to suffer stiffness caused by posttraumatic capsular contracture after elbow injury. Nonsurgical treatment consists mainly of stretching exercises and splinting, whether static progressive or dynamic, under the direction of a physical or occupational therapist. The most effective nonsurgical treatment for a specific patient was sought.

> *Case Report.*—Man, 21, suffered a closed dislocation of his right elbow when he fell on his extended arm during a college basketball game. The elbow was reduced and assessed radiographically in the emergency department, finding no fractures. A splint was applied to hold the arm in 90° of elbow flexion and neutral rotation of the forearm. When the splint was removed 10 days later, range of motion exercises were begun. Twelve weeks later the patient still complained of stiffness, with 45° to 110° of flexion possible. No signs of ulnar neuropathy or other radiographic abnormalities were seen. The treatment chosen was the application of a custom-made turnbuckle type orthosis and exercises under the supervision of an occupational therapist. These included a static progressive stretch every 5 minutes for 30 minutes three times a day with the arm in both flexion and extension. The patient was told that the rate of gain in motion would be highest in the first 3 months, but improvement could continue for up to 1 year. Depending on his progress, surgical contracture release could be required after 3 to 6 months of splinting.

Assessment of Evidence.—The principal treatment choices were static progressive splinting and dynamic splinting. Only one prospective randomized controlled trial compared the two approaches. No statistically significant differences in outcomes were noted between the two approaches. Range of motion continued to improve for up to 1 year after injury, although the major gains were made in the first 3 months after instituting therapy, with slower but noticeable improvement for 9 months thereafter. One study also found that a protective attitude toward stretching exercises in the first month of rehabilitation was associated with less recovery of elbow motion. No studies indicated whether patient self-administered stretching, therapist-administered stretching, or time alone was the best approach to achieving improvement.

Conclusions.—Stretching exercises, joint mobilization, and heat are widely employed as methods to manage posttraumatic elbow stiffness. However, scientific data supporting any of these methods are lacking. Further study into the effectiveness of each approach is needed, along with investigation into the role of patients' perceptions about stretching and pain or tightness during rehabilitation.

▶ A literature review of the treatment for elbow stiffness reveals a paucity of low, moderate, and high levels of evidence for the usual intervention for stiff elbows. Although the usual approach after elbow trauma is active and active-assistive exercises (A/AAROM) with the use of static progressive or dynamic orthoses for both terminal elbow flexion and extension when there is a plateau of progress, the evidence is lacking for dosage frequency, timeframes, and outcomes of range of motion (ROM) to be expected within what timeframes.

Functional ROM of the elbow is generally accepted at 100°. Of the 7 studies reviewed, only 5 reported achieving this benchmark. However, the studies were not homogenous as to when to initiate orthotic intervention, or how many times per day, or optimal hours of wear. Of note, there is also no consensus for which therapeutic procedure achieves best ROM (ie, A/AAROM, joint mobilizations, therapeutic activities, participation in place of exercise, orthotic intervention).

The authors suggest a set of great research ideas that could propel our knowledge of stiff elbow intervention further: a prospective, multicenter cohort to study mean and standard deviations of final ROM gain; timeframes to expect the most ROM change and when gains of ROM will no longer change significantly; randomized controlled trials with at least 12 months follow-up, which have a comparison of exercises with and without therapy supervision, and inclusion of exercise programs that include orthoses.

V. H. O'Brien, OTD, OTR/L, CHT

Do blood growth factors offer additional benefit in refractory lateral epicondylitis? A prospective, randomized pilot trial of dry needling as a stand-alone procedure versus dry needling and autologous conditioned plasma
Stenhouse G, Sookur P, Watson M (West Middlesex Univ Hosp NHS Trust, Isleworth, UK)
Skeletal Radiol 42:1515-1520, 2013

Objective.—To evaluate whether autologous conditioned plasma offers any therapeutic advantage over ultrasound-guided dry needling as a stand-alone procedure in the treatment of refractory lateral epicondylitis.

Materials and Methods.—Prospective, randomized pilot study of 28 patients (11 men, 17 women, mean age, 49.1 years) with refractory lateral epicondylitis (mean symptom duration, 19.1 months) who underwent either dry needling ($n = 13$) or dry needling combined with autologous conditioned plasma (ACP) injection ($n = 15$). Each patient received two separate injections (0 weeks and 1 month) and analysis of visual analogue pain scores (VAS) and Nirschl scores were performed pre-procedure, at 2 months and final evaluation at 6 months. Successful treatment was defined as more than a 25 % reduction in pain scores without re-intervention. Data was analyzed using the Mann—Whitney test and local research ethics committee approval was obtained.

Results.—At 2 months, the mean VAS improvement was 0.85 (12.3 %) in the dry needling group compared to 2.19 (27.1 %) in the ACP group ($p = 0.76$) and there was a 5.83-point and 20.3-point Nirschl score improvement respectively ($p = 0.72$). At the final follow-up of 6 months, the mean VAS improvement was 2.37 (34 %) in the dry needling group compared to 3.92 (48.5 %) in the ACP group ($p = 0.74$) and there was a 22.5-point and 40-point Nirschl score improvement, respectively ($p = 0.82$).

Conclusions.—There is a trend to greater clinical improvement in the short term for patients treated with additional ACP, however no significant difference between the two treatment groups was demonstrated at each follow-up interval. A larger, multicenter, randomized controlled trial is required to corroborate the results of this pilot study.

▶ The authors of this study compared treatment of refractory lateral epicondylitis (symptoms of at least 6 months duration and failure of conservative treatments) using ultrasound-guided dry needling alone versus dry needling with administration of autologous conditioned plasma (ACP). A prospective randomized trial was conducted, enrolling 28 consecutive patients. Each patient underwent 2 separate treatments, spaced 1 month apart. The authors found an improvement in the Visual Analog Scale (VAS) scores of both treatment groups as at 6 months, with a trend toward greater improvement in the ACP group. It is difficult to draw conclusions regarding the efficacy of these treatment strategies based on such a small sample size. The natural history of lateral epicondylitis is often spontaneous resolution over time. An additional comparison between a placebo group that underwent ultrasound scan and local anesthetic injection into the deep fascia without dry needling, dry needling alone, and dry needling and ACP is needed, with a larger patient sample, to confidently report that dry needling alone shows clinical efficacy.

F. G. Fishman, MD

Efficacy of Platelet-Rich Plasma for Chronic Tennis Elbow: A Double-Blind, Prospective, Multicenter, Randomized Controlled Trial of 230 Patients
Mishra AK, Skrepnik NV, Edwards SG, et al (Stanford Univ Med Ctr, Menlo Park, CA; Tucson Orthopaedic Inst, AZ; Georgetown Univ Hosp, Washington, DC; et al)
Am J Sports Med 42:463-471, 2014

Background.—Elbow tenderness and pain with resisted wrist extension are common manifestations of lateral epicondylar tendinopathy, also known as tennis elbow. Previous studies have suggested platelet-rich plasma (PRP) to be a safe and effective therapy for tennis elbow.

Purpose.—To evaluate the clinical value of tendon needling with PRP in patients with chronic tennis elbow compared with an active control group.

Study Design.—Randomized controlled trial; Level of evidence, 2.

Methods.—A total of 230 patients with chronic lateral epicondylar tendinopathy were treated at 12 centers over 5 years. All patients had at least 3 months of symptoms and had failed conventional therapy. There were no differences in patients randomized to receive PRP (n = 116) or active controls (n = 114). The PRP was prepared from venous whole blood at the point of care and contained both concentrated platelets and leukocytes. After receiving a local anesthetic, all patients had their extensor tendons needled with or without PRP. Patients and investigators remained blinded to the treatment group throughout the study. A successful outcome was defined as 25% or greater improvement on the visual analog scale for pain.

Results.—Patient outcomes were followed for up to 24 weeks. At 12 weeks (n = 192), the PRP-treated patients reported an improvement of 55.1% in their pain scores compared with 47.4% in the active control group ($P = .163$). At 24 weeks (n = 119), the PRP-treated patients reported an improvement of 71.5% in their pain scores compared with 56.1% in the control group ($P = .019$). The percentage of patients reporting significant elbow tenderness at 12 weeks was 37.4% in the PRP group versus 48.4% in the control group ($P = .143$). Success rates for patients at 12 weeks were 75.2% in the PRP group versus 65.9% in the control group ($P = .104$). At 24 weeks, 29.1% of the PRP-treated patients reported significant elbow tenderness versus 54.0% in the control group ($P = .009$). Success rates for patients with 24 weeks of follow-up were 83.9% in the PRP group compared with 68.3% in the control group ($P = .037$). No significant complications occurred in either group.

Conclusion.—No significant differences were found at 12 weeks in this study. At 24 weeks, however, clinically meaningful improvements were found in patients treated with leukocyte-enriched PRP compared with an active control group.

▶ Lateral epicondylitis commonly presents to the upper extremity surgeon's office. Because it is unclear what treatment, if any, is effective, management can be frustrating to patient and physician.

This report describes 230 patients treated with either platelet-rich plasma (PRP) or control needling followed up over 12 or 24 weeks. Successful treatment was defined as a 25% reduction in the visual analog scale (VAS) score. Although the study reports a significant difference between PRP and the control group, there are limitations to the study, including imputed but not actual follow-up VAS scores over divergent time periods and a large number of patients at variable time points or excluded in addition to what may be a small clinical difference (ie, 25% reduction in VAS, which may well fit within the margin of error).

J. E. Adams, MD

Change in Quality of Life and Cost/Utility Analysis in Open Stage-related Surgical Treatment of Elbow Stiffness

Giannicola G, Bullitta G, Sacchetti FM, et al (Univ of Rome "La Sapienza," Italy)

Orthopedics 36:e923-e930, 2013

The goals of this study were to examine the improvement in quality of life achieved after open surgical treatment of elbow stiffness and to verify the cost/utility ratio of surgery. Thirtythree patients (22 men and 11 women) underwent surgery. The etiologies of elbow stiffness were posttraumatic conditions (n = 26), primary osteoarthritis (n = 5), and rheumatoid arthritis (n = 2). Surgery included 14 ulnohumeral arthroplasties, 6 ulnohumeral arthroplasties associated with radiocapitellar replacement, 5 ulnohumeral arthroplasties associated with radial head replacement, and 8 total elbow arthroplasties. All patients were evaluated pre- and postoperatively with the Mayo Elbow Performance Score, the Mayo Elbow Performance Index, the modified American Shoulder and Elbow Surgeons score, the Quick Disabilities of the Arm, Shoulder and Hand score, and the Short Form 36 after a mean follow-up of 26 months. Possible variables affecting clinical outcome and quality of life improvement were assessed. The cost/utility ratio was evaluated as diagnosis-related group reimbursement per quality-adjusted life year. Mayo Elbow Performance Scores and modified American Shoulder and Elbow Surgeons scores increased, on average, by 43 and 41 points, respectively ($P < .0001$). Quick Disabilities of the Arm, Shoulder and Hand scores decreased, on average, by 44 points ($P < .0001$). The improvement in the SF-36 physical and mental component summary score was 7.6 and 7, respectively ($P = .0001$ and .0018). The cost/utility ratio ranged between 670 and 817 Euro/quality-adjusted life year. A significant correlation was found between pain score and quality of life improvement. An inverse correlation emerged between pre- and postoperative quality of life score. The current study shows that open surgery significantly improves quality of life and elbow function. Selecting the surgical procedure that most effectively reduces pain appears to be the most relevant variable responsible for quality of life improvement. Surgery shows a satisfactory cost/utility ratio, justifying a health spending increase to reduce the social costs resulting from lingering elbow stiffness.

▶ The goal of this study was to evaluate whether open, stage-related surgical treatment for elbow stiffness improves quality of life and elbow function and to analyze the cost/utility ratio of surgery. Evaluation of quality of life after management of stiffness has only been assessed previously by a single study. The authors of this study found a significant improvement in quality-of-life values for patients with lower quality-of-life values preoperatively. Additionally, all patients who did not obtain significant quality-of-life improvements had comorbidities. There was a positive cost utility ratio, suggesting a benefit to surgery in terms of the benefit to society. This is the first time this has been studied for the condition of elbow stiffness. Although the patient population was heterogeneous, related to cause of stiffness and procedure performed, this study supports surgical management of elbow stiffness as a valid means of improving quality of life and having a favorable cost/utility ratio.

T. J. Payne, MD

17 Pediatric Trauma

Intrafocal Pinning for Distal Radius Metaphyseal Fractures in Children
Parikh SN, Jain VV, Youngquist J (Cincinnati Children's Hosp Med Ctr, OH;
Univ of Cincinnati, OH)
Orthopedics 36:783-788, 2013

The purpose of this retrospective case control study was to evaluate the results of intrafocal pinning for distal radius metaphyseal fractures in children and to compare these results with conventional pinning. Data were collected from medical records and radiographs from patients who underwent closed reduction and percutaneous pinning for distal radius fracture in a Level I trauma center at the authors' institution between 2008 and 2010. Inclusion criteria included a dorsally angulated metaphyseal fracture without physeal involvement, an open distal radius physis, and a follow-up to radiographic union.

A total of 10 patients with intrafocal pinning were compared to 26 patients with conventional pinning. Preoperatively, angulation was greater in patients who received intrafocal pinning than conventional pinning based on anteroposterior radiographs. Postoperatively, the 2 groups did not differ in angulation on either anteroposterior or lateral radiographs. One malunion and 2 pin-related complications occurred in the conventional pinning group, and 1 pin-related complication occurred in the intrafocal pinning group. The 2 groups did not differ by age, sex, side of injury, days to surgery, or initial shortening.

This study affirms that the intrafocal pinning technique is an alternative to the conventional pinning technique for the stabilization of displaced metaphyseal distal radius fractures in children. Intrafocal pinning can also be used as a reduction tool for fractures that cannot be reduced by closed manipulation. The complications are comparable between the 2 techniques.

▶ Distal forearm metaphyseal fractures in children are fairly tolerant of angulation, provided that the distal radial ulnar joint is not disturbed. In cases in which an adequate reduction cannot be maintained by closed means, percutaneous pinning has become the standard for treatment of reducible fractures. Intrafocal pinning has a long-established track record in the distal radius and elsewhere for both assisting with fracture reduction and for providing definitive fixation as an adjunct to plaster. This study found no difference in outcomes or complications with either intrafocal or interfragmentary pinning for metaphyseal distal radius fractures with or without concomitant distal ulnar fractures. However, the study was underpowered to detect a clinically significant difference.

The study does highlight the technique of intrafocal pinning as both an alternative and a compliment to interfragmentary pinning. This is a valuable technique that may be used to avoid the need for an open reduction in some cases.

D. A. Zlotolow, MD

Pediatric Terrible Triad Elbow Fracture Dislocations: Report of 2 Cases

Dailiana ZH, Papatheodorou LK, Michalitsis SG, et al (Univ of Thessaly, Larissa, Greece)
J Hand Surg 38A:1774-1778, 2013

An elbow dislocation associated with radial head and coronoid process fractures, the terrible triad injury, has an unpredictable outcome in adults and is rare in children. We present 2 such injuries in children, 1 combined with an olecranon fracture, and both with good early clinical outcomes. However, in 1 of the 2 cases, avascular necrosis of the proximal radius was evident on radiographs.

▶ Terrible triad of the elbow (elbow dislocation, coronoid fracture, and radial head fracture) is a rare injury in adults and exceptionally rare in children. This article reports on 2 such injuries in a 4.5-year-old girl and an 11-year-old boy with short-term follow-up.

This article outlines the pattern of injury in 2 skeletally immature patients. Although they can be justifiably classified as terrible triad, the authors highlight the ways in which these injuries are unique. First, it is notable that the skeletal maturity of the 2 children is disparate. The 4.5-year-old girl had a fall from a small height. Furthermore, she had an associated proximal ulna fracture. Finally, she reportedly had medial collateral ligament avulsion (rather than the expected avulsion of the unossified apophysis). In contrast, the 11-year-old boy had a potentially high-energy injury (fall from bicycle). His case serves to remind us of the high risk of osteonecrosis of the radial head in displaced fractures treated with open reduction.

This case series alerts the physician treating pediatric elbow injuries to the fact that residual instability after closed reduction of a dislocation may be associated with similar injuries as seen in adults, particularly in difficult-to-interpret pediatric elbow films. Furthermore, application of the same principles used in adults seems to be effective in treating these injuries in children.

D. Bohn, MD

Confirmed Specific Ultrasonographic Findings of Pulled Elbow
Dohi D (Dohi Orthopaedic Hosp, Higashi, Hiroshima, Japan)
J Pediatr Orthop 33:829-831, 2013

Background.—Pulled elbow is a disorder commonly observed in children in routine medical practice; however, when the circumstances involved in the injury are unknown, difficulty has been encountered in differential diagnosis whether it is a bone fracture or pulled elbow. One of the reasons involved has been the unavailability of diagnostic imaging in confirming the diagnosis of the pulled elbow. Therefore, the author had performed ultrasonography for the pulled elbow and studied the specific ultrasonographic findings of the same.

Methods.—Using as subjects a total of 70 cases of pulled elbow, with their age ranging from 4 months to 6 years, ultrasonography was performed from September 2010 to February 2013 with the use of Hitachi EUB 7500 ultrasonographic apparatus with a 12 MHz transducer. Careful observation was made of the specific ultrasonographic images of anterior long-axis view of the radiohumeral joint before and after the manipulation.

Results.—Before the manipulation in all the cases, both the supinator muscle originating from the annular ligament and the annular ligament itself were entrapped within the radiohumeral joint, and a hypoechoic image of J-shape (J-sign) was observed. After the manipulation, the hypoechoic image of the J-shape disappeared and normal annular ligament image was observed.

Conclusions.—Accurate diagnosis of the pulled elbow can be done by ultrasonography through the confirmation of this specific J-sign.

Level of Evidence.—Level IV—diagnostic studies.

▶ Pulled elbow (aka nursemaid's elbow) is a common problem affecting toddlers. Although it is typically successfully treated with a simple reduction maneuver, diagnosis is occasionally difficult, especially when symptoms of immobility and pain don't resolve immediately after reduction. Differential diagnoses may include nondisplaced fracture or septic arthritis, in which cases repeated attempts at reduction are distressing to all involved in the child's care.

This report describes a novel way of verifying both the diagnosis and successful treatment of pulled elbow. The authors review a series of 70 patients who had ultrasound (US)-guided identification of the pathologic anatomy (supinator muscle and annular ligament interposition in the radiohumeral joint) and its resolution back to normal anatomy after reduction maneuver. They describe and demonstrate with photographs the appearance of the abnormal and normal anatomy on US. The test is painless and done with the elbow in the extended position.

Ultrasonography is becoming increasingly available in emergency departments and has the added advantage of being inexpensive and operated/interpreted by the physician on duty rather than depending on availability of a qualified US technician. This article could be practice changing for emergency care providers, especially in ambiguous cases in which symptoms don't resolve quickly.

D. Bohn, MD

Acute Compartment Syndrome After Intramedullary Nailing of Isolated Radius and Ulna Fractures in Children

Blackman AJ, Wall LB, Keeler KA, et al (Washington Univ School of Medicine, St Louis, MO)
J Pediatr Orthop 34:50-54, 2014

Background.—There exist varying reports in the literature regarding the incidence of compartment syndrome (CS) after intramedullary (IM) fixation of pediatric forearm fractures. A retrospective review of the experience with this treatment modality at our institution was performed to elucidate the rate of postoperative CS and identify risk factors for developing this complication.

Methods.—In this retrospective case series, we reviewed the charts of all patients treated operatively for isolated radius and ulnar shaft fractures from 2000 to 2009 at our institution and identified 113 patients who underwent IM fixation of both-bone forearm fractures. There were 74 closed fractures and 39 open fractures including 31 grade I fractures, 7 grade II fractures, and 1 grade IIIA fracture. If the IM nail could not be passed easily across the fracture site, a small open approach was used to aid reduction.

Results.—CS occurred in 3 of 113 patients (2.7%). CS occurred in 3 of 39 (7.7%) of the open fractures compared with none of 74 closed fractures ($P = 0.039$), including 45 closed fractures that were treated within 24 hours of injury. An open reduction was performed in all of the open fractures and 38 (51.4%) of the closed fractures. Increased operative time was associated with developing CS postoperatively (168 vs. 77 min, $P < 0.001$). CS occurred within the first 24 postoperative hours in all 3 cases.

Conclusion.—CS was an uncommon complication after IM fixation of pediatric diaphyseal forearm fractures in this retrospective case series. Open fractures and longer operative times were associated with developing CS after surgery. None of 45 patients who underwent IM nailing of closed fractures within 24 hours of injury developed CS; however, 51.4% of these patients required a small open approach to aid reduction and nail passage. We believe that utilizing a small open approach for reduction of one or both bones, thereby avoiding the soft-tissue trauma of multiple attempts to reduce the fracture and pass the nail, leads to decreased soft-tissue trauma and a lower rate of CS. We recommend a low threshold for converting to open reduction in cases where closed reduction is difficult (Table 3).

▶ Compartment syndrome (CS) complicating treatment of both-bone forearm fracture (BBFF) in children is relatively rare but devastating. This article

TABLE 3.—Comparison of Studies Reporting CS in Patients After Intramedullary Nailing of Pediatric Both-Bone Forearm Fractures

	Current	Yuan et al[19]	Flynn et al[5]
No. patients	113	80	103
CS incidence [n (%)]			
Overall	3/113 (2.7)	6/80 (7.5)	2/103 (1.9)
Open fractures	3/39 (7.7)	3/50 (6)	NR
Closed fractures	0/74 (0)	3/30 (10)	NR
Treated <24 h	3/84 (3.6)	NR	2/30 (6.7)
Treated >24 h	0/29 (0)	NR	0/73 (0)

CS indicates compartment syndrome; NR, not required.
Editor's Note: Please refer to original journal article for full references.

retrospectively reviews 113 patients treated with intramedullary (IM) fixation over a 10-year period in an attempt to identify risk factors for CS in such patients.

The authors found that there was an overall rate of CS of 2.7% (3/113). No children with closed injuries developed compartment syndrome after IM fixation (0/74). Three of 39 (7.7%) children with open fractures (all Gustilo type I) developed compartment syndrome. Independent risk factors associated with development of CS in this cohort were open fracture and increased surgical time.

It is notable that these authors describe a regimen for minimizing soft tissue trauma by limiting attempts to pass the rod to the distal fragment to 3 before open reduction is performed. Thus, 51% of the patients with closed fractures had open reduction. They offer this as an explanation for their very low (0/113) rate of CS in closed BBFF in contrast to the series reported by Yuan et al (Table 3), who reported a CS rate of 10% in closed fractures with IM fixation. The authors also cite a report by Flynn et al in which there was a 1.9% rate of CS (2/103 patients). That series found that the 2 patients who developed CS were treated within 24 hours of injury, and no patients treated > 24 hours after injury developed CS.

Although a missed compartment syndrome should be a "never" event, it appears that the rate of CS in pediatric patients with closed BBFFs treated with IM fixation > 24 hours after injury with short surgical times and minimal soft tissue trauma may be low enough to warrant routine outpatient management.

D. Bohn, MD

18 Congenital

Thumb Hypoplasia
Soldado F, Zlotolow DA, Kozin SH (Universitat Autonoma de Barcelona, Spain; Shriners Hosp for Children, Philadelphia, PA)
J Hand Surg 38A:1435-1444, 2013

Thumb hypoplasia, congenital underdevelopment of the thumb, can range from a slight decrease in thumb size to complete absence of the thumb. As part of the radial longitudinal deficiency spectrum, other organ systems may be affected as well. Hence, the global health of the child should be addressed before focusing on the thumb. The decision of whether to reconstruct the existing thumb or to ablate the thumb and perform a pollicization of the index finger hinges primarily on the examination of trapeziometacarpal joint stability. Ultrasound imaging may play a role in decision making in borderline cases. The ultimate goal of surgical treatment is to provide a stable and functional thumb.

▶ Thumb hypoplasia is a complex congenital abnormality for which there is not a universally applicable treatment for all patients. This article clearly defines the nature and classification of the progressive severity of thumb hypoplasia and guides the surgeon in treating each subset of patients with the most current concepts available. The authors introduce the technique of using ultrasound scan to evaluate carpometacarpal joint stability and the opponens pollicis to determine the need for pollicization or opposition transfer, respectively. This step is critical in embarking down the correct treatment pathway, and this article may help guide further research into the use of ultrasound scan in congenital hand surgery. The article includes many helpful patient photographs and roentograms to aid in diagnosis. Surgical technique guides are also included with step-by-step imagery. This article is a succinct yet comprehensive review of the management of thumb hypoplasia and is a worthwhile addition to any hand surgeon's library.

R. Endress, MD

Classification of Congenital Anomalies of the Hand and Upper Limb: Development and Assessment of a New System
Tonkin MA, Tolerton SK, Quick TJ, et al (Royal North Shore Hosp, St. Leonards, New South Wales, Australia; The Children's Hosp at Westmead, New South Wales, Australia; Univ of Sydney, New South Wales, Australia)
J Hand Surg 38A:1845-1853, 2013

The Oberg, Manske, and Tonkin (OMT) classification of congenital hand and upper limb anomalies was proposed in 2010 as a replacement for the Swanson International Federation of Societies for Surgery of the Hand classification system, which has been the accepted system of classification for the international surgical community since 1976. The OMT system separates malformations from deformations and dysplasias. Malformations are subdivided according to the axis of formation and differentiation that is primarily affected and whether the anomalies involve the whole limb or the hand plate. This review outlines the development of classification systems and explores the difficulty of incorporating our current knowledge of limb embryogenesis at a molecular level into current systems. An assessment of the efficacy of the OMT classification demonstrates acceptable inter- and intraobserver reliability. A prospective review of 101 patients confirms that all diagnoses could be classified within the OMT system. Consensus expert opinion allowed classification of those conditions for which there is not a clear understanding of the mechanism of dysmorphology. A refined and expanded OMT classification is presented.

▶ Classification systems are only valuable if they help guide treatment, predict a patient's prognosis, or assist in clarifying a patient's condition for research or for interphysician communication. The advantage of a morphologic classification system is that morphology does not change over time. Surely, variations in the presentation (ie, morphology) of congenital differences will continue to exist and challenge any classification system, but most cases will remain classifiable over time.

One of the problems with an etiologically based classification system is that the system needs to change to accommodate new understanding in the mechanisms of disease. Although there is much that we know about the mechanism of congenital differences, many conditions such as amyoplasia remain a mystery.

The Oberg, Manske, and Tonkin classification, although relatively reliable in terms of inter- and intraobserver variability, may or may not be accurate. Few people in the world understand congenital differences as well as the authors of this study, and their efforts to refine the classification scheme are certainly on the right track. However, until we have a better understanding of how these differences arise, and until the authors can show that the new classification system can better guide treatment and prognostication, it is unlikely that this new scheme will be adopted for widespread use.

D. A. Zlotolow, MD

Type II and IIIA Thumb Hypoplasia Reconstruction

Christen T, Dautel G (Centre Hospitalier Universitaire Vaudois, Lausanne, Switzerland; Univ Hosp of Nancy, France)
J Hand Surg 38A:2009-2015, 2013

Thumb hypoplasia treatment requires considering every component of the maldevelopment. Types II and IIIA hypoplasia share common features such as first web space narrowing, hypoplasia or absence of thenar muscles and metacarpophalangeal joint instability. Many surgical techniques to correct the malformation have been described. We report our surgical strategy that includes modifications of the usual technique that we found useful in reducing morbidity while optimizing the results. A diamond-shape kite flap was used to widen the first web space. Its design allowed primary closure of the donor site using a Dufourmentel flap. The ring finger flexor digitorum superficialis was transferred for opposition transfer, and the same tendon was used to stabilize the metacarpophalangeal joint on its ulnar and/or radial side depending on a uniplanar or more global instability. An omega-shaped K-wire was placed between the first and second metacarpals to maintain a wide opening of the first web space without stressing the reconstructed ulnar collateral ligament of the MCP joint. We report a

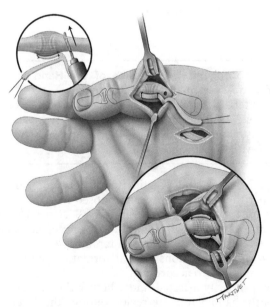

FIGURE 9.—Illustration depicting the fixation of the tendinous slips on the metacarpal head and the base of the proximal phalanx. The transosseous tunnel is drilled at a safe distance from the growth plate. (Reprinted from Christen T, Dautel G. Type II and IIIA thumb hypoplasia reconstruction. *J Hand Surg.* 2013;38A:2009-2015, with permission from the American Society for Surgery of the Hand.)

clinical series of 15 patients (18 thumbs) who had this reconstructive program (Fig 9).

▶ The authors present an alternative approach to children with Blauth type II to IIIa thumbs in which there is a tight first web space, hypoplastic or absent thenar muscles, and an unstable metacarpophalangeal (MCP) joint. In addition, in type IIIa, there may be extrinsic tendon abnormalities. These 2 types are grouped together because reconstruction is possible and pollicization is not necessary.

The authors have presented alternatives to each of the reconstructive steps. I am not convinced of the advantage of their approach and will itemize why. The authors chose a diamond flap over a 4-flap z-plasty for the first web space contracture. Their results show fairly minimal improvement because of the small flap inset. Also, the additional incisions do not seem worth the proposed gains. I feel that a big 4-flap z-plasty with wide release is indicated here.

The authors chose an flexor digitorum superficialis (FDS) transfer for thumb opposition and later comment that many parents were not satisfied with the size of the thumb. I prefer the standard Huber transfer so that at least some of the muscle bulk of the abductor digiti minimi will be at the base of the thumb.

The omega-shaped K-wire requires the child to have another anesthetic for removal; this does not seem to be worth it compared with the risk and cost of anesthesia. I do like how the authors attempt to stabilize the multidirectional instability of the metacarpophalangeal joint. To me, this has been the most unsatisfying part of my technique. I will now use a free graft to pass around the joint as they have elegantly shown (Fig 9).

J. Chang, MD

Classification of Congenital Anomalies of the Hand and Upper Limb: Development and Assessment of a New System
Tonkin MA, Tolerton SK, Quick TJ, et al (Royal North Shore Hosp, St. Leonards, New South Wales, Austral; The Children's Hosp at Westmead, Sydney, New South Wales, Australia; Univ of Sydney, New South Wales, Australia)
J Hand Surg 38A:1845-1853, 2013

The Oberg, Manske, and Tonkin (OMT) classification of congenital hand and upper limb anomalies was proposed in 2010 as a replacement for the Swanson International Federation of Societies for Surgery of the Hand classification system, which has been the accepted system of classification for the international surgical community since 1976. The OMT system separates malformations from deformations and dysplasias. Malformations are subdivided according to the axis of formation and differentiation that is primarily affected and whether the anomalies involve the whole limb or the hand plate. This review outlines the development of classification systems and explores the difficulty of incorporating our current knowledge of limb embryogenesis at a molecular level into current systems.

An assessment of the efficacy of the OMT classification demonstrates acceptable inter- and intraobserver reliability. A prospective review of 101 patients confirms that all diagnoses could be classified within the OMT system. Consensus expert opinion allowed classification of those conditions for which there is not a clear understanding of the mechanism of dysmorphology. A refined and expanded OMT classification is presented.

▶ The authors of this study sought to show that the Oberg, Manske, and Tonkin (OMT) classification of congenital hand and upper limb anomalies has significant advantages over the currently utilized modified Swanson/International Federation of Societies for Surgery of the Hand (IFSSH) Classification. Unlike the Swanson/IFSSH classification, which is based on a morphologic system, the OMT classification integrates morphology and our current understanding of the etiologies of these conditions. Using a framework that includes malformations, dysplasias, and deformations, they showed that the diagnoses could be successfully transferred from the Swanson/IFSSH classification to the OMT classification. Syndromes were classified separately secondary to the possible presence of multiple anomalies within a single syndrome. They reported an intraobserver reliability of the OMT system of 85% to 99%, which also correlated highly with the level of experience of the clinician. Most experts in the field of congenital hand surgery expressed preference for the OMT classification over the Swanson/IFSSH. As our understanding of limb embryogenesis and the molecular genetic basis of congenital upper extremity anomalies evolves, it seems appropriate that the system with which we classify these differences would also evolve. The OMT has been further refined based on the analysis of this study and is currently under review by the Congenital Hand Surgery Scientific Committee of the IFSSH for its use in the future.

F. G. Fishman, MD

Epidemiology of Congenital Upper Limb Anomalies in Stockholm, Sweden, 1997 to 2007: Application of the Oberg, Manske, and Tonkin Classification
Ekblom AG, Laurell T, Arner M (Karolinska Institutet, Stockholm, Sweden)
J Hand Surg Am 39:237-248, 2014

Purpose.—To investigate the epidemiology of congenital upper limb anomalies (CULA) based on the newly proposed Oberg, Manske, and Tonkin (OMT) classification, to compare this classification with the International Federation of Societies for Surgery of the Hand (IFSSH) classification, and to provide incidence rates of the different CULA.

Methods.—In this study, the same 562 individuals with a CULA who were analyzed in a previous epidemiologic study based on the IFSSH classification were reclassified according to the OMT classification. All children identified with CULA and born in Stockholm County between January 1, 1997 and December 31, 2007 were included in the study. During the period there were 261,914 live births in Stockholm County, and the population of Stockholm County was 1,949,516 inhabitants at the end of the period. From medical records and available radiographs, all cases were analyzed regarding type of CULA, sex, affected side, associated non-hand anomalies, and occurrence among relatives. Individuals with right and left side anomalies belonging to different OMT subgroups were counted as 2 anomalies; thus, the material consisted of 577 CULA in 562 children.

Results.—It was possible to organize all CULA into the OMT classification. The largest main category was malformations (429 cases), followed by deformations (124 cases), dysplasias (10 cases), and syndromes (14 cases). We present the relation between the IFSSH and OMT classifications, elucidate difficulties within the OMT classification, and propose additions to the classification.

Conclusions.—This study confirms that the OMT classification is useful and accurate, but also points out difficulties. With further refinements, we regard the OMT classification as a needed and appropriate replacement for the IFSSH classification.

Type of Study/Level of Evidence.—Diagnostic III.

▶ All children born with congenital upper limb anomalies (CULA) in Stockholm, Sweden, between 1997 and 2007 were categorized according to the Oberg, Manske, and Tonkin (OMT) classification. This same cohort was previously classified under the International Federation of Societies for Surgery of the Hand, which has fallen out of favor because of our increased knowledge on limb development. The OMT classification continues to be refined with the ultimate goal of obtaining a system that is easy to apply and allows for comparison of studies between different populations and time periods. A common language will help formulate appropriate treatment guidelines. For those who treat patients with CULA, this study provides the incidence, relative frequency, sex, affected side, associated nonhand anomalies, and occurrence among relatives, which can be useful when counseling our patients and their families. There may be regional differences that limit the applicability of the data, but the Swedish registries provide some of the most comprehensive epidemiologic information available. As the authors propose, continued modifications of the classification's imperfections will ultimately lead to a useful tool for all physicians treating patients with CULA.

A. Moeller, MD

19 Shoulder: Rotator Cuff

Biomechanical Comparison of Single-Row, Double-Row, and Transosseous-Equivalent Repair Techniques after Healing in an Animal Rotator Cuff Tear Model

Quigley RJ, Gupta A, Oh J-H, et al (Univ of California, Irvine, CA)
J Orthop Res 31:1254-1260, 2013

The transosseous-equivalent (TOE) rotator cuff repair technique increases failure loads and contact pressure and area between tendon and bone compared to single-row (SR) and double-row (DR) repairs, but no study has investigated if this translates into improved healing in vivo. We hypothesized that a TOE repair in a rabbit chronic rotator cuff tear model would demonstrate a better biomechanical profile than SR and DR repairs after 12 weeks of healing. A two-stage surgical procedure was performed on 21 New Zealand White Rabbits. The right subscapularis tendon was transected and allowed to retract for 6 weeks to simulate a chronic tear. Repair was done with the SR, DR, or TOE technique and allowed to heal for 12 weeks. Cyclic loading and load to failure biomechanical testing was then performed. The TOE repair showed greater biomechanical characteristics than DR, which in turn were greater than SR. These included yield load ($p < 0.05$), energy absorbed to yield ($p < 0.05$), and ultimate load ($p < 0.05$). For repair of a chronic, retracted rotator cuff tear, the TOE technique was the strongest biomechanical construct after healing followed by DR with SR being the weakest.

▶ Rotator cuff repair techniques have evolved. Yet, retear rates have been reported to occur in between 20% and 70%, depending on various factors such as age, tear size, and presence of fatty atrophy. Studies have found that healing potential is related to the amount of tendon-to-bone contact area created by the repair. This study compared the transosseous equivalent (TOE) repair, with its improved contact area and pressure, with single row (SR) and double row (DR) repairs in terms of biomechanical properties after a period of tendon healing in vivo using a rabbit chronic subscapularis tear model. Previous work from this group showed at time zero the TOE had a 38.5% increase in ultimate load compared with the DR group. In this study, the TOE repair group had an ultimate load that was 89% higher than that of the DR group. This higher in vivo value at a later time point compared with time zero suggests that the TOE group was not just stronger because of the repair construct used but also that an additive effect existed, that is, the stronger construct led to an improved healing environment.

These results suggest that the improved contact area and mean pressure of the tendon to the footprint of the TOE technique led to better healing. Also, at yield and ultimate loads, the strain on the tendon was greater for the TOE than the SR, indicating that under higher loads a greater distribution of stress occurred between the repair construct and the intact tendon for the TOE.

Because of these data, in addition to the growing body of literature to support the superior biomechanical strength of double row TOE repairs, many surgeons have incorporated this repair method in their common practice.

E. Cheung, MD

Partial Articular-sided Rotator Cuff Tears: In Situ Repair Versus Tear Completion Prior to Repair
Sethi PM, Rajaram A, Obopilwe E, et al (ONS Foundation for Clinical Res and Education, Greenwich; Yale Univ School of Medicine, New Haven, CT; Univ of Connecticut, Farmington)
Orthopedics 36:771-777, 2013

Uncertainty exists over the ideal surgical treatment method for partial articular-sided rotator cuff tears, with options ranging from debridement to in situ repair to tear completion prior to repair. The purpose of this study was to determine whether in situ repair was a viable biomechanical treatment option compared with tear completion prior to repair of partial articular-sided rotator cuff tears.

Fourteen fresh-frozen cadaveric shoulders were dissected. Partial articular-sided tears were created and repaired using in situ repair or tear completion prior to the repair. Strain and displacement were measured at 45°, 60°, and 90° of glenohumeral abduction. Testing was performed with a load of 100 N applied for 30 cycles. Data from the biomechanical testing displayed 4 conditions that showed improved characteristics of in situ repair over completion and repair: bursal-sided strain anteriorly at 45°, bursal-sided strain anteriorly at 90°, bursal-sided displacement anteriorly at 45°, and bursal-sided displacement anteriorly at 90°.

The data indicate that in situ repair is a viable biomechanical treatment option compared with tear completion prior to repair of partial articular-sided rotator cuff tears. When clinically appropriate, the in situ repair may offer some biomechanical advantages, with lower strain and displacement observed on the bursal side compared with tear completion prior to repair.

▶ The treatment of partial-thickness rotator cuff is controversial. These types of tears can be treated with debridement or repair. The 50% rule may be the best general guideline for treatment, in which tears smaller than 50% of the tendon's thickness are debrided and tears larger than 50% of the tendon's thickness are repaired. In some clinical situations, in situ repair may be a surgical option, such as in younger symptomatic athletes or laborers because of the loss of tissue integrity upon completion of the tear and the violation of previously intact tissue. The purpose of this study was to determine whether the in situ repair was a viable biomechanical treatment option compared with tear completion before repair. The authors hypothesized that the in situ repair would create strain characteristics that were improved from those achieved with repair after completion of a partial tear. When in situ repair was compared with tear completion, 4 conditions displayed statistically significant differences for improved strain and displacement characteristics of in situ repair over completion and repair: bursal-sided strain in the anterior section of the tendon at both 45° and 90° of abduction and bursal-sided displacement in the anterior section of the tendon at both 45° and 90° of abduction. The improved anterior tendon strain with in situ repair may be clinically relevant because this region of the rotator cuff is the first to experience load with physiologic motion. In addition, the data indicated that completion of the tear and subsequent repair created an increased amount of anterior strain on the bursal surface when compared with in situ repair at 45° and 90° of abduction. Nonetheless, clinical correlation has yet to support these findings, and this clinical problem remains controversial.

E. Cheung, MD

Calcific Tendinitis of the Rotator Cuff: A Randomized Controlled Trial of Ultrasound-Guided Needling and Lavage Versus Subacromial Corticosteroids
de Witte PB, Selten JW, Navas A, et al (Univ Med Ctr, Leiden, the Netherlands; et al)
Am J Sports Med 41:1665-1673, 2013

Background.—Calcific tendinitis of the rotator cuff (RCCT) is frequently diagnosed in patients with shoulder pain, but there is no consensus on its treatment.

Purpose.—To compare 2 regularly applied RCCT treatments: ultrasound (US)-guided needling and lavage (barbotage) combined with a US-guided corticosteroid injection in the subacromial bursa (subacromial bursa injection [SAI]) (group 1) versus an isolated SAI (group 2).

Study Design.—Randomized controlled trial; Level of evidence, 1.

Methods.—Patients were randomly assigned to the 2 groups. Shoulder function was assessed before treatment and at regular follow-up intervals (6 weeks and 3, 6, and 12 months) using the Constant shoulder score (CS, primary outcome), the Western Ontario Rotator Cuff Index (WORC), and the Disabilities of the Arm, Shoulder and Hand questionnaire (DASH). Additionally, calcification location, size, and Gärtner classification were assessed on radiographs. Results were analyzed using the t test, linear regression, and a mixed model for repeated measures.

Results.—This study included 48 patients (25 female, 52.1%; mean age, 52.0 ± 7.3 years; 23 patients in group 1) with a mean baseline CS of 68.7 ± 11.9. No patients were lost to follow-up. Four patients in group 1 and 11 in group 2 ($P = .06$) had an additional barbotage procedure or surgery during the follow-up period because of persisting symptoms and no resorption. At 1-year follow-up, the mean CS in group 1 was 86.0 (95% CI, 80.3-91.6) versus 73.9 (95% CI, 67.7-80.1) in group 2 ($P = .005$). The mean calcification size decreased by 11.6 ± 6.4 mm in group 1 and 5.1 ± 5.7 mm in group 2 ($P = .001$). There was total resorption in 13 patients in group 1 and 6 patients in group 2 ($P = .07$). With regression analyses, correcting for baseline CS and Gärtner type, the mean treatment effect was 20.5 points ($P = .05$) in favor of barbotage. Follow-up scores were significantly influenced by baseline scores. Results for the DASH and WORC were similar.

Conclusion.—On average, there was improvement at 1-year follow-up in both treatment groups, but clinical and radiographic results were significantly better in the barbotage group.

▶ This study is a well-constructed randomized, controlled trial. The authors had the objective of comparing ultrasound-guided steroid injection alone or in combination with ultrasound-guided barbotage (needling of the calcific deposit with normal saline lavage) for calcific tendonitis of the rotator cuff. The construction of this study was optimized to measure for response to each of the interventions. Findings of improvement at 1 year in both groups were present; however, the patients who had barbotage combined with steroid injection were significantly better in terms of resorption of the calcifications and higher clinical scores. The authors of the study point out that few randomized controlled trials compare treatment for calcific tendonitis of the rotator cuff and that this study validates the efficacy of barbotage combined with steroid injection in the treatment of this condition at 1-year follow-up. This study is an excellent example of design and execution and effectively answered the question that was posed by the investigators.

T. J. Payne, MD

Arthroscopic Repair of Massive Rotator Cuff Tears: Outcome and Analysis of Factors Associated With Healing Failure or Poor Postoperative Function
Chung SW, Kim JY, Kim MH, et al (Konkuk Univ Med Ctr, Seoul, Korea; Myongji Hosp, Goyang, Korea; Seoul Natl Univ Hosp, Seoul, Korea; et al)
Am J Sports Med 41:1674-1683, 2013

Background.—Many patients with an unhealed cuff after repair show functional improvement.

Purpose.—To evaluate outcomes of arthroscopically repaired massive rotator cuff tears and to identify prognostic factors affecting rotator cuff healing and functional outcome, especially in patients with failed rotator cuff healing.

Study Design.—Case series; Level of evidence, 4.

Methods.—Among 173 patients who underwent arthroscopic repair of a massive rotator cuff tear, 108 patients with a mean age of 63.7 years were included. Outcome evaluation was completed both anatomically (CT arthrography or ultrasonography) and functionally at a minimum of 1 year postoperatively; mean follow-up period was 31.68 ± 15.81 months. Various factors affecting cuff healing were analyzed, and factors affecting functional outcome were evaluated in patients with failed repairs using both univariate and multivariate analyses.

Results.—The anatomic failure rate was 39.8% in arthroscopically repaired massive rotator cuff tears; however, functional status significantly improved regardless of cuff healing ($P < .05$). Several factors were associated with failure of cuff healing in the univariate analysis, but only fatty infiltration (FI) of the infraspinatus was significantly related to healing failure in the multivariate analysis ($P = .04$). Among patients with failed rotator cuff healing, only reduced postoperative acromiohumeral distance (AHD) was related to poor functional outcome in the multivariate analysis ($P = .01$), with a cutoff value of 4.1 mm.

Conclusion.—Despite a high rate of healing failures, arthroscopic repair can be recommended in patients with massive rotator cuff tears because of the functional gain at midterm follow-up. Higher FI of the infraspinatus was the single most important factor negatively affecting cuff healing. In cases of failed massive rotator cuff repair, no preoperative factor was able to predict poor functional outcome; reduced postoperative AHD was the only relevant functional determinant in the patients' eventual functional outcome and should be considered when ascertaining a prognosis and planning further treatment strategies.

▶ This study evaluated the outcomes after arthroscopic repair of a large cohort of patients with massive rotator cuff tears. It evaluated many different pre- and postoperative findings and tried to correlate them with eventual patient outcomes. Their overall retear rate was roughly 40%, but patients were significantly improved in terms of pain and function irrespective of cuff integrity. Functionally, forward elevation was improved but external rotation was not. The authors' multivariate analysis indicated that fatty infiltration was associated with failure to heal. On univariate analysis, failure to heal was associated with female sex, longer symptom duration, lower bone mineral density, higher fatty infiltration of all rotator cuff muscles, bigger tear size (AP and retraction), and smaller pre- and postoperative acromiohumeral distance (AHD). Among those patients with failed rotator cuff healing, only postoperative AHD less than 4.1 mm correlated with poor outcomes. This study adds to the existing literature (including a recent meta-analysis that did not include this study[1]) that shows that patient outcomes improve after shoulder surgery for rotator cuff tears. This seems to be true even when the rotator cuff does not heal or heals incompletely.

J. Braman, MD

Reference

1. Russell RD, Knight JR, Mulligan E, Khazzam MS. Structural integrity after rotator cuff repair does not correlate with patient function and pain: a meta-analysis. *J Bone Joint Surg Am.* 2014;96:265-271.

Effect of Postoperative Repair Integrity on Health-Related Quality of Life After Rotator Cuff Repair: Healed Versus Retear Group
Yoo JH, Cho NS, Rhee YG (Kyung Hee Univ, Seoul, Korea)
Am J Sports Med 41:2637-2644, 2013

Background.—Although rotator cuff repair is performed to improve health-related quality of life (HRQL) by reducing pain and improving shoulder function, it has not been clearly demonstrated that HRQL is improved in retear cases.

Purpose.—To compare HRQL outcomes after rotator cuff repair between patients with healed cuffs and those with retears using the Short Form—36 Health Survey (SF-36).

Study Design.—Cohort study; Level of evidence, 3.

Methods.—A total of 81 patients who underwent rotator cuff repair were enrolled in this study. There were 56 patients in the healed group and 25 patients in the retear group. The mean age at the time of surgery was 56 years (range, 35-73 years) in the healed group and 59.7 years (range, 45-74 years) in the retear group. The mean follow-up period was 29.7 months (range, 14-95 months) and 26.4 months (range, 13-101 months) in the healed and retear groups, respectively.

Results.—At final follow-up, the SF-36 scores for physical and mental component summaries (PCS and MCS, respectively) revealed significant improvement, from 36.6 to 51.2 (PCS) and 34.4 to 51.6 (MCS) in the healed group ($P < .0001$ in both cases) and from 34.2 to 49.4 (PCS) and 33.4 to 53.2 (MCS) in the retear group ($P < .0001$ in both cases). Mean scores on the SF-36 subscale for role limitations because of physical health problems (RP) were 52.3 in the healed group and 50.6 in the retear group. The RP and PCS scores were significantly higher in the healed group ($P = .007$ and $P = .025$, respectively). All domains and component summaries also had a fair to moderate correlation (range, 0.296-0.496) with the SF-36 score.

Conclusion.—Although clinical shoulder outcome measures (University of California, Los Angeles [UCLA] and American Shoulder and Elbow Surgeons [ASES] scores) and all dimensions of the SF-36 showed significant improvement in both groups after rotator cuff repair, scores were significantly higher in the healed group on RP and PCS of the SF-36 as well as on the UCLA and ASES. There was no significant difference in MCS scores between the 2 groups. Despite similar improvements in the MCS scores, there were apparent objective differences between the groups. The values were statistically significant but clinically not significant for some of these measures.

▶ This cohort study of 81 patients evaluates healing of a rotator cuff repair on health-related quality of life. Improvement in patient outcome, despite healing of the rotator cuff tendon, has previously been reported. However, comparisons between both shoulder functional outcome measures like the UCLA or ASES scores, as well as health-related quality of life scores have not previously been reported in patients with healed rotator cuffs and those with a retear of the rotator cuff. In this study, 56 patients with healed rotator cuff and 25 patients with a retear of the rotator cuff were followed up for at least 2 years. American Shoulder and Elbow Surgeons (ASES), University of California, Los Angeles (UCLA), visual analog scale, and Short Form-36 Health Survey (SF-36) outcome measures were completed. The patients with a healed rotator cuff had significantly increased functional outcome scores on ASES, UCLA, and the role physical (RP) and physical component summaries (PCS) components of the SF-36. The RP component evaluates problems with activities because of physical health, whereas the PCS is a summary of components of which one is the RP. Ultimately, this study found that eventual healing of the rotator cuff tendons compared with retear is associated with improvement in shoulder functional outcome scores and health-related quality of life components of the SF-36.

J. Macalena, MD

Fatty degeneration of the rotator cuff muscles on pre- and postoperative CT arthrography (CTA): is the Goutallier grading system reliable?
Lee E, Choi J-A, Oh JH, et al (Seoul Natl Univ Bundang Hosp, Republic of Korea)
Skeletal Radiol 42:1259-1267, 2013

Objectives.—To retrospectively evaluate fatty degeneration (FD) of rotator cuff muscles on CTA using Goutallier's grading system and quantitative measurements with comparison between pre- and postoperative states.

Materials and Methods.—IRB approval was obtained for this study. Two radiologists independently reviewed pre- and postoperative CTAs of 43 patients (24 males and 19 females, mean age, 58.1 years) with 46 shoulders confirmed as full-thickness tears with random distribution. FD of supraspinatus, infraspinatus/teres minor, and subscapularis was assessed using Goutallier's system and by quantitative measurements of Hounsfield units (HUs) on sagittal images. Changes in FD grades and HUs were compared between pre- and postoperative CTAs and analyzed with respect to preoperative tear size and postoperative cuff integrity. The correlations between qualitative grades and quantitative measurements and their inter-observer reliabilities were also assessed.

Results.—There was statistically significant correlation between FD grades and HU measurements of all muscles on pre- and postoperative CTA ($p < 0.05$). Inter-observer reliability of fatty degeneration grades were excellent to substantial on both pre- and postoperative CTA in supraspinatus (0.8685 and 0.8535) and subscapularis muscles (0.7777 and 0.7972), but fair in infraspinatus/teres minor muscles (0.5791 and 0.5740); however, quantitative Hounsfield units measurements showed excellent reliability for all muscles (ICC: 0.7950 and 0.9346 for SST, 0.7922 and 0.8492 for SSC, and 0.9254 and 0.9052 for IST/TM). No muscle showed improvement of fatty degeneration after surgical repair on qualitative and quantitative assessments; there was no difference in changes of fatty degeneration after surgical repair according to preoperative tear size and post-operative cuff integrity ($p > 0.05$). The average dose-length product (DLP, mGy·cm) was 365.2 mGy·cm (range, 323.8-417.2 mGy·cm) and estimated average effective dose was 5.1 mSv.

Conclusions.—Goutallier grades correlated well with HUs of rotator cuff muscles. Reliability was excellent for both systems, except for FD grade of IST/TM muscles, which may be more reliably assessed using quantitative measurements.

▶ This study evaluated the important problem of evaluating fatty degeneration in patients with full-thickness rotator cuff tears. Fatty degeneration has been found to be a predictor of clinical outcome in patients with rotator cuff tears. The most widely utilized grading system for assessing fatty infiltration has been the Goutallier system (0, no fat; 1, fatty streaks; 2, less fat than muscle; 3, fat equal to muscle; 4, fat greater than muscle). The Goutallier system is qualitative by definition. This study compares the Goutallier system of grading fatty atrophy with a quantitative measure of Housfield units on preoperative and postoperative computed tomography (CT) scans. Good correlation was noted for both the qualitative measure of the Goutallier system and the quantitative measure of the Housfield units on patients before and after surgery. Measurements of the infraspinatus were somewhat more accurately measured quantitatively. Both of these systems utilized CT arthrograms as the index study. Future studies using magnetic resonance imaging to assess fatty infiltration, which is more commonly obtained than CT scan, will be necessary.

J. Braman, MD

Failure With Continuity in Rotator Cuff Repair "Healing"
McCarron JA, Derwin KA, Bey MJ, et al (Cleveland Clinic, OH; Bone and Joint Ctr, Detroit, MI)
Am J Sports Med 41:134-141, 2013

Background.—Ten to seventy percent of rotator cuff repairs form a recurrent defect after surgery. The relationship between retraction of the repaired tendon and formation of a recurrent defect is not well defined.

Purpose/Hypotheses.—To measure the prevalence, timing, and magnitude of tendon retraction after rotator cuff repair and correlate these outcomes with formation of a full-thickness recurrent tendon defect on magnetic resonance imaging, as well as clinical outcomes. We hypothesized that (1) tendon retraction is a common phenomenon, although not always associated with a recurrent defect; (2) formation of a recurrent tendon defect correlates with the timing of tendon retraction; and (3) clinical outcome correlates with the magnitude of tendon retraction at 52 weeks and the formation of a recurrent tendon defect.

Study Design.—Case series; Level of evidence, 4.

Methods.—Fourteen patients underwent arthroscopic rotator cuff repair. Tantalum markers placed within the repaired tendons were used to assess tendon retraction by computed tomography scan at 6, 12, 26, and 52 weeks after operation. Magnetic resonance imaging was performed to assess for recurrent tendon defects. Shoulder function was evaluated using the Penn score, visual analog scale (VAS) score for pain, and isometric scapular-plane abduction strength.

Results.—All rotator cuff repairs retracted away from their position of initial fixation during the first year after surgery (mean [standard deviation], 16.1 [5.3] mm; range, 5.7-23.2 mm), yet only 30% of patients formed a recurrent defect. Patients who formed a recurrent defect tended to have more tendon retraction during the first 6 weeks after surgery (9.7 [6.0] mm) than those who did not form a defect (4.1 [2.2] mm) ($P = .08$), but the total magnitude of tendon retraction was not significantly different between patient groups at 52 weeks. There was no significant correlation between the magnitude of tendon retraction and the Penn score ($r = 0.01$, $P = .97$) or normalized scapular abduction strength ($r = -0.21$, $P = .58$). However, patients who formed a recurrent defect tended to have lower Penn scores at 52 weeks ($P = .1$).

Conclusion.—Early tendon retraction, but not the total magnitude, correlates with formation of a recurrent tendon defect and worse clinical outcomes. "Failure with continuity" (tendon retraction without a recurrent defect) appears to be a common phenomenon after rotator cuff repair. These data suggest that repairs should be protected in the early postoperative period and repair strategies should endeavor to mechanically and biologically augment the repair during this critical early period.

▶ This study evaluated the role that tendon retraction—after repair—has in the role of outcomes after arthroscopic rotator cuff repair. The authors enrolled 14 patients with rotator cuff tears in a study that used tantalum (metal) balls implanted in the rotator cuff after repair as markers to allow computed tomography (CT) scanning measurements of the tendon location postoperatively. They did serial CT scans and magnetic resonance imaging scans at regular intervals (6, 12, 26, 52 weeks after surgery) to assess for cuff integrity and movement of the markers. Their results showed that early movement of the tendon (before 6 weeks) was associated with recurrent defect formation. In all patients, the distance between the anchors and the beads increased. However, in those patients (4 of 14) who had recurrent defects, the distance increased rapidly (in the first 6 weeks). Interestingly, the rest of the patients still had an increase in the distance between the beads and the rotator cuff footprint over the first year postoperatively despite having intact rotator cuff tendon by magnetic resonance imaging. This led the authors to describe "failure with continuity" of the cuff—patients who had significant retraction but still had an intact cuff repair by imaging study. Finally, because approximately 80% of the retraction in their cohort occurred in the first 12 weeks, the authors advocate slow rehabilitation.

J. Braman, MD

Advantages of Arthroscopic Transosseous Suture Repair of the Rotator Cuff without the Use of Anchors

Kuroda S, Ishige N, Mikasa M (Matsudo Orthopaedic Hosp, Japan)
Clin Orthop Relat Res 471:3514-3522, 2013

Background.—Although arthroscopic anchor suturing is commonly used for rotator cuff repair and achieves good results, certain shortcomings remain, including difficulty with reoperation in cases of retear, anchor dislodgement, knot impingement, and financial cost. In 2005, we developed an anchorless technique for arthroscopic transosseous suture rotator cuff repair.

Description of Technique.—After acromioplasty and adequate footprint decortication, three K-wires with perforated tips are inserted through the inferior margin of the greater tuberosity into the medial edge of the footprint using a customized aiming guide. After pulling the rotator cuff stump laterally with a grasper, three K-wires are threaded through the rotator cuff and skin. Thereafter, five Number 2 polyester sutures are passed through three bone tunnels using the perforated tips of the K-wires. The surgery is completed by inserting two pairs of mattress sutures and three bridging sutures.

Methods.—We investigated the retear rate (based on MR images at least 1 year after the procedure), total score on the UCLA Shoulder Rating Scale, axillary nerve preservation, and issues concerning bone tunnels with this

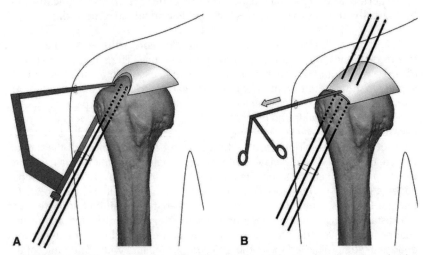

FIGURE 1.—(A) The aiming tip of the drill guide passing through the anterolateral portal was placed on the medial edge of the footprint and three K-wires with perforated tips were inserted through the inferior margin of the greater tuberosity. (B) The rotator cuff stump was pulled laterally, and the K-wires were threaded through the rotator cuff and skin posterior to the acromioclavicular joint. (With kind permission from Springer Science+Business Media. Kuroda S, Ishige N, Mikasa M. Advantages of arthroscopic transosseous suture repair of the rotator cuff without the use of anchors. *Clin Orthop Relat Res.* 2013;471:3514-3522, with permission from The Author(s).)

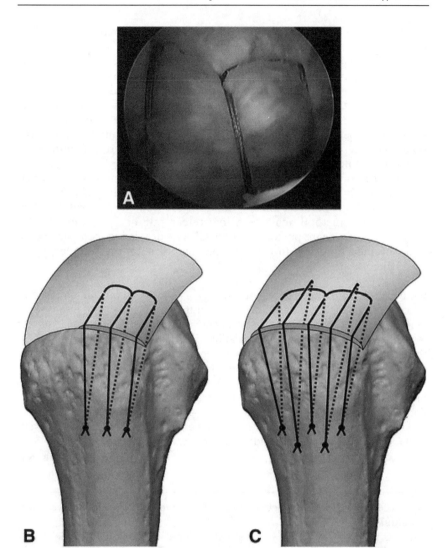

FIGURE 10.—(A) An intraoperative view and (B) a diagram shows the rotator cuff securely fixed to the footprint with two mattress sutures and three bridging sutures. (C) When the AP diameter of the rotator cuff tear exceeded 3 cm, we added two bridging sutures. (With kind permission from Springer Science+Business Media. Kuroda S, Ishige N, Mikasa M. Advantages of arthroscopic transosseous suture repair of the rotator cuff without the use of anchors. *Clin Orthop Relat Res*. 2013;471:3514-3522, with permission from The Author(s).)

technique in 384 shoulders in 380 patients (174 women [175 shoulders] and 206 men [209 shoulders]). Minimum followup was 2 years (mean, 3.3 years; range, 2–7 years). Complete followup was achieved by 380 patients (384 of 475 [81%] of the procedures performed during the period in question). The remaining 91 patients (91 shoulders) do not have 1-year postsurgical MR images, 2-year UCLA evaluation or intraoperative tear measurement, or they have previous fracture, retear of the rotator cuff, preoperative cervical radiculopathy or axillary nerve palsy, or were lost to followup.

Results.—Retears occurred in 24 patients (24 shoulders) (6%). The mean overall UCLA score improved from a preoperative mean of 19.1 to a score of 32.7 at last followup (maximum possible score 35, higher scores being better). Postoperative EMG and clinical examination showed no axillary nerve palsies. Bone tunnel-related issues were encountered in only one shoulder.

Conclusions.—Our technique has the following advantages: (1) reoperation is easy in patients with retears; (2) surgical materials used are inexpensive polyester sutures; and (3) no knots are tied onto the rotator cuff. This low-cost method achieves a low retear rate and few bone tunnel problems, the mean postoperative UCLA score being comparable to that obtained by using an arthroscopic anchor suture technique (Figs 1 and 10).

▶ The authors present an excellent review of a novel technique for arthroscopic rotator cuff repair. Some of the benefits that the authors highlight of this technique are the absence of expensive anchors, not having knots tied onto the rotator cuff, and an ease of reoperation if necessary. This study highlights their experience with 475 rotator cuff repairs. They were able to follow up with more than 80% of these patients to 2 years. They found a 6% retear rate and no evidence of nerve injury. UCLA score improved from 19.1 to 32.7 at final follow-up. Fig 1A, B show the placement of the guide wires, and Fig 10A through C show final construct. Considerable suture management and familiarity with advanced arthroscopic techniques may be necessary to replicate the clinical results reported in this article.

J. Macalena, MD

Is Ultrasound-Guided Injection More Effective in Chronic Subacromial Bursitis?

Hsieh L-F, Hsu W-C, Lin Y-J, et al (Shin Kong Wu Ho-Su Memorial Hosp, Taipei, Taiwan; Natl Taiwan Univ of Science and Technology, Taipei; et al)
Med Sci Sports Exerc 45:2205-2213, 2013

Purpose.—Although ultrasound (US)-guided subacromial injection has shown increased accuracy in needle placement, whether US-guided injection produces better clinical outcome is still controversial. Therefore, this study aimed to compare the efficacy of subacromial corticosteroid injection under US guidance with palpation-guided subacromial injection in patients with chronic subacromial bursitis.

Methods.—Patients with chronic subacromial bursitis were randomized to a US-guided injection group and a palpation-guided injection group.

The subjects in each group were injected with a mixture of 0.5 mL dexamethasone suspension and 3 mL lidocaine into the subacromial bursa. The primary outcome measures were the visual analog scale for pain and active and passive ranges of motion of the affected shoulder. Secondary outcome measures were the Shoulder Pain and Disability Index, the Shoulder Disability Questionnaire, and the 36-item Short-Form Health Survey (SF-36). The primary outcome measures were evaluated before, immediately, 1 wk, and 1 month after the injection; the secondary outcome measures were evaluated before, 1 wk, and 1 month after the injection.

Results.—Of the 145 subjects screened, 46 in each group completed the study. Significantly greater improvement in passive shoulder abduction and in physical functioning and vitality scores on the SF-36 were observed in the US-guided group. The pre- and postinjection within-group comparison revealed significant improvement in the visual analog scale for pain and range of motion, as well as in the Shoulder Pain and Disability Index, Shoulder Disability Questionnaire, and SF-36 scores, in both groups.

Conclusions.—The US-guided subacromial injection technique produced significantly greater improvements in passive shoulder abduction and in some items of the SF-36. US is effective in guiding the needle into the subacromial bursa in patients with chronic subacromial bursitis.

▶ The authors prospectively studied, randomized, and compared outcomes of injections for subacromial bursitis between ultrasound-guided and palpation-guided injections. The outcome measures included range of motion, pain, and patient-related outcomes (Shoulder Pain and Disability Index, the Shoulder Disability Questionnaire, and the 36-item Short-Form Health Survey [SF-36]).

The ultrasound-guided group had the advantage of identifying bursitis and increased fluid (effusion), and, when present, drainage before injection was performed. Whereas the nonultrasound group simply underwent injection.

The injection mixture was 0.5 mL of (5 mg/mL) dexamethasone and 3 mL of 1% lidocaine.

Outcomes were measured immediately, at 1 week, and at 1 month after injection. Forty-eight patients were collected in each group, and 46 were available for follow-up analysis.

Results showed that the ultrasound injection group had better passive shoulder abduction and some aspects of SF-36.

Despite the fact that patient bias may occur with the ultrasound group, as these patients may perceive that they are getting a better treatment with the ultrasound scan, the results in the ultrasound group were superior. Perhaps the precision of injection and the ability to drain before injection with ultrasound technique helps patients get better sooner. Longer-term outcomes would be helpful.

M. Rizzo, MD

Effect of Diet-Induced Vitamin D Deficiency on Rotator Cuff Healing in a Rat Model

Angeline ME, Ma R, Pascual-Garrido C, et al (Hosp for Special Surgery, NY)
Am J Sports Med 42:27-34, 2014

Background.—Few studies have considered hormonal influences, particularly vitamin D, on healing.

Hypothesis.—Vitamin D deficiency would have a negative effect on the structure of the healing tendon-bone interface in a rat model and would result in decreased tendon attachment strength.

Study Design.—Controlled laboratory study.

Methods.—Vitamin D deficiency was induced in 28 male Sprague-Dawley rats using a specialized vitamin D–deficient diet and ultraviolet light restriction. Serum levels of vitamin D were measured after 6 weeks. These vitamin D–deficient animals (experimental group) plus 32 rats with normal vitamin D levels (controls) underwent unilateral detachment of the right supraspinatus tendon from the greater tuberosity of the humerus, followed by immediate repair using bone tunnel suture fixation. The animals were sacrificed at 2- and 4-week intervals after surgery for biomechanical analysis. A paired *t* test was used to compare serum vitamin D levels at day 0 and at 6 weeks. A nonparametric Mann-Whitney *U* test was used to compare load-to-failure and stiffness values between the experimental group and controls. Bone density and new bone formation at the tendon insertion site on the greater tuberosity were assessed with micro–computed tomography (CT). The organization of collagen tissue, new bone formation, vascularity at the tendon-bone interface, fibrocartilage at the tendon-bone interface, and collagen fiber continuity between the tendon and bone tissue were evaluated with safranin O and picrosirius red staining.

Results.—Blood draws confirmed vitamin D deficiency at 6 weeks compared with time zero/baseline for rats in the experimental group (10.9 ng/mL vs 6.5 ng/mL, respectively; $P < .001$). Biomechanical testing demonstrated a significant decrease in load to failure in the experimental group compared with controls at 2 weeks (5.8 ± 2.0 N vs 10.5 ± 4.4 N, respectively; $P < .006$). There was no difference in stiffness at 2 weeks between the control and experimental groups. At 4 weeks, there was no significant difference in load to failure or stiffness between the control and experimental groups. Histological analysis showed less bone formation and less collagen fiber organization in the vitamin D–deficient specimens at 4 weeks as compared with controls. Micro-CT analysis showed no significant difference between groups for total mineral density and bone volume fraction of cortical, whole, or trabecular bone at 4 weeks.

Conclusion.—The biomechanical and histological data from this study suggest that low vitamin D levels may negatively affect early healing at the rotator cuff repair site.

Clinical Relevance.—It is estimated that 1 billion people worldwide are vitamin D deficient. In the deficient state, acutely injured rotator cuffs may have a reduced ability for tendon healing. Further studies are needed to determine the exact mechanism by which vitamin D affects tendon healing and whether vitamin D supplementation can improve rotator cuff tendon healing and reduce the incidence of retears.

▶ The authors proposed an intriguing research question and subsequently developed a basic laboratory method to investigate the effect of vitamin D levels on the tendon-bone enthesis in rotator cuff repair. Although direct application of a rat model to the human population may have flaws, this study illustrates the importance of sufficient vitamin D levels in the acute phase of tendon-to-bone healing. They have shown differences in both the biomechanical strength and the histological data. The body of knowledge regarding vitamin D metabolism and its physiologic implications continues to expand. I have been mindful of obtaining vitamin D levels in fracture patients but until this study had not considered preoperative assessment of vitamin D levels in patients scheduled for tendon-to-bone repair (ie, biceps tendon). As the authors point out, the study implicates vitamin D in the tendon-to-bone healing process, yet many questions remain unanswered. Evidence to support oral supplementation of vitamin D in tendon-to-bone repair may be lacking. However, I am inclined to consider preoperative assessment and oral supplementation of vitamin D. Many of my patients are likely deficient because of lack of sun exposure and would benefit from supplementation, if not for tendon-to-bone healing, then for their overall bone health.

A. Moeller, MD

20 Shoulder: Miscellaneous

Glenohumeral Findings on Magnetic Resonance Imaging Correlate With Innings Pitched in Asymptomatic Pitchers

Lesniak BP, Baraga MG, Jose J, et al (Univ of Miami Miller School of Medicine, FL; Univ of Miami, FL; et al)

Am J Sports Med 41:2022-2027, 2013

Background.—In recent years, there has been a documented increase in the number of professional baseball players on the disabled list and the total number of days on the disabled list. Pitchers account for the largest number of disabled list reports.

Purpose.—To examine the relationship between magnetic resonance imaging (MRI) findings in asymptomatic professional pitchers and subsequent time on the disabled list (DL).

Study Design.—Cohort study (Prognosis); Level of evidence, 2.

Methods.—A total of 21 asymptomatic professional pitchers from a single Major League Baseball (MLB) organization underwent preseason MRIs of their dominant shoulder from 2001 to 2010. Asymptomatic was defined as no related DL stays in the 2 seasons before the MRI. These studies were reevaluated by a fellowship-trained musculoskeletal radiologist who was blinded to patient name, injury history, and baseball history. A second investigator who was blinded to the MRI results collected demographic data, total career number of innings pitched, and any subsequent DL reports for each subject.

Results.—The mean age at the time of MRI was 29.04 years (range, 20-39 years). Eleven of 21 pitchers had a rotator cuff tear (RCT): 9 had an articular surface tear (AST), and 2 had a full-thickness rotator cuff tear (FTT). Ten had superior labral anterior posterior (SLAP) tears, and 13 had either anterior or posterior labral tears. There was a statistically significant relationship between the number of innings pitched and presence of an RCT (AST + FTT). The mean number of career innings pitched by those with an RCT was 1014 compared with a mean of 729 innings pitched in pitchers without an RCT ($P < .01$). In addition, the number of career innings pitched was moderately correlated with presence of RCT ($r = 0.46$) and presence of superior and anterior/posterior labral tears ($r = 0.43$). There were no statistically significant findings between any single preseason MRI finding and subsequent time on the DL.

Conclusion.—The MRI findings in asymptomatic MLB pitchers do not appear to be related to near future placement on the DL. However, there was a significant difference in numbers of innings pitched between pitchers who had an RCT and those who did not and a moderate correlation between innings pitched and the presence of RCT as well as the presence of labral lesions. This finding supports the notion that RCT and labral injury in pitchers may result from repetitive overhead motion with subsequent strain on the rotator cuff tendons and glenoid labrum. Asymptomatic shoulder lesions in professional baseball pitchers appear to be more frequent than previously thought.

▶ In this study, 21 major league pitchers without prior injury to their shoulder underwent magnetic resonance imaging. The presence of rotator cuff tears, articular cartilage injuries, superior labral anterior posterior (SLAP) tears, and labral tears were correlated with innings pitched and subsequent shoulder injuries. Interestingly, 20 of 21 pitchers had evidence of rotator cuff tendinosis, 11 of 21 had evidence of rotator cuff tears, and 2 of 21 had full-thickness tears. Ten of 21 SLAP tears and 13 of 21 anterior or posterior labral tears were present. These are strikingly high rates of identifiable pathology in an otherwise asymptomatic population of overhead athletes. It is also interesting to note the likelihood of having a cuff tear or a labral tear was correlated positively with career innings pitched. There was not a correlation between identification of shoulder pathology and a future trip to the disabled list. No players in this study underwent shoulder surgery in the timeframe of the study. Although no direct correlation is present, the increasing frequency of shoulder injuries with innings pitched is a concerning trend. Future studies will be necessary to identify its clinical significance.

J. Macalena, MD

Selective Activation of the Infraspinatus Muscle

Ha S-M, Kwon O-Y, Cynn H-S, et al (Baekseok Univ, Republic of Korea; Yonsei Univ, Kangwon-do, Republic of Korea; et al)
J Athl Train 48:346-352, 2013

Context.—To improve selective infraspinatus muscle strength and endurance, researchers have recommended selective shoulder external-rotation exercise during rehabilitation or athletic conditioning programs. Although selective strengthening of the infraspinatus muscle is recommended for therapy and training, limited information is available to help clinicians design a selective strengthening program.

Objective.—To determine the most effective of 4 shoulder external-rotation exercises for selectively stimulating infraspinatus muscle activity while minimizing the use of the middle trapezius and posterior deltoid muscles.

Design.—Cross-sectional study.

Setting.—University research laboratory.

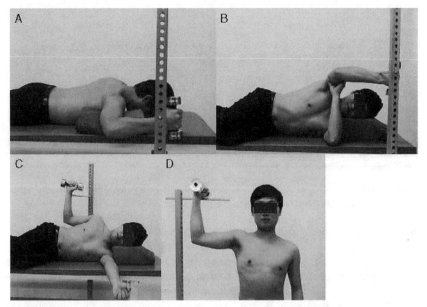

FIGURE 1.—Four types of exercise. A, Prone external-rotation exercise. B, Side-lying wiper exercise. C, Side-lying external-rotation exercise. D, Standing external-rotation exercise. (Reprinted from Ha S-M, Kwon O-Y, Cynn H-S, et al. Selective activation of the infraspinatus muscle. *J Athl Train.* 2013;48:346-352, with permission from the National Athletic Trainers' Association, Inc.)

Patients or Other Participants.—A total of 30 healthy participants (24 men, 6 women; age = 22.6 ± 1.7 years, height = 176.2 ± 4.5 cm, mass = 65.6 ± 7.4 kg) from a university population.

Intervention(s).—The participants were instructed to perform 4 exercises: (1) prone horizontal abduction with external rotation (PER), (2) side-lying wiper exercise (SWE), (3) side-lying external rotation (SER), and (4) standing external-rotation exercise (STER).

Main Outcome Measure(s).—Surface electromyography signals were recorded from the infraspinatus, middle trapezius, and posterior deltoid muscles. Differences among the exercise positions were tested using a 1-way repeated-measures analysis of variance with Bonferroni adjustment.

Results.—The infraspinatus muscle activity was greater in the SWE (55.98% ± 18.79%) than in the PER (46.14% ± 15.65%), SER (43.38% ± 22.26%), and STER (26.11% ± 15.00%) ($F_{3,87} = 19.97$, $P < .001$). Furthermore, the SWE elicited the least amount of activity in the middle trapezius muscle ($F_{3,87} = 20.15$, $P < .001$). Posterior deltoid muscle activity was similar in the SWE and SER but less than that measured in the PER and STER ($F_{3,87} = 25.10$, $P < .001$).

Conclusions.—The SWE was superior to the PER, SER, and STER in maximizing infraspinatus activity with the least amount of middle trapezius

TABLE 1.—Electromyographic Activation for Each Exercise

| Muscle | Exercise, % Maximal Voluntary Isometric Contraction (Mean ± SD) | | | | $F_{3,87}$ | P |
	Prone Horizontal Abduction With External Rotation	Side-Lying Wiper	Side-Lying External Rotation	Standing External Rotation		
Infraspinatus	46.14 ± 15.65	55.98 ± 18.79	43.38 ± 22.26	26.11 ± 15.00	19.97	<.001
Middle trapezius	19.14 ± 14.85	6.55 ± 6.87	24.14 ± 21.57	19.21 ± 11.90	20.15	<.001
Posterior deltoid	15.31 ± 10.76	7.01 ± 9.26	4.11 ± 4.08	13.09 ± 12.91	25.10	<.001

and posterior deltoid activity. These findings may help clinicians design effective exercise programs (Fig 1, Table 1).

▶ This cross-sectional study aimed to determine the most functional activation of the infraspinatus muscle to inform clinicians in their design of the most effective and selective activation of this important component of the rotator cuff. The infraspinatus is key in controlling external rotation and the distraction of the glenohumeral joint in general functional use and overhead throwing use, respectively, of the shoulder. The selective purpose was to find the position of the shoulder that most effectively selects the infraspinatus with the least amount of cocontraction of the deltoid and middle trapezius. Literature does not yet support the most effective functional activation of the infraspinatus.

The study compares external rotation force in 4 body and shoulder combined positions as described (Fig 1). To test their hypothesis, a novel position, side-lying external rotation (SWE), is presented by the authors as being the most selective exercise for infraspinatus strengthening. Surface electromyography was used to measure force output over the infraspinatus, middle trapezius, and deltoid. Isometric contraction was used for each position, with a positional jig set to allow the subject to hold a 1-kg free weight, pushing against a rod with the radial aspect of the wrist. Each contraction was held for 5 seconds, and the mean force measure of 3 repetitions was used. Appropriate rest periods between each repetition and between each set of exercises was used.

The results of the study showed that in the novel position of SWE, the infraspinatus had the most selective and greatest isometric muscle activity compared with the 3 other positions. The middle trapezius and deltoid fired in all 4 positions yet fired the least in this SWE position (Table 1). Thus, this study suggests this SWE may be the best position to selectively strengthen this important muscle of the rotator cuff, the infraspinatus. However, the authors note the study was on healthy young students with no prior injury. Further research is required for persons with shoulder pain.

V. H. O'Brien, OTD, OTR/L, CHT

Histomorphologic Changes of the Long Head of the Biceps Tendon in Common Shoulder Pathologies

Mazzocca AD, McCarthy MBR, Ledgard FA, et al (Univ of Connecticut Health Ctr, Farmington; et al)
Arthroscopy 29:972-981, 2013

Purpose.—To assess molecular and histologic differences between the proximal (intra-articular) and distal (extra-articular) portions of the long head of the biceps (LHB) tendon in 3 different disease states (biceps instability, tendinosis, and degenerative joint disease [DJD]) compared with a healthy tendon (fresh frozen).

Methods.—We used 32 LHB tendons of patients undergoing tenodesis (mean age, 54.7 ± 10.1 years) and 9 harvested tissue donors. Tendons were divided according to 4 diagnostic groups: (1) biceps instability, (2) tendinosis, (3) DJD, and (4) normal control. After sectioning, tendons were fixed in formalin and stained with H&E and alcian blue for histologic analysis. Measurements of collagen organization by use of polarized light microscopy was then performed, and protein expression for type I and type III collagen, tenascin C, and decorin was determined.

Results.—There were no statistical differences found for protein expression of type I or type III collagen, tenascin C, or decorin. The proximal and distal regions of the tendons had statistically significant differences in alcian blue staining, with the proximal portion containing a higher amount of proteoglycan (instability, $P = .001$; tendinosis, $P = .005$; DJD, $P = .008$; control, $P = .011$). When compared with the nonpathologic control tendons, a significant increase in alcian blue staining for the proximal region was seen in all 3 groups. Total polarized light analysis showed that the distal tendon had a significantly higher intensity (organization) compared with the proximal tendon ($P < .001$); this was also seen in all of the diagnostic groups (instability, $P = .010$; tendinosis, $P = .013$; DJD, $P = .07$; control, $P = .028$).

Conclusions.—This study showed a greater degree of degeneration of the proximal (intra-articular) regions of the LHB tendon when compared with the distal regions in all pathologic groups. However, no major differences at the cellular level were found among groups.

Clinical Relevance.—The pathomechanisms of the various forms of known LHB diagnoses are not yet fully understood and basic science studies may help in understanding their etiology and therefore optimizing treatment options.

▶ The long head of the biceps tendon has long been thought related to shoulder pain. Current treatment options, including tenotomy and biceps tenodesis, are frequently undertaken either in isolation or in concert with other procedures. This study evaluated the staining characteristics of the long head of the biceps tendon and compared it with those of control samples. Increased degeneration was noted in the proximal aspect of all tendons compared with the distal aspect of the tendons. No distinct changes in the cellular makeup of the proximal and distal aspects of the tendons were appreciated. This study evaluated only the cellular makeup of the tendon. All clinical symptoms may not be explained by only cellular degeneration, mechanical forces such as instability within the groove, or compression within the bicipital groove. Further, this study does not address the effect of the biceps tendon on the superior labrum. Certainly, future work will be necessary to further identify the relationship of the biceps tendon and shoulder pain.

J. Macalena, MD

Arthroscopic Capsulolabral Reconstruction for Posterior Instability of the Shoulder: A Prospective Study of 200 Shoulders
Bradley JP, McClincy MP, Arner JW, et al (Burke and Bradley Orthopedics, Pittsburgh, PA; Univ of Pittsburgh Med Ctr, PA; et al)
Am J Sports Med 41:2005-2014, 2013

Background.—There are few reports in the literature detailing the arthroscopic treatment of unidirectional posterior shoulder instability.

Hypothesis.—Arthroscopic capsulolabral reconstruction is effective in restoring stability and function and alleviating pain in athletes with symptomatic unidirectional posterior instability.

Study Design.—Cohort study; Level of evidence, 2.

Methods.—One hundred eighty-three athletes (200 shoulders) with unidirectional recurrent posterior shoulder instability were treated with arthroscopic posterior capsulolabral reconstruction and underwent an evaluation at a mean of 36 months postoperatively. A subset of 117 shoulders of contact athletes was compared with the entire group of 200 shoulders. Patients were evaluated prospectively with the American Shoulder and Elbow Surgeons (ASES) scoring system. Stability, strength, and range of motion were evaluated preoperatively and postoperatively with standardized subjective scales. Methods of intraoperative soft tissue fixation as well as anchorless (n = 44) and anchored (n = 156) plications were recorded for each patient.

Results.—At a mean of 36 months postoperatively, the mean ASES score improved from 45.9 to 85.1 ($P < .001$). There were also significant improvements in stability, pain, and function based on previously used scales ($P < .001$). The contact athletes did not demonstrate any significant differences when compared with the entire cohort for any outcome measure. With regard to the method of internal fixation, patients who underwent capsulolabral plications with suture-anchors showed significantly greater improvement in ASES scores ($P < .001$) and a higher rate of return to play ($P < .05$) when compared with patients with anchorless capsulolabral plications.

Conclusion.—Arthroscopic capsulolabral reconstruction is an effective, reliable treatment for symptomatic, unidirectional recurrent posterior glenohumeral instability in an athletic population. Overall, 90% of patients were able to return to sport, with 64% of patients able to return to the same level postoperatively. With the incorporation of bone suture-anchors in capsulolabral reconstruction, patients had greater improvements in ASES scores and a higher rate of return to play.

▶ Arthroscopic instability repair has evolved as a much less morbid technique for stabilization of the posteriorly unstable shoulder. This problem, although less common than anterior instability, is still found relatively frequently in the athletic population, particularly in collision athletes. This study evaluated the postoperative outcomes of patients treated with plication alone vs plication with suture anchors. The authors were able, in this series, to achieve significant improvements in American Shoulder and Elbow Scores (ASES; from 45.9 to 85.1) overall. In subset analysis, they found that contact athletes did not have different outcomes from the rest of the cohort. Additionally, they found that there was a significantly better ASES outcome and return to play rate with the use of anchors for plication vs plication alone. Finally, they showed a 90% return-to-sport rate overall, with 64% returning to the same level of participation as before surgery. This article adds to the literature showing that arthroscopic posterior instability repair can be effective at improving shoulder function even in collision athletes. Even with good results, however, less than two-thirds of athletes were able to participate at the same level as preoperatively.

J. Braman, MD

Footprint Contact Restoration Between the Biceps-Labrum Complex and the Glenoid Rim in SLAP Repair: A Comparative Cadaveric Study Using Pressure-Sensitive Film

Kim S-J, Kim S-H, Lee S-K, et al (Yonsei Univ College of Medicine, Seoul, South Korea)
Arthroscopy 29:1005-1011, 2013

Purpose.—To compare pressurized footprint contact and interface pressure between the biceps-labrum complex and the superior glenoid rim after SLAP repair using 3 different techniques.

Methods.—Twenty-four fresh-frozen human cadaveric shoulders were divided into 3 groups. SLAP lesions were repaired by (1) 2 single-loaded anchors in a simple suture configuration (group T), (2) a double-loaded anchor in a simple suture configuration in a V shape (group V), or (3) a double-loaded anchor by use of a hybrid simple and mattress suture configuration (group H). Pressure-sensitive film quantified pressurized contact areas and interface pressures between the biceps-labrum complex and the glenoid rim after SLAP repair.

Results.—Groups T and V showed significantly larger contact areas than group H ($P < .0001$). However, there was no significant difference between groups T and V. Despite a substantial contact area around the biceps-labrum complex in group T, there was a lack of sufficient contact area just below the biceps anchor. Group V showed a uniform contact area around the entire biceps-labrum complex, but in group H the contact area was concentrated only around the posterior superior labrum, where the simple suture was used.

Conclusions.—The methods using 2 single-loaded suture anchors and using 1 double-loaded suture anchor with a simple suture configuration showed significantly larger pressurized contact areas than the method using 1 double-loaded suture anchor with both a simple and mattress suture configuration. The interface pressure was not significantly different among groups.

Clinical Relevance.—Although there have been several kinds of repair techniques and biomechanical studies for the type II SLAP lesion, there has been no study about footprint restoration on the superior glenoid rim. This study analyzed and compared the footprint contact restoration after type II SLAP repair among 3 different techniques.

▶ This is a cadaveric study of 3 repair techniques for small superior labral from anterior to posterior (SLAP) tears. It used pressure-sensitive film to determine the compressive force and area of force concentration for the repairs. The authors used 1 repair type that had an anchor anterior and 1 with an anchor posterior to the biceps origin, each with simple sutures (group T). The second type was double loaded at the biceps origin with 1 strand anterior and 1 strand posterior to the biceps (group V). The final construct evaluated used a double-loaded suture anchor with 1 simple stitch posterior to the biceps origin and 1 mattress at the biceps origin. They found that the area of compression was better for 2-anchor constructs and that the 2-anchor constructs did not differ from each other. The authors did not comment on the amount of displacement of the biceps origin from the anatomic position that occurred with any of their repair constructs. Although this study shows that footprint compression improves with dual-loaded anchor placement in a cadaver, the correlation with clinical outcomes remains unclear.

J. Braman, MD

21 Rehabilitation

Effectiveness of cast immobilization in comparison to the gold-standard self-removal orthotic intervention for closed mallet fingers: a randomized clinical trial
Tocco S, Boccolari P, Landi A, et al (Studio Terapico Kaiser, Parma, Italy; Policlinico of Modena, Italy; et al)
J Hand Ther 26:191-201, 2013

Study Design.—Randomized clinical trial.

Introduction.—Although orthotic immobilization has become the preferable treatment choice for closed mallet injuries, it is unclear whether orthosis self-removal has an impact on the final outcome.

Purpose.—To evaluate the treatment efficacy of cast immobilization of closed mallet fingers using Quickcast® (QC) compared to a removable, lever-type thermoplastic orthosis (LTTP).

Methods.—57 subjects were randomized in 2 groups. DIPj extensor lag and the Gaberman success scale were used as primary outcomes.

Results.—LTTP subjects resulted in greater extensor lag than QC subjects ($x = 5$; $p = 0.05$) at 12 weeks from baseline, and high edema and older age negatively affected DIPj extensor lag. No other differences were found between groups.

Conclusion.—Cast immobilization seems to be slightly more effective than the traditional approach probably for its greater capacity to reduce edema.

Level of Evidence.—1B.

▶ This article is based on a randomized, clinical trial comparing 2 orthosis, the removable lever-type thermoplastic orthosis to cast immobilization of closed mallet fingers. The conservative orthotic treatment consisting of immobilizing the distal interphalangeal joint for a number of weeks is a standard treatment. The authors did a good job citing literature reviews on wear schedules and the limited information on postimmobilization phase of rehabilitation and concluded that it is still unclear which aspect of treatment have the most impact on the final outcome of mallet finger injury. The authors' hypothesis stating conservative treatment outcomes would be better if patients were not able to remove their orthoses during the immobilization phase. Methods and design of the study were well stated as was the exact treatment protocol. The authors reported outcome measures, complications, and details of the data analysis through tables and a flow chart in a relatively easy-to-interpret way. Success rate reported was favorable as 19% for the nonremovable quick cast orthosis; however, this statistic was quantified by identifying the limitation of the small sample size. Also, the success rate in this clinical trial could not be compared with that of other studies simply because they had used personal outcome measures. Based on the literature review, the authors then attempted to use recommended detailed scales, which clearly defined range of motion and pain levels for their study. I found the study limitations of time constraints and limited economic resources to be realistic and agree with the authors that this would provide additional strength to the study. It was reassuring to clinicians like this reviewer, to have a clinical trial conclude that edema and age of the patient still continues to have the greatest impact on success of conservative treatment of a mallet injury.

S. Kranz, OTR/L, CHT

Is the UNB test reliable and valid for use with adults with upper limb amputation?

Resnik L, Baxter K, Borgia M, et al (Providence VA Med Ctr, RI; Premier Orthopaedics and Work Rehabilitation, North Kingstown, RI; et al)
J Hand Ther 26:353-359, 2013

Study Design.—Clinical measurement.

Introduction.—The University of New Brunswick (UNB) Test of Prosthetic Function was developed for children. No studies have examined its use with adults.

Purpose of the Study.—Our purposes were to utilize the UNB with adults to examine test—retest, inter-rater reliability and examine validity.

Methods.—The UNB was administered to 51 subjects. Forty-five completed it twice within 1 week. Internal consistency was examined. Test—retest reliability and inter-rater reliability were estimated. ANOVAs compared scores by prosthetic use. Correlations between UNB scales, 2 dexterity tests (the Modified Box and Block Test, the modified Jebsen—Taylor Hand Function Test), and the self-reported Upper Extremity Functional Scale (UEFS) were examined.

Results.—Alphas were 0.74—0.75 and 0.69—9.79 for spontaneity and skill respectively. ICCs for test—retest reliability and inter-rater reliability were 0.73, 0.76 for spontaneity and 0.76 and 0.79 for skill. There were no differences in scores by prosthetic experience. UNB correlations with dexterity measures were moderate, and correlations with UEFS were weak for spontaneity and non-significant for skill.

Conclusions.—UNB scales had acceptable reliability and preliminary evidence of validity for adults.

Level of Evidence.—IIb.

▶ The aim of this study was to establish psychometrics of the University of New Brunswick (UNB) test of prosthetic function for adults. This test is currently validated only for children ages 2 through 13 years. Currently, there are no prosthetic use functional tests validated for the adult age group. The UNB tests the spontaneity and skilled use of a prosthesis during bimanual tasks. Spontaneity refers to how readily the prosthesis is used, rated from 0 to 4: not used at all, use of the proximal portion of the prosthesis, very delayed use of the terminal device, slightly delayed use, and immediate or automatic use of the device. The skilled use of the prosthetic device is also scored on a 0 to 4 scale: the prosthesis is not used, no active use or passive use of the device, attempted active use of device, some degree of slowness or uncertain active use of the terminal device, and quick and skilled active use of the device (see Table 1 in the article for the full definition). The UNB test is divided into meaningful tasks for 4 pediatric age groups: 2 through 4, 5 through 7, 8 through 10, and 11 through 13. The authors chose to use the tasks from the tests from the 11- through 13-year group, as these were found to be close to adult functional items. These items are to cut paper, use a tape dispenser, tie a package, thread a needle, cut thread, sew a button, dry dishes, cut meat, sweep the floor, and sweep up a pile of dust.

The subjects, all of whom were patients of 4 Veterans Affairs (VA) Hospitals with unilateral amputation using the DEKA[1] prosthesis, were part of an ongoing study to optimize the DEKA prosthetic arm across the 4 specific sites of the VA system. The UNB was administered as a test of function and to proceed to validate its use in adults. The testing was scored twice in one week, called visits 1 and 2. Visit 1 tested 51 subjects, and visit 2 tested 45 subjects. All subjects were tested with raters in person. Fifty subjects were rated via videotape by blinded raters. No delineation was made of the level of the amputation, the years of use, or the frequency of use: full or part time. However, the groups were stratified for years and frequency of use. The authors sought to find test-retest and intrarater reliability, and they hypothesized that there would be a difference in subjects with more years of use and greater frequency of use in the scoring for spontaneity and skills. Dexterity and function were also tested and correlated with well-known and validated tests: the Box and Block test, the modified Jebsen—Taylor Test of Hand Function, and a self-reported functional measure, the Upper Extremity Functional Scale (UEFS).

The results found the test-retest and interrater reliability were moderately high with ICCs for each respectively at 0.75 and 0.79. For the spontaneity and skill summary scores, the interraters ICCs were 0.72 and 0.73, with high correlation between spontaneity and skill summary scores at 0.92. Through analyses of variance, it was found that subjects with full-time use of the prosthesis had higher scores in both spontaneity and skill, yet no difference was found for either years of use or for loss of the dominant extremity. It is noted that all subjects with loss of the dominant extremity changed hand dominance. The UNB skills test had moderate correlation to the dexterity tests. Scores between the UNB skills and the UEFS were not significant.

A strong correlation was found between both spontaneity and skill mean summary scores, meaning one test is a strong predictor of the other. Therefore, they recommend, and the results demonstrate an indication that the UNB test has acceptable reliability with preliminary evidence for the use of the skill test for adults, with more scoring criteria testing needed to refine the scoring rules.

V. H. O'Brien, OTD, OTR/L, CHT

Reference

1. DEKA arm. http://www.dekaresearch.com/founder.shtml. Accessed February 15, 2014.

Is Diagrammatic Goniometry Feasible for Finger ROM Evaluation and Self-evaluation?
Macionis V (Vilnius Univ Faculty of Medicine, Lithuania)
Clin Orthop Relat Res 471:1894-1903, 2013

Background.—While "diagrammatic" evaluation of finger joint angles using two folded paper strips as goniometric arms has been proposed and could be an alternative to standard goniometry and a means for self-evaluation, the measurement differences and reliability are unknown.

Questions/Purposes.—This study assessed the standard and diagrammatic finger goniometry performed by an experienced examiner on patients in terms of (1) intragoniometer and intergoniometer (ie, intrarater) differences and reliability; (2) interrater differences and reliability relative to patients' diagrammatic self-evaluation; and (3) the interrater differences related to patient's hand dominance.

Methods.—Sixty-one patients without previous training self-evaluated active extension of all joints of the fifth finger of one hand once using two rectangular strips of paper. A practitioner used a goniometer and a diagram to perform parallel evaluations once in 12 patients and three times in 49 patients. The diagrams were scanned and measured. All evaluations and proportions of differences between the paired measurements of 5° or less were combined for analysis.

Results.—Intrarater intraclass correlation coefficients (ICC) based on the second and third practitioner's trials for the proximal interphalangeal joint were greater than 0.99. Reliability was poor when calculations involved the first measurement of the practitioner (ICCs < 0.38). Interrater reliability was poor regardless of the practitioner's trial (ICCs < 0.033). The proportions of the absolute differences of 5° or less between all paired practitioner's measurements were similar. The proportions of the acceptable differences between paired practitioner's and patients' measurements were nonequivalent for the interphalangeal joints. The interrater differences did not depend on patients' handedness.

Conclusions.—In experienced hands both techniques produce clinically comparable reliability, but patients' performance in extempore diagrammatic self-evaluation is inadequate. Further studies are necessary to explore whether appropriate training of patients can improve consistency of diagrammatic self-evaluation.

Level of Evidence.—Level III, diagnostic study. See Guidelines for Authors for a complete description of levels of evidence.

▶ The author takes on a difficult topic here and is to be commended. The objective results of hand surgery studies rely on the ability to measure joint motion accurately and reproducibly. Goniometric measurements are the standard but rely on an experienced observer. The authors look at the intrarater reliability of goniometer measurements and patient diagrammatic self-evaluation. A novel technique previously reported by the author uses paper strips to assess the range of motion of a joint. The angle subtended by the strips is then traced and measured. The results show that while an experienced examiner has reproducible results, the patient, although able to demonstrate apparently acceptable technique, does not. The strength of the study is its novelty and simplicity of a single examiner. The principal weakness, stated by the author, is the lack of expertise in the patient evaluators. Still, the author has taken on a difficult and potentially useful project—to be able to get measurements of joint motion from the patients themselves. The use of nearly ubiquitous cell phone cameras seems to be a logical next step in development of this measurement technique. I hope he will continue to develop new novel techniques for patient self-evaluation and reporting.

D. J. Mastella, MD

Do patient-reported outcome measures capture functioning aspects and environmental factors important to individuals with injuries or disorders of the hand?
Coenen M, Kus S, Rudolf K-D, et al (Ludwig-Maximilians-Universität (LMU), Munich, Germany; BG Trauma Hosp Hamburg, Germany; et al)
J Hand Ther 26:332-342, 2013

Study Design.—Qualitative study.

Introduction.—Clinical outcome evaluation needs to consider the patient perspective for an in-depth understanding of functioning and disability.

Purpose of the Study.—To explore whether patient-reported outcome measures (PROMs) used in the field of hand injuries or hand disorders, capture functioning aspects and environmental factors important to the patients.

Methods.—We performed a qualitative study and a systematic literature review. The focus group sessions were recorded, transcribed verbatim, and the identified concepts were linked to the ICF. We searched in MEDLINE for reviews, related to injuries or disorders of the hand, reporting on PROMs. We linked the items of the identified PROMs to the ICF and compared the qualitative data with the content of the PROMs.

Results.—Statements from 45 individuals who participated in eight focus groups were linked to 97 categories of the ICF. From 15 reviews included, eight PROMs were selected. The selected PROMs capture 34 of the categories retrieved from the qualitative data.

Conclusions.—PROMs used in the context of hand injuries or hand disorders capture only in parts the functioning aspects important to the patients.

▶ The purpose of this well-designed qualitative study was to ascertain whether currently utilized patient-reported outcome measures (PROM) adequately capture the environmental and functional aspects, which are important to the client being treated. The authors combined an extensive systematic literature search to identify reports about outcome measures related to hand injuries or disorders with well-organized focus groups to gather the patient perspective. The authors used recognized methods of data analysis for qualitative studies and linked their finding to the International Classification of Functioning, Disability and Health categories. They found that the final 8 PROM identified in their study as the most comprehensive did adequately capture most components of activity and participation but omitted many of the concepts identified by the focus group participants as important to them, including emotional functions such as handling stress and environmental and body structures.

With the increasing pressures in our profession to validate our treatment programs and assure compensation for our services as well as to promote and ensure validity of our field of hand therapy, it is essential that clinicians are able to objectively provide specific measures that can best document ones' physical and emotional capacity to return to life skills after an upper extremity injury. It is clear from the extensive research performed by the authors in this study that several PROM that we use in our clinical practice can help us assess our level of success with therapeutic treatment. What we can take away is that there is not one sole instrument that can assess all of the constructs raised by a patient that will truly determine ones' ability to function after injury. We need to develop assessment tools that are more comprehensive and patient focused that will include the areas identified by the focus group such as environmental and emotional factors.

C. Gordon, OTR/L, CHT

Patterns of research utilization among Certified Hand Therapists
Groth GN, Farrar-Edwards D (UW Hosps and Clinics, Madison; Univ of Wisconsin-Madison)
J Hand Ther 26:245-254, 2013

Study Design.—Mixed methods, cross-sectional.

Introduction.—Nearly 30% of Certified Hand Therapists rarely or never use research findings when treating carpal tunnel syndrome.

Purpose of the Study.—To identify groups of CHTs with common research utilization patterns.

Methods.—National randomized mail survey of 600 CHTs ($n = 308$, RR = 55%). Latent class and thematic analysis of eight questions assessing research use and beliefs.

TABLE 5.—Explanatory Quotes by Group

Group	Illustrative Quotes
Analytic ($n = 135$; 45%)	• I use research findings when it is a good study—double blind, sample size, etc. I use old research that has not been disputed. • I like to search databases. A big stopping point is not having free and convenient access to the articles when one is not affiliated w/a university or hospital. • ...I take data presented with a grain of salt. The proof is in the practice.
Pragmatic ($n = 53$; 18%)	• [My] treatment approach is very individualized and whole body oriented and therefore difficult to study with evidenced-based methodology. One could say that now I practice results-based therapy. • I have found that so many of the research articles for hand therapy do not change my approach to splinting, pain control, edema control, or home programs for many diagnoses.
Skeptic ($n = 65$; 22%)	• I am slow to "jump on the bandwagon" concerning new treatment techniques, especially if they contradict my own experience. • Research methodology sometimes goes over my head, but I do love to read the latest research studies affecting our professional work.
Traditional ($n = 46$; 15%)	• I... rely on anecdotal information. • I have a pretty eclectic approach to treating CTS... • Research is often not conclusive, usually suggesting more research needs to be done. • I have been a therapist a long time and remember when I would treat CTS conservatively with 6 wks of phono/iontophoresis, ROM, massage, splinting, etc. and didn't see good results.
Common themes Rarity of diagnosis	• We see very little CTS for conservative management. Other diagnoses would push me to do more evidence-based research. • I don't routinely see CTS patients.
Low cognitive demand	• Due to limited time and access, I tend to look for current research in areas that tend to have increased complications and decreased results i.e. lateral epicondylitis. • I use EBM for my practice, however, CTS is such a basic topic that I usually do not research it on a regular basis. • I don't consider CTS complex in any way. I get good outcomes. Don't feel I have the need.

Results.—Four groups of CHT research users were identified: *Analytic* ($n = 135, 45\%$); *Skeptic* ($n = 65, 22\%$); *Pragmatic* ($n = 53, 18\%$); and *Traditional* ($n = 46, 15\%$). Highest research use was reported among Analytics and Pragmatics although Skeptics willingly relied on research evidence when it contradicted other sources of knowledge. Age, not experience or population density, was a significant covariate of group membership.

Conclusions.—Empowering CHTs to use research findings by increased understanding of their group membership, and understanding others' groups, may increase progress toward evidence-based practice (Table 5).

▶ Evidence-based practice (EBP) has become the standard of care in health care, demanding that therapists understand and implement research findings in developing their treatments. The authors of this study determined the use of EBP among health care professionals by researching the current scientific evidence and found that as many as 30% were not using research evidence in their clinical practice. To determine how to influence Certified Hand Therapists (CHTs) to use EBP the authors chose to identify groups of CHTs with similar research utilization patterns and beliefs so that strategies can be developed to facilitate increased use of EBP. Much effort was put forth to collect data from a random sample of CHTs through mail survey. In the end they identified 4 groups of research users: analytic, pragmatic, skeptic, and traditional (Table 5). Of interest, the group that was least likely to use research had the youngest mean age.

It is difficult to know how accurately the results of this study reflect the CHT population. The authors chose a common diagnosis of carpal tunnel syndrome to use in their survey study with many of the respondents indicating both a rarity of this population in their practice and low cognitive demand regarding treatment of this diagnosis, thus, limiting the need to rely on research. Because of the survey nature of this study, the authors may not have had a true cross section of the CHT profession and had to rely on self-report for research use.

As a hands-on clinician, although this type of research is of interest, it is not as applicable to my practice. The leaders and educators of hand therapists will appreciate this detailed study as they work to teach the relevance and methods of using research for EBP. By identifying research styles in CHTs, they may better influence increased use of research data for EBP. Because all of the data used in this report were gathered in 2009, it is my hope that in the ensuing 5 years, more therapists have implemented research findings in their clinical decisions.

S. J. Clark, OTR/L, CHT

22 Miscellaneous

A Novel Technique for Ligamentous Reconstruction of the Sternoclavicular Joint
Gaines RJ, Liporace FA, Yoon RS, et al (Naval Med Ctr, Portsmouth, VA; Univ of Medicine and Dentistry of New Jersey, Newark)
J Orthop Trauma 28:e65-e69, 2014

The technique presented is a departure from previous attempts to standardize the treatment of sternoclavicular dislocations. It offers stability without requiring extra dissection around vital intrathoracic structures and greatly decreases the risk of migration of the implant used for fixation.

▶ The authors describe a novel treatment method for sternoclavicular dislocations. It has been performed in 4 cases over the last several years in the military population.

The method involves the use of a zip loop (Biomet, Warsaw, IN) and a doubled gracilis graft. First, the dislocation is reduced by pulling the proximal clavicle anteriorly. With a 3.5-mm drill, an antegrade hole is drilled from the intramedullary proximal aspect of the clavicle through the anteromedial cortex. The manubrium also requires 2 holes created with a 3-mm burr: first, 1 cm from the superior manubrial margin and, second, 1 cm from the lateral border of the manubrium.

The zip loop is used to anchor the construct with the button at the clavicle and function as a one-way pulley to advance the 2 limbs of the gracilis (one limb through each hole of the manubrium). The 2 limbs are then tied to each other in a square knot fashion.

This technique appears safe and reliable. It is important to have thoracic surgeons available and scrubbed in (especially when reducing the dislocation and creating the holes for tendon passage). This method utilizes the newer technology of the zip loop in a creative way to help with the treatment of this problem in hopes to minimize its already high potential of morbidity.

M. Rizzo, MD

One-per-Mil Tumescent Technique for Upper Extremity Surgeries: Broadening the Indication
Prasetyono TOH, Biben JA (Univ of Indonesia, Jakarta)
J Hand Surg Am 39:3-12.e7, 2014

Purpose.—We studied the effect of 1:1,000,000 epinephrine concentration (1 per mil) to attain a bloodless operative field in hand and upper extremity surgery and to explore its effectiveness and safety profile.

Methods.—This retrospective observational study enrolled 45 consecutive patients with 63 operative fields consisting of various hand and upper extremity problems. One-per-mil solution was injected into the operative field with tumescent technique to create a bloodless operating field without tourniquet. The solution was formulated by adding a 1:1,000,000 concentration of epinephrine and 100 mg of lidocaine into saline solution to form 50 mL of tumescent solution. Observation was performed on the clarity of the operative field, which we described as totally bloodless, minimal bleeding, acceptable bleeding, or bloody. The volume of tumescent solution injected, duration of surgery, and surgical outcome were also reviewed.

Results.—The tumescent technique with 1-per-mil solution achieved 29% totally bloodless, 48% minimal bleeding, 22% acceptable bleeding, and 2% bloody operative fields in cases that included burn contracture and congenital hand and upper extremity surgeries.

Conclusions.—One-per-mil tumescent solution created a clear operative field in hand and upper extremity surgery. It proved safe and effective for a wide range of indications.

Type of Study/Level of Evidence.—Therapeutic IV.

▶ So-called WALANT (wide awake, local anesthesia, no tourniquet) technique is gaining popularity. Large volumes of low-concentration lidocaine mixed with epinephrine improve the visibility of the operative field through the mechanical tumescence of the small vessels and the vasoconstrictive effect of the epinephrine, obviating the need for a tourniquet to control intraoperative bleeding. There are clear benefits in some instances to having patients awake without a tourniquet and able to participate in the procedure. Flexor tendon tenolyses, tendon transfers, or procedures at or proximal to the tourniquet are such examples. Many of the procedures performed in this study do not require the active participation of the patient during the procedure (eg, Apert hand reconstruction, syndactyly release, or burn contracture releases) and required general anesthesia. This leaves the primary potential benefit in the fact that no tourniquet was used. Less than one-third of these patients had a bloodless operative field (something easily achieved with use of a tourniquet), all to save a .04% rate of reported complications caused by the tourniquet itself. Although this study gives us an alternative option if tourniquets are not available, I am not convinced that this offers any advantage over what I currently use, especially in the congenital population.

A. Daluiski, MD

Essential Hand Surgery Procedures for Mastery by Graduating Plastic Surgery Residents: A Survey of Program Directors
Noland SS, Fischer LH, Lee GK, et al (Stanford Univ Hosp, Seattle, WA; Univ of Washington Med Ctr, Seattle)
Plast Reconstr Surg 132:977e-984e, 2013

Background.—This study was designed to establish the essential hand surgery procedures that should be mastered by graduating plastic surgery residents. This framework can then be used as a guideline for developing Objective Structured Assessment of Technical Skill to teach technical skills in hand surgery.

Methods.—Ten expert hand surgeons were surveyed regarding the essential hand surgery procedures that should be mastered by graduating plastic surgery residents. The top 10 procedures from this survey were then used to survey all 89 Accreditation Council for Graduate Medical Education—approved plastic surgery program directors.

Results.—There was a 69 percent response rate to the program director survey (*n* = 61). The top nine hand surgery procedures included open carpal tunnel release, open A1 pulley release, digital nerve repair with microscope, closed reduction and percutaneous pinning of metacarpal fracture, excision of dorsal or volar ganglion, zone II flexor tendon repair with multistrand technique, incision and drainage of the flexor tendon sheath for flexor tenosynovitis, flexor tendon sheath steroid injection, and open cubital tunnel release.

Conclusions.—Surgical educators need to develop objective methods to teach and document technical skill. The Objective Structured Assessment of Technical Skill is a valid method for accomplishing this task. There has been no consensus regarding which hand surgery procedures should be mastered by graduating plastic surgery residents. The authors have identified nine procedures that are overwhelmingly supported by plastic surgery program directors. These nine procedures can be used as a guideline for developing Objective Structured Assessment of Technical Skill to teach and document technical skills in hand surgery.

▶ The authors of this study aimed to identify the 10 most essential operations in hand surgery that a plastic surgery resident should master during his training. These top hand operations were identified by evaluating surveys that were sent out to plastic surgery program directors, in which they were asked which of the operations they found most important. The ranking of operations according to their priority did not differ significantly between program directors with different personal backgrounds (with or without hand fellowship training). There was also only a slight difference according to the availability of a hand fellowship at their current institution.

The study group has published a similar report on the same topic with orthopedic surgery program directors as targets instead of plastic surgeons.[1] A broad consensus between hand surgeons of plastic and orthopedic surgical background was seen when comparing the results of the 2 studies.

The authors suggest that these core procedures favored by both groups could be used as a guideline for a combined training prerequisite curriculum for hand surgery.

The results of this study can be useful for the reorganization of any resident program that contains hand surgery as one of many other components, no matter if it is plastic surgery, orthopedic surgery, or trauma surgery.

M. Choi, MD

Reference

1. Noland SS, Fischer LH, Lee GK, Hentz VR. Essential hand surgery procedures for mastery by graduating orthopedic surgery residents: a survey of program directors. *J Hand Surg Am.* 2013;38:760-765.

Outcomes of Single-Stage Grip-Release Reconstruction in Tetraplegia
Reinholdt C, Fridén J (Univ of Gothenburg, Göteborg, Sweden)
J Hand Surg 38A:1137-1144, 2013

Purpose.—To evaluate the outcomes of our technique for single-stage grip-release reconstruction and compare it with previous 1- and 2-stage grip reconstructions in tetraplegia.

Methods.—A total of 14 patients (16 hands) with tetraplegia underwent a single-stage combination of operations to provide pinch, grip, and release function. We compared the study group with a historical control group of 15 patients (18 hands) who had been treated with staged flexion-extension grip-release reconstructions. Both groups were classified as ocular cutaneous 4. Assessment parameters included grip and pinch strength, maximal opening of the first webspace, and Canadian Occupational Performance Measurement. Both groups were rehabilitated with early active mobilization beginning the first day after surgery.

Results.—Grip strength and opening of the first webspace were significantly greater in the single-stage group than in the comparative group. Pinch strength was not significantly different between groups. On the Canadian Occupational Performance Measurement score, patients belonging to the single-stage group were highly satisfied (increase of 3.7 points) and could perform several of their self-selected goals (3.5 points of improvement).

Conclusions.—The single-stage grip-release reconstruction provides people who have spinal cord injuries and tetraplegia with improved and reliable grip function; active finger flexion, active thumb flexion, passive thumb extension, and passive interossei function can all be achieved through this procedure. Early active mobilization is particularly important in improving functional outcome after this combination of grip reconstruction procedures.

Type of Study/Level of Evidence.—Therapeutic III.

▶ This article from the busy Swedish group reports on their current approach to the care of the tetraplegic upper limb. The article focuses on the outcomes of their current approach in which multiple tendon transfers are performed in one setting using the alphabet procedure.[1] This combining of procedures that were traditionally staged is based on the group's previous work, which showed that a side-to-side tendon repair provided greater pullout strength than the traditional Pulvertaft weave.[2] The theoretical advantage of this new repair was that tendon transfer patients could have earlier mobilization, shortening down time, and more done in one operative setting. This report shows excellent results with their current regimen with strong grasp strength (6.53 ± 0.69 kg) and appropriate pinch 2.8 ± 0.36 kg.

Beyond showing the feasibility of performing multiple procedures in one setting followed by early mobilization, this article also provides clinical wisdom from this experienced group. The pearls in the article include the team's approach to the intrinsic minus hand. They have changed from the Zancolli lasso to the House procedure to restore intrinsic balance, because they found that the House procedure provided better opening for the patient with tetraplegia. The group also has changed their approach to the thumb carpometacarpal (CMC). Currently, the group fuses the CMC in most patients, and they now use a locking T-plate instead of k-wires or staples. This has reduced their nonunion rate.

Overall, this report provides a guide to a state-of-the-art approach to the tetraplegic limb and is a useful read for anyone interested in these procedures.

C. Curtin, MD

References

1. Fridén J, Reinholdt C, Turcsányii I, Gohritz A. A single-stage operation for reconstruction of hand flexion, extension, and intrinsic function in tetraplegia: the alphabet procedure. *Tech Hand Up Extrem Surg.* 2011;15:230-235.
2. Brown SH, Hentzen ER, Kwan A, Ward SR, Fridén J, Lieber RL. Mechanical strength of the side-to-side versus Pulvertaft weave tendon repair. *J Hand Surg Am.* 2010;35:540-545.

Patient Perception of Physician Reimbursement for Common Hand Surgical Procedures
Fowler JR, Buterbaugh GA (Univ of Pittsburgh, PA; Hand & UpperEx Ctr, Wexford, PA)
Orthopedics 36:e1149-e1154, 2013

Health care—related costs have been the focus of intense scrutiny in politics and in the media. However, public perception of physician reimbursement is poorly understood. The purpose of this study was to determine patient perception of physician reimbursement for 2 common hand surgery procedures: carpal tunnel release and open reduction and internal fixation of a distal radius fracture.

Anonymous surveys were completed by 132 patients in an outpatient hand and upper-extremity practice. The surveys asked patients to estimate reasonable surgeon fees and actual Medicare reimbursement for 2 common hand surgery procedures (carpal tunnel release and internal fixation of a distal radius fracture) and 2 common surgical procedures (coronary artery bypass and appendectomy). On average, patients estimated that a reasonable surgeon fee for carpal tunnel release and 90 days of postoperative care was $2629 and that actual Medicare reimbursement was $1891. Patients estimated that a reasonable surgeon fee for internal fixation of an extra-articular distal radius fracture and 90 days of postoperative care was $3874 and that actual Medicare reimbursement was $2671. Higher level of education, annual household income, and insurance status had no statistically significant effect on patient estimates of reimbursement.

Patients in an outpatient hand and upper extremity practice believe that surgeons are reimbursed at a rate 3.6 to 4.7 times greater than actual reimbursement. These misperceptions highlight the lack of understanding and transparency in health care costs and may interfere with the ability of patients to make well-informed decisions about health care.

▶ This article is significant because it attempts to highlight the discrepancy in patient perception of physician reimbursement for 2 common hand surgery procedures: carpal tunnel release and open reduction and internal fixation of a distal radius fracture. I did not find this discrepancy surprising at all, given the ever-decreasing reimbursement of hand surgery procedures and the lack of understanding by many Americans of our highly complex health care system.

Strengths of this study are the simple format and straightforward questions in the survey used to gather the data. Weaknesses include the relatively low completion rate (44%), the fact that most (76%) of the respondents were of one insurance group (private insurance versus Medicare and Medicaid), and the low power (52%) of the study.

Despite the study's shortcomings, I believe it demonstrates well that our patients really have no idea how much we are reimbursed for our surgical procedures, and, therefore, may be misinformed when it comes to discussing where dollars need to be saved with regard to the sky-rocketing costs of our health care system. I would love to see a study looking at patients' perceptions of the costs of implants used in surgical procedures or one looking at patients' perceptions of what an insurance company's margin is on an average patient's annual health care costs versus premiums paid. I'll bet there would be large discrepancies for both as well!

Rarely I'll get a patient who questions his explanation of benefits after a surgical procedure but not for the reason you might think. Usually they wonder why I got paid so little for the surgery I performed for them. Then I explain to them that that payment also includes all office visits for 90 days after the surgery, and then they are genuinely shocked. Not only do our patients need to be more educated on the financial aspects of our health care system, the system itself needs to be greatly simplified.

S. S. Shin, MD, MMSc

Using the Strengthening the Reporting of Observational Studies in Epidemiology (STROBE) Statement to Assess Reporting of Observational Trials in Hand Surgery

Sorensen AA, Wojahn RD, Manske MC, et al (Washington Univ School of Medicine, St Louis, MO)

J Hand Surg 38A:1584-1589, 2013

Purpose.—To use the Strengthening the Reporting of Observational Studies in Epidemiology (STROBE) statement checklist to critically evaluate the change in quality of observational trial reporting in the *Journal of Hand Surgery American* between 2005 and 2011.

Methods.—A cross-sectional analysis of observational studies published in the *Journal of Hand Surgery American* was designed to sample 2 6-month periods of publication (March 2005 to August 2005 and June 2011 to November 2011). Fifty-one items were extracted from the STROBE statement for evaluation. Overall STROBE compliance rates for articles and specific checklist items were determined. Final compliance percentages from each period were compared by Student *t*-testing. Changes in item compliance over time were quantified.

Results.—Overall compliance with the STROBE statement was 38% (range, 10%—54%) in 2005 and 58% (range, 39%—85%) for 2011 manuscripts representing a significant improvement. Seventy-five percent or greater of articles (2005/2011) provided the explicit reporting of background (100%/97%), follow-up time (85%/94%), overall interpretation of data (100%/94%), and results of similar studies (95%/89%). Twenty-five percent or less of articles provided the study design in the abstract (10%/20%), a clear description of the study's setting (10%/ 23%), the handling of missing data (0%/6%), the potential directions of bias (5%/11%), and the use of a power analysis (0%/17%). Eighty-six percent (44/51) of items were more frequently satisfied in 2011 articles than in 2005 publications. Absolute increases in compliance rates of 40% or greater were noted in 10 items (20%) with no worsening in compliance for an individual item over 6%.

Conclusions.—The overall quality of the reporting of observational trials in the *Journal of Hand Surgery American* improved from 2005 to 2011. Current observational trials in hand surgery could still benefit from increased reporting of methodological details including the use of power analyses, the handling of missing data, and consideration of potential bias.

Level of evidence.—Diagnostic III.

▶ Unlike the medical literature, the surgical literature has few large-scale randomized trials but does have a large number of observational studies. Having a standardized method of conducting and reporting observational research allows for more accurate critical appraisal of the results. This study takes a close look at the change in quality of reports between 2005 and 2011 in a prominent hand surgery journal. Each study was systematically reviewed by 2 observers and consensus achieved. The cross-sectional design, however, may have resulted in some bias, as only a small number of studies were included (2 six-month periods). The studies included may or may not be representative of the hand surgery literature as a whole, and the possibility of sampling error leading to selection bias does exist. Overall, I was pleased that the authors found that the quality has improved over time; however, a compliance rate of 58% indicates there is still room for improvement. Many of the common areas in which the literature was lacking included a description of the study setting, handling of missing data, and a power analysis. I feel that these areas can potentially be easily improved as awareness of the STROBE statement guidelines is increased. As the quality of the hand surgery literature continues to improve, we will help advance the field of hand surgery into the future.

R. Grewal, MD

Does the Gatekeeper Model Work in Hand Surgery?

Hartzell TL, Shahbazian JH, Pandey A, et al (Faith Regional Health Services, Norfolk, NE; David Geffen School of Medicine at the Univ of California, Los Angeles; Univ of Southern California; et al)

Plast Reconstr Surg 132:381e-386e, 2013

Background.—Most managed care plans use a physician "gatekeeper" to control referrals to hand surgeons. The appropriateness of this model for upper extremity complaints has never been challenged. The purpose of this study was to evaluate the prior management of patients with elective hand disorders who present to a hand surgery clinic.

Methods.—All patients presenting to a tertiary, academic medical center for a new-patient hand surgery evaluation from February 3, 2011, to June 15, 2011, were prospectively enrolled. Patients were evaluated for prior provider, diagnosis, treatment, and complications. Actual diagnosis, recommended workup, and appropriate treatment were determined independently by two experienced hand examiners. Traumatic injuries and surgeon disagreements in diagnosis and treatment were excluded, leaving 125 patients.

Results.—Ninety-eight percent of patients had been evaluated by a primary care provider. Overall, the correct diagnosis was established 34 percent of the time. Nerve compression syndromes were diagnosed with the greatest accuracy (64 percent), whereas stenosing tenosynovitis was diagnosed correctly only 15 percent of the time. Before presentation, 74 percent of patients had undergone a study or intervention. On review, 70 percent of studies/interventions were deemed unnecessary. Advanced imaging was unwarranted in 90 percent of patients who received it. Seventeen percent of patients experienced a complication. Most (67 percent) were caused by a delay in diagnosis, whereas 33 percent resulted from an intervention.

Conclusions.—Health care providers less familiar with an examination of the hand often misdiagnose and mistreat common problems. A referral system may not be the most efficient means of delivering care to patients with elective hand maladies.

▶ The authors have evaluated what many hand surgeons perceive and documented that many patients present to a hand specialist in a delayed manner, often with the incorrect diagnosis and possibly with unnecessary tests. This is an important article, as it documents the current problem. For any change to occur, the problem must be documented, and reporting in the peer-reviewed literature is an important first step. The study is well designed and gives meaningful information when advocating for change.

Musculoskeletal education is sparse in many medical schools as well as primary care, emergency medicine, and internal medicine residency programs. In spite of a high number of presenting complaints to emergency rooms and primary care physicians being related to upper extremity conditions, they are not life or limb threatening and, therefore, are often underappreciated. The appeal of caring for a patient after a myocardial infarction or cerebrovascular accident is greater than for a patient with wrist tendonitis.

Data such as these will hopefully help change the paradigm of upper extremity musculoskeletal care. The urgent care model can be used successfully for these conditions, often providing a diagnosis and treatment in one appointment rather than multiple physician visits and the possibility of unnecessary tests during the process. Unfortunately, it is difficult to change culture, and, if this is to happen, it will be a slow process, but the data provided in this paper are an important first step.

W. C. Hammert, MD

Does the Gatekeeper Model Work in Hand Surgery?

Hartzell TL, Shahbazian JH, Pandey A, et al (David Geffen School of Medicine at the Univ of California, Los Angeles; Univ of Southern California, Los Angeles, CA; Univ of Maryland Med Ctr, Baltimore)
Plast Reconstr Surg 132:381e-386e, 2013

Background.—Most managed care plans use a physician "gatekeeper" to control referrals to hand surgeons. The appropriateness of this model for upper extremity complaints has never been challenged. The purpose of this study was to evaluate the prior management of patients with elective hand disorders who present to a hand surgery clinic.

Methods.—All patients presenting to a tertiary, academic medical center for a new-patient hand surgery evaluation from February 3, 2011, to June 15, 2011, were prospectively enrolled. Patients were evaluated for prior provider, diagnosis, treatment, and complications. Actual diagnosis, recommended workup, and appropriate treatment were determined independently by two experienced hand examiners. Traumatic injuries and surgeon disagreements in diagnosis and treatment were excluded, leaving 125 patients.

Results.—Ninety-eight percent of patients had been evaluated by a primary care provider. Overall, the correct diagnosis was established 34 percent of the time. Nerve compression syndromes were diagnosed with the greatest accuracy (64 percent), whereas stenosing tenosynovitis was diagnosed correctly only 15 percent of the time. Before presentation, 74 percent of patients had undergone a study or intervention. On review, 70 percent of studies/interventions were deemed unnecessary. Advanced imaging was unwarranted in 90 percent of patients who received it. Seventeen percent of patients experienced a complication. Most (67 percent) were caused by a delay in diagnosis, whereas 33 percent resulted from an intervention.

Conclusions.—Health care providers less familiar with an examination of the hand often misdiagnose and mistreat common problems. A referral system may not be the most efficient means of delivering care to patients with elective hand maladies.

▶ The authors analyze the gatekeeper model by examining prior treatment of patients who present elective hand pathologies. The study was performed by prospectively enrolling all referred patients over a 4-month period, excluding traumatic injuries or those in which surgeons disagreed in diagnosis. A total of 125 patients were included, mostly from primary care physicians (PCPs). The correct diagnosis was made 34% of the time, with 70% of prior diagnostic or treatment interventions, including unnecessary advanced imaging, 90% of the time. Almost 1 of 5 patients experienced a complication, with two-thirds from a delay in diagnosis and one-third from an intervention. Overall, the authors concluded there are high rates of misdiagnosis and mistreatment of elective hand maladies by non-hand specialist care providers.

Strengths of this study are the large number of patients from a single center prospectively analyzed with a relatively uniform elective patient referral population. However, it is limited by the very small overall percentage of patients with hand pathologies being treated by PCPs. This sampling bias is furthered by the inclusion of only a single institution. Finally, technically, a "gatekeeper model" refers to a managed care organization, yet many of these patients were from preferred provider organizations. Regardless, the patients did all see a PCP before hand surgery referral, thus, showing the importance of their role in all aspects of our health care system.

This is an important study, as it highlights multiple important aspects of the landscape of our evolving health care system. First, medical school and nonorthopedic residencies lack musculoskeletal education. PCPs are the foundation of our health care system. Their wide diversity of knowledge and expertise enables patients to be evaluated and triaged to the appropriate specialist. However, this study highlights that general PCPs might not be the ideal candidates for these referrals but instead there should be "gatekeepers" with some basic orthopedic or hand training. Given that a musculoskeletal complaint is the most common reason for a primary care appointment, a system with specialty trained orthopedic primary care providers and therapists would provide better care, at potentially less cost, with quicker and more accurate diagnoses.

As changes in our health care system occur, from the reimbursement structures to insurance plans, to regulations, this article highlights the importance of reforms in musculoskeletal education and design in the referral landscape. It reinforces the findings of many of its predecessors, highlighting the problems with the current gatekeeper system and the need for a more orthopedic specialty-driven model.

E. R. Wagner, MD

Factitious Hand Disorders: Review of 29 Years of Multidisciplinary Care
O'Connor EA, Grunert BK, Matloub HS, et al (Med College of Wisconsin, Milwaukee)
J Hand Surg 38A:1590-1598, 2013

Purpose.—To improve our understanding of factitious hand disorders with a review of our experience over 29 years in a multidisciplinary hand center.

Methods.—A retrospective chart review was performed to identify workers' compensation patients treated for factitious hand disorders in the multidisciplinary hand center between January 1981 and September 2010. Multidisciplinary evaluation at this center involved evaluation by hand surgeons, occupational therapists, and psychologists. Data collected include age, sex, race, educational level, clinical presentation, number of diagnostic tests, number of surgeries, time to referral to the multidisciplinary center, direct cost of care, psychological diagnosis, Minnesota Multiphasic Personality Inventory, treatment modalities, and work status.

Results.—We identified 174 workers' compensation patients with factitious hand disorders. Presentation was used to classify patients into 1 of 4 categories: psychopathological dystonia, factitious edema, psychopathological complex regional pain syndrome, and factitious wound creation and manipulation. There were statistically significant differences between the 4 categories in demographics, utilization of medical resources, psychopathology, treatment modalities, and return-to-work status. Patients with factitious wounds were more educated, used more medical resources, demonstrated an angry or hostile profile, and experienced a lower return-to-work rate. Patients with dystonia were less educated, used less medical resources, demonstrated a hypochondriasis or depressed profile, and experienced a higher return-to-work rate.

Conclusions.—Treatment of factitious hand disorders remains frustrating and costly due to failure or recurrence after traditional approaches. This review is a large-scale examination of the factitious hand disorder population that demonstrates the unique pathology involved in each of the 4 categories. There is a specific association between the category of hand disorder and the underlying pathology and prognosis.

Type of Study/Level of Evidence.—Prognostic IV (Table 1).

▶ Factitious problems of the hand present several unique problems for the practicing surgeon. First, Burke[1] suggests that hand surgeons are not usually

TABLE 1.—Clinical Signs Suspicious for Factitious Disorder

Physical Presentation	Patient	Psychopathology
Accessible site	Predict outcomes	Recent stress
Nondominant side	Worsen at time of discharge or stress	Multiple somatic complaints
Patterned injury	Conservative management refused	Psychiatric illness
Cyclical	Vague history	History of secondary gain
Sterile cultures	Refusal to obtain outside records	History of childhood illness
Multiple symptoms	Noncompliance	Symptom modeling
Unusual course	Excessive medical knowledge	Family history of factitious disorder
Multiple invasive procedures		
Multiple medical consults		

formally trained to deal with such problems and that the aptitudes that preselect surgeons may not be the best to address such problems. In addition, because it is a diagnosis requiring a high index of suspicion and often requires exclusion of organic problems, confirmation of diagnosis is often difficult. Finally, there is a paucity of information about the prevalence, epidemiology, and prognosis of factitious hand problems.

The first and second issues are clinical case problems involving specific patients. They are addressed by a multidisciplinary approach to the patient involving a hand surgeon, hand therapist, and psychologist. This report also covers the spectrum of factitious disorders with relevant references to other clinical case series and a table of clinical signs suspicious for such disorders (Table 1) to help clinicians better recognize the possibility of such a diagnosis when confronted with such patients.

This review of a group of such disorders diagnosed in a multidisciplinary care center over a long period sheds some light into a third issue. While the costs and difficulty of treating such conditions have been described in prior literature, there is almost no published information on a large series of cases looking at the different pathologies and relating them with patient characteristics and prognosis.

Based on the groupings of such disorders, the authors found differences in areas such as educational levels, resource use, and return to work depending on the types of disorders. This information is useful on multiple fronts, such as using it as a basis to predict outcomes after specific pathologies and as a starting point to develop strategies to better manage such problems.

A. K. S. Chong, MD

Reference

1. Burke FD. Factitious disorders of the upper limb. *J Hand Surg Eur Vol.* 2008;33: 103-109.

Hand Surgery After an Episode of Disproportionate Pain and Disability

Matzon J, Lutsky K (Thomas Jefferson Univ, Philadelphia, PA; Rothman Inst, Philadelphia, PA)
J Hand Surg Am 38:2454-2456, 2013

Background.—Disproportionate pain and disability is labeled variously, including causalgia, reflex sympathetic dystrophy, allodynia, sympathetically maintained pain, and complex regional pain syndrome. Psychologists and psychiatrists may view this as catastrophic thinking or hyperprotectiveness, whereas medical doctors may view it as an as-yet-unknown pathophysiological process. Elective surgery on a limb is often avoided for patients who had disproportionate pain and disability previously, even if the symptoms resolved completely or the occurrence was in the distant past. The concern is that the patient will have a maladaptive physiological response to pain, a maladaptive psychological response to pain, or the two combined. There has been little confidence that treatment will be successful after an experience labeled as disproportionate.

> *Case Report.*—Man, 34, served as a Special Weapons and Tactics (SWAT) officer and developed swelling, stiffness, and diffuse pain on light touch after having a cast placed on a nondisplaced small finger metacarpal shaft fracture. Stellate ganglion blocks and physical therapy allowed him to return to work 6 months after the fracture on light duty, but he had radial-side wrist pain, focal tenderness over the first dorsal compartment, and a positive Finkelstein test. The diagnosis was de Quervain tendinopathy, which was managed initially with local corticosteroid injections, but the patient wanted a surgical treatment. It was decided to address the pathophysiology of the first dorsal compartment, which appeared to be the focus of his symptoms and disability. In a detailed discussion with the patient, the clinician explained the risks of surgical intervention. About 3 months after the disproportionate pain resolved, he had a first dorsal compartment release under regional (axillary) block and recovered without any adverse consequences, returning to work 6 weeks postoperatively.

Discussion.—The current evidence regarding disproportionate pain and disability suffers from small numbers of patients and the fact that researchers involved in several studies have been found guilty of scientific misconduct. This undermines the findings in most studies. Additionally, there is no consensus reference standard to diagnose disproportionate pain and disability or differentiate proportionate from disproportionate responses. No reliable and valid test objectively distinguishes between the two experiences. Human illness behavior is better considered on a continuum that includes both biological and psychosocial factors associated with increased pain and disability. The goal is to limit pain intensity and magnitude of disability for all patients.

Conclusions.—Patients need to be counseled that there is a definite but as yet unquantified risk for developing disproportionate pain and disability postoperatively. It appears wise to wait until these symptoms resolve before undertaking any discretionary surgery. General anesthesia should be avoided when possible, and motion exercises should be initiated as soon as possible postoperatively to diminish the possibility of recurrent stiffness.

▶ The authors address a common concern among hand surgeons regarding the risks of operating on patients with pain out of proportion to the clinical diagnosis or presentation. Often, we as surgeons have concerns when patients present with exaggerated symptoms and conditions, such as causalgia, reflex sympathetic dystrophy, allodynia, sympathetically maintained pain, or complex regional pain syndrome (CRPS), that enter into the differential diagnosis. In addition to questioning the efficacy of surgical intervention, the possibility of worsening or creating a flare of conditions such as CRPS adds to the complexity of these cases.

The authors do an admirable job of informing us that there is little science to guide us as surgeons, and although there remains a risk of recurrence of disproportionate pain and disability after discretionary surgery, the magnitude of the risk is unclear. Furthermore, there is little evidence regarding the optimal timing or methods to help decrease that risk. I agree with the authors' conclusion of the importance of counseling patients of these risks in hopes that (when all conservative treatments are exhausted) if the patient pursues surgery, it will yield the desired outcome. Ideally, it is best if the out-of-proportion pain resolves before surgery, but unfortunately occasionally the condition (ie, DeQuervain's in this example) is the presumed root of the problem, and the pain does not subside until it is treated.

M. Rizzo, MD

In Vivo Gliding and Contact Characteristics of the Sigmoid Notch and the Ulna in Forearm Rotation

Chen YR, Tang JB (Affiliated Hosp of Nantong Univ, Jiangsu, China)
J Hand Surg 38A:1513-1519, 2013

Purpose.—To investigate shifting of the contact center over the surfaces of 2 opposing bones of the distal radioulnar joint during forearm rotation.

Methods.—We recruited 8 volunteers and used their right wrists. Serial computed tomography scans were obtained with the forearm at neutral position and 6 other positions of forearm rotation. We reconstructed 3-dimensional images and mapped contact regions of both the sigmoid notch and ulnar head by calculating the shortest distance between the 2 opposing bones. The center of contact was also defined and plotted against the distal radioulnar joint rotation to determine the sliding distance over the surfaces of the 2 bones.

Results.—During forearm rotation, the maximal sliding of the sigmoid notch over the ulnar head was 7.4 mm in forearm pronation and 9.2 mm in forearm supination, which occurred in volar-dorsal direction primarily. Sliding of the ulnar head over the sigmoid notch was more limited, measuring 4.7 mm during pronation and 2.3 mm during supination. Most of the motion occurred between 30° pronation and 60° supination. In the proximal-distal direction, the contact site of the sigmoid notch with the ulnar head translated distally 1.6 mm during pronation and proximally 0.7 mm during supination.

Conclusions.—During forearm rotation, the sigmoid notch slides substantially against the ulnar head at each part of the forearm rotation arc. The sliding of the ulnar head over the sigmoid notch is smaller, most of which is at the range from moderate forearm pronation to slight supination. The contact site of the sigmoid notch with the ulnar head moves slightly distally during forearm pronation and proximally during supination.

Clinical Relevance.—The *in vivo* findings provide more detailed information and insight into distal radioulnar joint motion kinematics.

▶ This article from *The Journal of Hand Surgery* uses computed tomography (CT) scans taken at different positions of pronosupination in young, healthy volunteers. The purpose of the study was to evaluate in detail a well-known characteristic of the distal radial ulnar joint: that the point of contact between the distal radius and ulna seems to change with motion. It has long been known that the radii of curvature of the distal ulna and the sigmoid notch of the radius differ and that this difference allows the radius to translate on the ulna in terms of its point of contact.

The authors' assumption that there is a uniformity of cartilage thickness in the sigmoid notch and the distal ulna head allowed them to estimate the contact areas, but the contact areas are not the key focus of this investigation. The authors instead focused on the point of minimal distance between the radius and ulna to estimate the point of maximum contact. That point represents the center of the contact area, independent of how large the contact area is. They note that the point of contact of the radius on the ulna seems to translate on the ulna to a greater degree than the point of contact of the ulna on the radius. This was evaluated in great detail. It seems as if the radius slides along the ulna in the pronosupination arc to a greater extent than the ulna slides on the radius. This may be the basis for the variability in the shape of the radial sigmoid notch because relatively little distance of the sigmoid notch is contacted maximally in the pronosupination arc.

Although not directly applicable to clinical practice, it is clear that this advanced study offers a glimpse into how one might actively investigate the change in the point of maximal contact with range of motion in a small joint. It turns out that the biomechanics of small joints are notoriously difficult to investigate because it is impossible to interpose sensitive materials in these joints without significantly altering their characteristics. In this study, CT scans performed in 7 specific positions allow a relatively detailed picture of where the radius and ulna interact. It is also notable that the proximodistal shift of the radius on the ulna was also directly investigated and found to be relatively small. The entire translation of this point of contact is less than 3 mm, a key fact when considering that the average ulnar shortening osteotomy done for ulnar impaction syndrome is about 3 mm. This distance has been shown to be adequate for clinical resolution of ulnar impaction syndrome symptoms. It is notable that this distance was found to be small in this study.

Although the authors are quick to point out the limitations of their study, they have contributed to this limited picture a detailed understanding of the way that the point of maximal contact between the ulna and the radius moves with routine forearm pronosupination in an elegant way using 3-dimensional reconstructions from CT scans. Their study further underlines the immense complexity of the distal radial ulnar joint and may serve as a basis for why arthroplasties designed on allowing some loose translation of the ulna on the radius may be more successful by limiting shear forces on the prosthetic than those that commit the radius and ulna to a strict, nonmoving relationship.

J. Elfar, MD

Biomechanical Analysis of the Distal Metaphyseal Ulnar Shortening Osteotomy
Greenberg JA, Werner FW, Smith JM (SUNY Upstate Med Univ, Syracuse, NY)
J Hand Surg 38A:1919-1924, 2013

Purpose.—To investigate the effect of a closing wedge osteotomy at the distal ulnar metaphysis on unloading the ulnar side of the wrist.

Methods.—Seven fresh frozen cadaver arms mounted in a wrist simulator were used for the analysis. A 6-degrees-of-freedom load cell was mounted on the distal radius and another on the distal ulna. Radioulnar carpal joint forces and transverse distal radioulnar joint (DRUJ) load were measured at static wrist positions and during dynamic wrist motions before and after the distal metaphyseal ulnar shortening osteotomy (DMUSO) was performed.

Results.—At each static position, significant decreases in ulnar load were noted after DMUSO. In addition, mean and maximum loads decreased for each dynamic wrist motion. There were no statistically significant differences in transverse forces across the DRUJ after DMUSO.

Conclusion.—This study showed that DMUSO is an effective way to decrease the load across the ulnocarpal joint. The geometry of the osteotomy and resultant change in the position of the ulnar head did not increase transverse joint reaction forces.

Clinical Relevance.—This technique is an alternative to open diaphyseal techniques or methods that damage the articular surface of the distal ulna. Clinical studies will be necessary to associate the biomechanical correction noted in this study with clinical symptom improvement.

▶ Ulnar impingement is a condition that all hand surgeons deal with and often with some level of trepidation. Greenburg and colleagues present an important biomechanical study aimed at helping define the effects and limitations of a distal metaphyseal ulnar shortening osteotomy (DMUSO) in a cadaveric model. The authors tested 7 fresh-frozen cadaver specimens with extensor and flexor tendon tensioning through flexion, extension, radial, and ulnar positioning while evaluating the data in 6 degrees of freedom. The authors noted an average correction in ulnar variance of 2.8 mm and a significant decrease in ulnar load in all statically tested positions. Interestingly, the authors found no significant increase in transverse forces across the distal radioulnar joint in static testing and dynamic wrist motions. This article helps lay the foundation of understanding the biomechanical effects of a DMUSO. As the authors note, there are limitations with this small cadaveric study, but the data help add biomechanical validity to a potentially more efficient way of addressing ulnocarpal impaction.

J. M. Froelich, MD

Factors Associated With Survey Response in Hand Surgery Research
Bot AGJ, Anderson JA, Neuhaus V, et al (Harvard Med School, Boston, MA; Massachusetts General Hosp, Boston)
Clin Orthop Relat Res 471:3237-3242, 2013

Background.—A low response rate is believed to decrease the validity of survey studies. Factors associated with nonresponse to surveys are poorly characterized in orthopaedic research.

Questions/Purposes.—This study addressed whether (1) psychologic factors; (2) demographics; (3) illness-related factors; and (4) pain are predictors of a lower likelihood of a patient returning a mailed survey.

Methods.—One hundred four adult, new or return patients completed questionnaires including the Pain Catastrophizing Scale, Patient Health Questionnaire-9 depression scale, Short Health Anxiety Index, demographics, and a pain scale (0–10) during a routine visit to a hand and upper extremity surgeon. Of these patients, 38% had undergone surgery and the remainder was seen for various other conditions. Six months after their visit, patients were mailed the DASH questionnaire and a scale to rate their satisfaction with the visit (0–10). Bivariate analysis and logistic regression were used to determine risk factors for being a nonresponder to the followup of this study. The cohort consisted of 57 women and 47 men with a mean age of 51 years with various diagnoses. Thirty-five patients (34%) returned the questionnaire. Responders were satisfied with their visit (mean satisfaction, 8.7) and had a DASH score of 9.6.

Results.—Compared with patients who returned the questionnaires, nonresponders had higher pain catastrophizing scores, were younger, more frequently male, and had more pain at enrollment. In logistic regression, male sex (odds ratio [OR], 2.6), pain (OR, 1.3), and younger age (OR, 1.03) were associated with not returning the questionnaire.

Conclusions.—Survey studies should be interpreted in light of the fact that patients who do not return questionnaires in a hand surgery practice differ from patients who do return them. Hand surgery studies that rely on questionnaire evaluation remote from study enrollment should include tactics to improve the response of younger, male patients with more pain.

Level of Evidence.—Level II, prognostic study. See Guidelines for Authors for a complete description of levels of evidence.

▶ This interesting report by Dr Bot and his colleagues confirms something most hand surgeons suspect. That postvisit surveys are biased by differences between respondents and nonrespondents. Young men seem to do the worst in replying to survey requests. This should be no surprise! Furthermore, it was interesting that those with higher pain catastrophizing scores and more pain at enrollment also were less likely to respond.

I think this report will often be quoted in the discussion of self-reported patient outcome surveys. Every study is vulnerable to a low return rate or a skewed distribution of outcomes. Perhaps incentives such as gift cards may help increase the yield to give hand surgeons greater returns and more objective data.

J. Chang, MD

Article Index

Chapter 1: Hand and Wrist Arthritis

Chapter 2: Wrist Arthroscopy

Chapter 3: Carpus

Chapter 4: Dupuytren's Contracture

Chapter 5: Compressive Neuropathies

Chapter 6: Nerve

Chapter 7: Brachial Plexus

Chapter 8: Microsurgery

Chapter 9: Tendon

Chapter 10: Trauma

Chapter 11: Distal Radius Fractures

Chapter 12: Tumor

Chapter 13: Vascular

Chapter 14: Diagnostic Imaging

Chapter 15: Elbow: Trauma

Chapter 20: Shoulder: Miscellaneous

Chapter 21: Rehabilitation

Chapter 22: Miscellaneous

Author Index

A

Akahane M, 153
Al-Qattan M, 87
Alkhalefah GK, 100
Almeida VW, 69
Altobelli GG, 127
Amadio PC, 112, 113
Amin N, 79
Amrami KK, 16
Anderson JA, 271
Angeline ME, 236
Arner JW, 244
Arner M, 221

B

Babinet A, 177
Bahrami F, 131, 132
Baraga MG, 239
Barbier O, 152
Barton E, 82
Bauer A, 92
Baxter K, 248
Beck JD, 50
Ben Salah Frih Z, 82
Beredjiklian P, 58
Bernstein J, 58
Berrocal YA, 69
Bey MJ, 230
Bhatt RA, 101
Biben JA, 256
Bither N, 196
Blackman AJ, 138, 214
Boccolari P, 121, 247
Boeckstyns MEH, 71, 77
Bogunovic L, 181
Borgia M, 248
Bot AGJ, 271
Bradley JP, 244
Broering CA, 95
Brouwers L, 22
Brown PJ, 114
Brown SH, 93
Bueno RA, 100
Bullitta G, 209
Burns PB, 12
Burton C, 169
Buterbaugh GA, 259

C

Calfee R, 178
Canham CD, 118
Capito AE, 26
Carballeira A, 182
Cavadas PC, 182
Cha S-M, 30
Chan R, 205
Chandra PS, 53
Chang H-C, 188
Chang J, 92
Charvet B, 110
Chatterton BD, 75
Chen S-C, 102
Chen YR, 268
Cheng M-H, 102
Chetta M, 12
Chikenji T, 54
Chilelli BJ, 120, 125
Cho NS, 228
Choi J-A, 229
Christen D, 170
Christen T, 219
Chung KC, 60, 97
Chung SW, 226
Clifford L, 183
Coenen M, 251
Coleman S, 36
Collis J, 40
Collocott S, 40
Conneely S, 127
Crosby SN, 163
Cutler L, 173
Cynn H-S, 240

D

D'Agostino P, 152
Dailiana ZH, 212
Damiano M, 66
Dautel G, 219
Davidge K, 57, 66
de Witte PB, 225
Deml C, 154
Derwin KA, 230
Dias JJ, 33, 43, 173
Didonna ML, 6
Dienstknecht T, 72
Diserens-Chew T, 169

Dohi D, 213
Dovi-Akue D, 201
Driessens S, 169
Duckworth AD, 55
Dy CJ, 123, 142, 148

E

Ebersole GC, 57, 66
Edwards SG, 207
Eilenberg WH, 81
Ek ETH, 143
Ekblom AG, 221
El Sallakh S, 198
Ercan EC, 107, 130

F

Farnebo S, 117
Farrar-Edwards D, 252
Ferreira LM, 200
Fischer LH, 257
Fletcher ND, 163
Flouzat-Lachaniette C-H, 177
Fowler JR, 51, 259
Fox PM, 117
Fridén J, 258
Friedrich JB, 104
Frihagen F, 164
Fujitani R, 153

G

Gaines RJ, 255
Gao K, 91
Garcia MJ, 39
Gateley D, 179
Gelberman RH, 181
Giannicola G, 209
Gilpin D, 36
Gingery A, 54
Gleiss A, 81
Glodny B, 154
Gold JE, 48
Goldfarb CA, 181
Gonzalez A, 105